T0211577

Lecture Notes in Computer Science 10554

Commenced Publication in 1973
Founding and Former Series Editors:
Gerhard Goos, Juris Hartmanis, and Jan van Leeuwen

More information about this series at http://www.springer.com/series/7412

M. Jorge Cardoso · Tal Arbel et al. (Eds.)

Fetal, Infant and Ophthalmic Medical Image Analysis

International Workshop, FIFI 2017
and 4th International Workshop, OMIA 2017
Held in Conjunction with MICCAI 2017
Québec City, QC, Canada, September 14, 2017
Proceedings

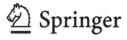 Springer

Editors
M. Jorge Cardoso
University College London
London, UK

Tal Arbel
McGill University
Montreal, Canada

Workshop Editors *see next page*

ISSN 0302-9743   ISSN 1611-3349   (electronic)
Lecture Notes in Computer Science
ISBN 978-3-319-67560-2   ISBN 978-3-319-67561-9   (eBook)
DOI 10.1007/978-3-319-67561-9

Library of Congress Control Number: 2017952887

LNCS Sublibrary: SL6 – Image Processing, Computer Vision, Pattern Recognition, and Graphics

Printed on acid-free paper

This Springer imprint is published by Springer Nature
The registered company is Springer International Publishing AG
The registered company address is: Gewerbestrasse 11, 6330 Cham, Switzerland

Workshop Editors

International Workshop on Fetal and Infant Image Analysis, FIFI 2017

Andrew Melbourne
University College London
London
UK

Michael Ebner
University College London
London
UK

Pim Moeskops
Eindhoven University of Technology
Eindhoven
The Netherlands

Antonios Makropoulos
Imperial College London
London
UK

Ernst Schwartz
Medical University of Vienna
Vienna
Austria

Adrien Desjardin
University College London
London
UK

Emma Robinson
Imperial College London
London
UK

Tom Vercauteren ⓘ
University College London
London
UK

4th International Workshop on Ophthalmic Medical Image Analysis, OMIA 2017

Hrvoje Bogunovic
Medical University of Vienna
Vienna
Austria

Emanuele Trucco
University of Dundee
Dundee
UK

Xinjian Chen
Soochow University
Suzhou
China

Yanwu Xu
A*STAR Institute for Infocomm
    Research
Singapore
Singapore

Mona K. Garvin
University of Iowa
Iowa City, IA
USA

Preface FIFI 2017

The application of sophisticated analysis tools to fetal, infant and paediatric imaging data is of interest to a substantial proportion of the MICCAI community. The main objective of this workshop is to bring together researchers in the MICCAI community to discuss the challenges of image analysis techniques as applied to the fetal and infant setting. Advanced medical image analysis allows the detailed scientific study of conditions such as prematurity and the study of both normal singleton and twin development in addition to less common conditions unique to childhood. This workshop brings together methods and experience from researchers and authors working on these younger cohorts and provides a forum for the open discussion of advanced image analysis approaches focused on the analysis of growth and development in the fetal, infant and paediatric period.

September 2017

Andrew Melbourne
Pim Moeskops
Ernst Schwartz
Emma Robinson
Michael Ebner
Antonios Makropoulos
Adrien Desjardins
Tom Vercauteren

Organization

Organizing Committee

Andrew Melbourne	University College London, London, UK
Pim Moeskops	Eindhoven University of Technology, Eindhoven, The Netherlands
Ernst Schwartz	Medical University of Vienna, Vienna, Austria
Emma Robinson	Imperial College London, London, UK
Michael Ebner	University College London, London, UK
Antonios Makropoulos	Imperial College London, London, UK
Adrien Desjardins	University College London, London, UK
Tom Vercauteren	University College London, London, UK

Program Committee

Andrew Melbourne	University College London, UK
Pim Moeskops	Eindhoven University of Technology, The Netherlands
Ernst Schwartz	Medical University of Vienna, Austria
Emma Robinson	Imperial College London, UK
Michael Ebner	University College London, UK
Antonios Makropoulos	Imperial College London, UK
Adrien Desjardins	University College London, UK
Tom Vercauteren	University College London, UK
Guotai Wang	University College London, UK
Nishikant Deshmukh	Johns Hopkins University, USA
Roxane Licandro	Medical University of Vienna, Austria
Sebastiano Ferraris	University College London, UK

Preface OMIA 2017

Age-related macular degeneration, diabetic retinopathy, and glaucoma are the main causes of blindness. Oftentimes blindness can be avoided by early intervention, making computer-assisted early diagnosis of retinal diseases a research priority. Related research is exploring retinal biomarkers for systemic conditions like dementia, cardiovascular disease, and complications of diabetes. Significant challenges remain, including reliability and validation, effective multimodal analysis (e.g., fundus photography, optical coherence tomography, and scanning laser ophthalmoscopy), more powerful imaging technologies, and the effective deployment of cutting-edge computer vision and machine learning techniques. The Fourth International Workshop on Ophthalmic Medical Image Analysis (OMIA-4) addresses all these aspects and more, this year in collaboration with the ReTOUCH retinal image challenge.

September 2017

Hrvoje Bogunovic
Xinjian Chen
Mona K. Garvin
Emanuele Trucco
Yanwu Xu

Organization

Organizing Committee

Hrvoje Bogunovic	Medical University of Vienna, Austria
Xinjian Chen	Soochow University, China
Mona K. Garvin	University of Iowa, USA
Emanuele Trucco	VAMPIRE project, University of Dundee, UK
Yanwu Xu	Institute for Infocomm Research, A*STAR, Singapore

Program Committee

Bashir Al-Diri	University of Lincoln, UK
Philippe Burlina	Johns Hopkins University, USA
Qiang Chen	Nanjing Science and Technology University, China
Jun Cheng	Institute for Infocomm Research, Singapore
Lixin Duan	University of Electronic Science and Technology of China
Huazhu Fu	Institute for Infocomm Research, Singapore
Andrea Giachetti	University of Verona, Italy
Huiying Liu	Institute for Infocomm Research, Singapore
Tom MacGillivray	University of Edinburgh, UK
Xianjing Meng	Shandong University, China
Fabio Scarpa	University of Padova, Italy
Abhay Shah	University of Iowa, USA
Fei Shi	Soochow University, China
Domenico Tegolo	University of Palermo, Italy
Jui-Kai Wang	University of Iowa, USA
Xiaoming Xi	Shandong University, China
Dehui Xiang	Soochow University, China
Mengdi Xu	Institute for Infocomm Research, Singapore
Xiayu Xu	Xi'an Jiaotong University, China
Xenophon Zabulis	Foundation for Research and Technology - Hellas, Greece
Yitian Zhao	Beijing Institute of Technology, China
Yalin Zheng	University of Liverpool, UK
Yuanjie Zheng	Shandong Normal University, China
Weifang Zhu	Soochow University, China

Contents

4th International Workshop on Ophthalmic Medical Image Analysis, OMIA 2017

International Workshop on Fetal and Infant Image Analysis, FIFI 2017

Template-Free Estimation of Intracranial Volume: A Preterm Birth Animal Model Study

Juan Eugenio Iglesias[1(✉)], Sebastiano Ferraris[1], Marc Modat[1], Willy Gsell[2],
Jan Deprest[2,3], Johannes L. van der Merwe[2], and Tom Vercauteren[2,3]

[1] Translational Imaging Group, University College London (UCL), London, UK
e.iglesias@ucl.ac.uk
[2] Biomedical Sciences Group, KU Leuven, Leuven, Belgium
[3] Wellcome/EPSRC Centre for Interventional and Surgical Sciences,
UCL, London, UK

Abstract. Accurate estimation of intracranial volume (ICV) is key in neuro-imaging-based volumetric studies, since estimation errors directly propagate to the ICV-corrected volumes used in subsequent analyses. ICV estimation through registration to a reference atlas has the advantage of not requiring manually delineated data, and can thus be applied to populations for which labeled data might be inexistent or scarce, e.g., preterm born animal models. However, such method is not robust, since the estimation depends on a single registration. Here we present a groupwise, template-free ICV estimation method that overcomes this limitation. The method quickly aligns pairs of images using linear registration at low resolution, and then computes the most likely ICV values using a Bayesian framework. The algorithm is robust against single registration errors, which are corrected by registrations to other subjects. The algorithm was evaluated on a pilot dataset of rabbit brain MRI ($N = 7$), in which the estimated ICV was highly correlated ($\rho = 0.99$) with ground truth values derived from manual delineations. Additional regression and discrimination experiments with human hippocampal volume on a subset of ADNI ($N = 150$) yielded reduced sample sizes and increased classification accuracy, compared with using a reference atlas.

1 Introduction

Background. Intracranial volume (ICV) is a crucial covariate in MRI-based neuroimaging studies. Correcting for ICV, by division or regression [1], is necessary for comparing volume estimates of brain structures from cases with different head sizes. While the automated segmentation of brain structures has received a considerable amount of attention in the literature, ICV estimation is often overlooked, despite the fact that a poor ICV estimate can have a very detrimental impact on the corrected volume of an otherwise very well segmented structure. Compared with skull stripping, ICV estimation needs to account for all the tissue and fluid inside the skull, not only the brain. Otherwise, atrophy or growth of brain structures would be partially explained by changes of the whole brain.

© Springer International Publishing AG 2017
M.J. Cardoso et al. (Eds.): FIFI/OMIA 2017, LNCS 10554, pp. 3–13, 2017.
DOI: 10.1007/978-3-319-67561-9_1

The literature of ICV estimation is dominated by methods designed for adult human brain MRI. Earlier approaches relied on simple thresholding and morphological operations [2]. In the 2000s, methods based on linear registration [3,4] gained popularity: scaling factors are derived from an affine registration to a reference atlas, and multiplied by the ground truth ICV of the atlas to yield the estimates. These methods are implemented in widespread neuroimaging packages (e.g., FreeSurfer [5], FSL [6]). Other approaches rely on explicit segmentation of the intracranial cavity, typically with supervised methods based on parametric or non-parametric models. Representative examples of the former are the Bayesian segmentation [7] implemented in the SPM package [8], or variants thereof [9]. Examples of the latter include multi-atlas methods [10] and patch matching [11].

Although supervised methods can potentially yield better results, registration-based algorithms for ICV estimation are still widely used in adult human brain MRI, e.g., in FreeSurfer and FSL. The reason is threefold: they are fast; they do not require multimodal MRI pulse sequences; and they do not require labeled training data. Even if no ground truth ICV is available for the reference atlas, the ICV can still be estimated up to a constant scaling factor, which has no impact on the subsequent ICV correction. The main drawback of registration-based ICV estimation is that it is very sensitive to registration errors, which reflect directly on the ICV estimates through the determinant of the transformation matrix.

Motivation: limitations in ICV computation for developing brain and animal models. The literature on ICV estimation in the developing human brain is very sparse, but it is possible to use registration-based methods based on existing atlases, such as those described in [12,13]. In animals, however, the availability of atlases – particularly for species other than mouse, rat and monkey – is very limited, especially for the developing brain. A particularly interesting case is rabbit models, which are increasingly important in neuroscience. One of the main application of rabbit models is the study of preterm birth, a problem with large economic and social impact [14,15], and which is difficult to study in humans [16]. The only available rabbit atlas [17] is for the adult brain, and has no ICV information, as it was created from *ex vivo* brains without the skull.

Contribution. In this paper, we address the problem of ICV estimation by computing the ICV of all subjects/cases in a study *simultaneously*. The method has two major advantages: it does not require any labeled data, which is costly to collect (which is why many methods rely on semiautomatically generated silver standards, e.g., [4,10,11]); and is agnostic to species. Therefore, the proposed method readily enables application to developing brain and animal studies.

More specifically, we propose a probabilistic framework, in which the true, underlying ICVs are assumed to be independent samples of a Gaussian distribution with unknown parameters, and in which pairwise registrations yield noisy measurements of the ratios between these ICVs. Within this framework, we use Bayesian inference to compute the most likely ICVs. The information in the registrations enables estimation up to a scaling factor, which is disambiguated by the model hyperparameters. The proposed method preserves the advantages of registration-based algorithms described above, while being more robust to registration errors. Such robustness translates into increased statistical power and reduced sample sizes in subsequent analyses, as shown in our experiments below.

2 Methods

2.1 Probabilistic Framework

The graphical model of our probabilistic framework is shown in Fig. 1. Let $v = [v_1, \ldots, v_N]^t$ be a vector of log-transformed ICVs from N subjects; since we work with ratios, the logarithmic domain is more appropriate. These ICVs are assumed to be independent samples of a Gaussian distribution with unknown mean and variance (μ, σ^2). Prior knowledge on these two parameters is encoded in the hyperparameters of their prior distribution, which we choose to be a Normal Inverse Gamma (NIG), parameterized by $[m, n, a, b]^t$. This is the conjugate prior of a Gaussian with unknown mean and variance, and can be decomposed into an Inverse Gamma (IG) distribution on σ^2 (parameterized by $[a, b]^t$) and a Gaussian distribution on μ, with mean m and variance σ^2/n.

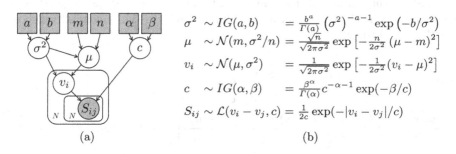

$$\sigma^2 \sim IG(a, b) = \frac{b^a}{\Gamma(a)} \left(\sigma^2\right)^{-a-1} \exp\left(-b/\sigma^2\right)$$

$$\mu \sim \mathcal{N}(m, \sigma^2/n) = \frac{\sqrt{n}}{\sqrt{2\pi\sigma^2}} \exp\left[-\frac{n}{2\sigma^2}(\mu - m)^2\right]$$

$$v_i \sim \mathcal{N}(\mu, \sigma^2) = \frac{1}{\sqrt{2\pi\sigma^2}} \exp\left[-\frac{1}{2\sigma^2}(v_i - \mu)^2\right]$$

$$c \sim IG(\alpha, \beta) = \frac{\beta^\alpha}{\Gamma(\alpha)} c^{-\alpha-1} \exp(-\beta/c)$$

$$S_{ij} \sim \mathcal{L}(v_i - v_j, c) = \frac{1}{2c} \exp(-|v_i - v_j|/c)$$

(a)   (b)

Fig. 1. Graphical model (a) and corresponding equations (b). Circles represent random variables, boxes represent hyperparameters, shaded elements are observed, and plates indicate replication. $\mathcal{N}$ is the Gaussian distribution, and $\mathcal{L}$ is the Laplace distribution.

Now, we assume that we have a set $\mathcal{S}$ of subject pairs (i, j) for which pairwise scaling factors S_{ij} have been computed. Factor S_{ij} corresponds to a noisy estimate of the difference in log-ICVs between subjects i and j, i.e., $v_i - v_j$. The set of measurements does not need to exhaustively cover every (i, j), but must ensure that the adjacency matrix $A_{ij} = \delta(S_{ij} \neq 0)$ corresponds to a fully connected graph, such that there is always a path of scaling factors available between any two subjects. We use the matrix $\boldsymbol{S}$ to represent the measured scaling factors, with diagonal $S_{ii} = 0, \forall i$, and $S_{ij} = $ NaN if the scaling factor is not available, i.e., $(i, j) \notin \mathcal{S}$. These measurements, which are computed with a linear registration algorithm, correspond to the logarithm of the determinant of the estimated transform matrices. Here we assume that the registration method is symmetric, which yields an antisymmetric S, i.e., $S_{ij} = -S_{ji}$. In order to make the algorithm robust against outliers, we further assume that the measurement errors are independent samples of a Laplace distribution (based on the robust ℓ_1 norm, rather than ℓ_2 that the Gaussian distribution relies on) with zero location and scale parameter c. Assuming zero location is appropriate, since the registration is symmetric. The scale parameter is unknown, but we place a conjugate prior distribution on it – the IG distribution, with hyperparameters α and β.

2.2   Bayesian Inference

Our goal is to find the value $\hat{v}$ that maximizes the posterior probability of the ICVs v, given the pairwise scaling measurements and the hyperparameters:

$$\hat{v} = \underset{v}{\operatorname{argmax}}\, p(v|S, m, n, a, b, \alpha, \beta) = \underset{v}{\operatorname{argmax}}\, p(S|v, \alpha, \beta)p(v|m, n, a, b)$$

$$= \underset{v}{\operatorname{argmax}} \int_c p(S|c, v)p(c|\alpha, \beta)dc \int_\mu \int_{\sigma^2} p(v|\mu, \sigma^2)p(\mu, \sigma^2|m, n, a, b)d\mu d\sigma^2. \quad (1)$$

Thanks to the conjugate priors, the two integrals in Eq. 1 have closed-form solutions, so we can easily consider all possible values of the model parameters – weighted by their probabilities – in the estimation. The negated logarithm of this expression is the cost function to minimize ($\mathcal{C}$). In the appendix, we show that $\mathcal{C}$ is equal to:

$$\mathcal{C}(v; S, m, n, a, b, \alpha, \beta) = (\alpha + |\mathcal{S}|)\log\left[\beta + \sum_{(i,j)\in\mathcal{S}} |S_{ij} - v_i + v_j|\right] + \dots$$

$$\frac{2a + N}{2}\log\left[b + \sum_{i=1}^{N} \frac{(v_i - \bar{v})^2}{2} + \frac{Nn(\bar{v} - m)^2}{2(N + n)}\right] + Z(\alpha, \beta, |\mathcal{S}|, n, a, b, N), \quad (2)$$

where Z is a term independent of v, and $\bar{v} = (1/N)\sum_{i=1}^{N} v_i$ is the sample mean of v. The final optimization problem is hence: $\operatorname{argmin}_v C(v; S, m, n, a, b, \alpha, \beta)$. This is an unconstrained problem, which can be efficiently solved with standard algorithms; we used conjugate gradient [18] initialized with $v_i = m$, $\forall i$. The final solution is obtained by exponentiating $\hat{v}$ to bring it back to the natural domain.

3   Experiments and Results

3.1   Data

We used two brain MRI datasets in this study: one of rabbits, and one of humans. The rabbit dataset was acquired as part of a study seeking to understand the effects of steroids on fetuses. Scans from 7 rabbits (5 preterm born, 2 term) were acquired *in vivo* on a Bruker 9.4 T animal scanner using a RARE T2 sequence (TR = 42 ms, TE = 1000 ms, 0.15 mm resolution isotropic). The intracranial cavity was manually delineated by S.F. on the images, providing a ground truth for the ICVs. Since the size of the rabbit dataset is limited, we also performed experiments on a larger, more conventional human dataset consisting of T1 scans of 150 subjects from the Alzheimer's Disease Neuroimaging Initiative (ADNI): 77 Alzheimer's disease (AD) patients and 73 age-matched controls (EC). No ground truth ICVs was available for this dataset, so we used indirect validation techniques. While direct validation is generally preferable, indirect methods make the evaluation independent of segmentation errors, and do not require manual delineation, which is prohibitive for large datasets.

3.2 Experiments on Rabbit Dataset

This experiment assesses the performance of the method in pediatric animal brain MRI, in which the availability of labeled data is extremely limited. We used correlation with ground truth volumes rather than absolute errors because the errors depend on m, whereas correlations do not, and also because ICV correction is based on correlation. We set the hyperparameters to $n = a = \alpha = 0.001$, $b = \beta = 0.1$, which represents very weak priors, such that the posterior distribution of the model parameters is mostly driven by the data. We set m to the mean value of the ground truth volumes, which has no effect on the correlation or ICV correction. For registration, we used a symmetric linear method based on block matching (NiftyReg [19]), applied to images downsampled by a factor of 4 in each dimension (for efficiency). Figure 2 shows sample MRI slices and the scatter plot for the ground truth and estimated ICVs, along with their linear regression. The correlation is very strong: $\rho = 0.996$, with p $\approx 10^{-6}$. These results are encouraging, but further validation is needed, given the small dataset.

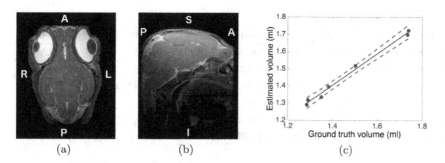

(a) (b) (c)

Fig. 2. (a) Sample axial and (b) sagittal slices from rabbit scans in our dataset; letters indicate orientation. (c) Scatter plot of ICVs: ground truth vs. estimated with our method, along with regression line (solid) and its 95% confidence interval (dashed).

3.3 Experiments on Human Dataset

We further evaluated our method indirectly with three experiments on the human dataset: we tested the strength of the correlation of hippocampal volume with age and ICV; we evaluated the ability of the ICV-corrected hippocampal volumes to discriminate EC from AD; and we tested the dependence of the performance on the set size $|\mathcal{S}|$.

We compared our proposed approach ("**PROP**") against performing no correction ("**NOCORR**") and four different methods: 1. FreeSurfer v5.3 [4] ("**FS**"): based on registration to a single template (MNI305) using cross-correlation; 2. Single atlas ("**SINGAT**"): a reimplementation of FS with NiftyReg at full resolution; 3. **SPM** [7]: we compute the ICV by summing the volumes of the gray matter, white matter and CSF, computed with SPM12 (default parameters); and 4. Non-linear ("**PROPNL**"): PROP with nonlinear registration [20] – we manually segmented the intracranial cavity in the atlas; nonlinearly propagated this mask to all subjects to create a silver standard; computed pairwise nonlinear registrations between subjects; propagated the silver standard masks; and computed S_{ij} as the difference in mask volume before and after registration.

By matching registration algorithms, SINGAT isolates the contribution of our framework to the improvement achieved over FS. SPM represents a much more complex, segmentation-based algorithm. PROPNL enables us to assess the potential improvement yielded by a more precise registration, which in principle could avoid bias from brain atrophy and disregard the contribution of extracranial regions. We used the same values of n, a, α, β as in the rabbit dataset, and set m to the mean ICV computed by FreeSurfer.

Table 1. Correlation coefficients (ρ) between hippocampal volume and age/ICV, with 95% confidence intervals and p-values (null hypothesis: $\rho = 0$). For age, we have included the required sample size to detect the effect of age on hippocampal volume, with significance level 0.01 and power 0.99. Bold font indicates the top performing method.

Method	ρ_{age} (95% C.I.)	p-value	Sample size	ρ_{icv} (95% C.I.)	p-value
NOCORR	-0.23 ([$-0.44, -0.01$])	0.0453	13	N/A	N/A
FS	-0.32 ([$-0.51, -0.10$])	0.0076	10	0.31 ([0.09,0.51])	0.009312
SINGAT	-0.38 ([$-0.56, -0.16$])	0.0014	9	0.47 ([0.27,0.63])	0.000042
SPM	-0.37 ([$-0.55, -0.15$])	0.0021	9	0.45 ([0.24,0.61])	0.000109
PROPNL	-0.32 ([$-0.51, -0.10$])	0.0067	10	0.40 ([0.19,0.58])	0.000615
PROP	**-0.40 ([$-0.58, -0.18$])**	**0.0008**	**8**	**0.51 ([0.32,0.67])**	**0.000007**

Effect of aging on hippocampal volume: Using only the healthy subjects, we first inspect the partial correlation between hippocampal volumes (computed with FreeSurfer, left-right averaged) and age/ICV, i.e., correcting for each other. For our method, we used all pairwise registrations. The results are shown in Table 1, and sample outputs in Fig. 3. All methods increase the correlations between hippocampal volume and age. SINGAT outperforms FreeSurfer, thanks to the more robust registration. Despite being a more complex method, the performance of SPM is on par with that of SINGAT, because SPM sometimes

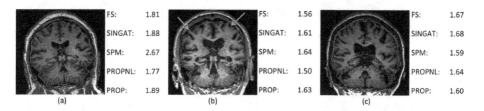

Fig. 3. Coronal slices of three subjects, and estimated ICVs (in liters). The intracranial cavity mask from SPM is contoured in red, and the one propagated from the reference atlas in blue. (a) Oversegmentation by SPM. (b) Good SPM segmentation, poor mask from reference (see areas pointed by arrows). (c) Good SPM segmentation; poor registration to the atlas negatively impacts the performance of all methods, except ours.

includes large portions of bone in the segmentation due to poor contrast in T1 MR (see Fig. 3a). We observed a similar effect in PROPNL, exacerbated by the fact that errors propagate along two registrations (see Fig. 3b). Our method produces the highest correlation, with a mild, borderline significant (Steiger's test [21]: p = 0.05) improvement over the second-to-best method (SINGAT). Compared with the widely used FreeSurfer, the improvement is noticeable: $\Delta\rho = 0.08$ (Steiger's p = 0.01), and sample size reduced from 10 to 8. A similar trend can be observed for the correlation between ICV and hippocampal volume.

Alzheimer's disease classification: We computed the area under the ROC curve (AUROC) and the accuracy at its elbow for classifiers based on thresholding ICV/age corrected hippocampal volumes. We used DeLong's test [22] to compare AUROCs. The results are shown in Table 2. Our method provides the highest AUROC, with significant improvement with respect to all others, except SPM. It also provides the second-to-best accuracy at elbow, after PROPNL.

Table 2. AD/EC classification: AUROC, accuracy at elbow and Delong's p for comparison of the AUROC with that of the method in the corresponding column.

Method	AUROC	Acc. Elbow	Vs.	FS	SINGAT	SPM	PROPNL	PROP
NOCORR	0.905	0.847	DeLong p	0.0311	0.0077	0.0052	0.0031	0.0008
FS	0.911	0.840		*	0.0193	0.0148	0.0045	0.0005
SINGAT	0.915	0.847		*	*	0.0716	0.0461	0.0004
SPM	0.921	0.873		*	*	*	0.9962	0.1052
PROPNL	0.921	**0.880**		*	*	*	*	0.0468
PROP	**0.927**	0.873		*	*	*	*	*

Performance as a function of the number of available registrations: Since the number of registrations increases quickly with N, it is useful to test how robust our algorithm is against missing scaling factors, to see if computational cost can be reduced by computing only a subset of the registrations, without

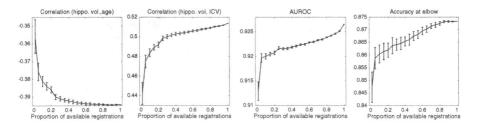

Fig. 4. Performance vs. % of maximum set size; error bars span two standard deviations

significant loss of accuracy. For a number of set sizes, we drew 100 random samples (with rejection to ensure fully connected graphs); computed the partial correlations, AUROCs and accuracies; and calculated their averages across the samples. The results are shown in Fig. 4. The correlations increase quickly in the beginning, and plateau at around 40–50% of the maximum set size. The AUROC and accuracy improve slowly until 100%, as they are more sensitive to volume estimate changes in samples closer to the decision boundary.

4   Discussion and Conclusion

We propose an ICV estimation method that does not require labeled data and is agnostic to the imaged species, and which inherits the advantages of registration-based ICV estimation – while being more robust against registration errors. This is despite using linear registration, which could be biased by extracranial and intracranial changes (e.g., neck size, atrophy); such bias was not observed in our experiments. Our approach can be combined with any registration method; we used a symmetric algorithm to save half of the registrations when building S.

Despite the high number of required registrations, our method is not too computationally expensive, as low-resolution registrations run in 3–4 s on a single core. Moreover, S can be precomputed such that, when a new scan arrives, only N new registrations are required. We also tested a non-linear version, but the increased flexibility did not compensate for the introduced registration errors and increased computational cost. The inference algorithm takes just a few seconds, which is negligible compared with the running time of the registrations.

The experiments in this paper have shown that our method outperforms single atlas ICV estimation in analyses like effect of age and AD classification. Moreover, it also outperforms the much more complex SPM, in spite of using linear registrations. Even though the contribution of the raw hippocampal volume is larger that of the ICV to such analyses, our method can still provide a moderate, statistically significant improvement. Future work will consider more complex distributions for the ICVs, e.g., conditioned on sex and gestational age.

Acknowledgement. Supported by ERC (677697), EPSRC (EP/L016478/1, EP/M506448/1), Wellcome/EPSRC (203145Z/16/Z, WT101957, NS/A000027/1).

Appendix: Details of the Inference Algorithm

Replacing $p(\boldsymbol{S}|c, \boldsymbol{v})$ and $p(c|\alpha, \beta)$ (Fig. 1b) in the first integral of Eq. 1:

$$\int_c (2c)^{-|S|} \exp\left(-\frac{1}{c} \sum_{(i,j)\in S} |S_{ij} - v_i + v_j|\right) \frac{\beta^\alpha}{\Gamma(\alpha)} c^{-\alpha-1} \exp(-\beta/c) dc. \quad (3)$$

Defining $\alpha' = \alpha + |S|$ and $\beta' = \beta + \sum_{(i,j)\in S} |S_{ij} - v_i + v_j|$, Eq. 3 becomes:

$$\frac{1}{2^{|S|}} \frac{\Gamma(\alpha')}{\Gamma(\alpha)} \frac{\beta^\alpha}{\beta'^{\alpha'}} \int_c \frac{\beta'^{\alpha'}}{\Gamma(\alpha')} c^{-\alpha'-1} \exp(-\beta'/c) dc = \frac{1}{2^{|S|}} \frac{\Gamma(\alpha')}{\Gamma(\alpha)} \frac{\beta^\alpha}{\beta'^{\alpha'}}, \quad (4)$$

as the integral is over the probability density of $IG(\alpha', \beta')$ and thus equal to 1.

For the second integral in Eq. 1 (over μ and σ^2), substitution of the expressions for the probabilities (again, see Fig. 1b in the paper) yields:

$$\int_\mu \int_{\sigma^2} \frac{1}{(2\pi\sigma^2)^{N/2}} \exp\left(-\frac{1}{2\sigma^2} \sum_{i=1}^N (v_i - \mu)^2\right) \ldots$$
$$\times \frac{b^a}{\Gamma(a)} (\sigma^2)^{-a-1} \exp(-b/\sigma^2) \frac{\sqrt{n}}{\sqrt{2\pi\sigma^2}} \exp\left[-\frac{n}{2\sigma^2} (\mu - m)^2\right] d\mu d\sigma^2. \quad (5)$$

We now define $m' = (nm + N\bar{v})/(n + N)$, $n' = n + N$, $a' = a + \frac{N}{2}$, and:

$$b' = b + \frac{1}{2} \sum_{i=1}^N (v_i - \bar{v})^2 + \frac{nN}{n + N} \frac{(\bar{v} - m)^2}{2},$$

where $\bar{v}$ is the average of $\boldsymbol{v}$. Then, Eq. 5 becomes:

$$\int_\mu \int_{\sigma^2} \frac{b'^{a'}}{\Gamma(a')} (\sigma^2)^{-a'-1} \exp(-b'/\sigma^2) \frac{\sqrt{n'}}{\sqrt{2\pi\sigma^2}} \exp\left[-\frac{n'}{2\sigma^2} (\mu - m')^2\right] d\mu d\sigma^2 \ldots$$
$$\times \frac{1}{(2\pi)^{N/2}} \sqrt{\frac{n}{n'}} \frac{b^a}{b'^{a'}} \frac{\Gamma(a')}{\Gamma(a)} = \frac{1}{(2\pi)^{N/2}} \sqrt{\frac{n}{n'}} \frac{b^a}{b'^{a'}} \frac{\Gamma(a')}{\Gamma(a)}, \quad (6)$$

since the integral is over the probability density function of $NIG(m', n', a', b')$ and hence equal to 1.

Combining Eqs. 4 and 6, the problem in Eq. 1 becomes:

$$\hat{\boldsymbol{v}} = \underset{\boldsymbol{v}}{\text{argmax}} \frac{1}{2^{|S|}} \frac{\Gamma(\alpha')}{\Gamma(\alpha)} \frac{\beta^\alpha}{\beta'^{\alpha'}} \frac{1}{(2\pi)^{N/2}} \sqrt{\frac{n}{n'}} \frac{b^a}{b'^{a'}} \frac{\Gamma(a')}{\Gamma(a)}$$
$$= \underset{\boldsymbol{v}}{\text{argmax}} \left(\beta'^{\alpha'} b'^{a'} z(\alpha, \beta, |S|, n, a, b, N)\right)^{-1},$$

where z groups the terms independent of $\boldsymbol{v}$. Taking the negated logarithm:

$$C = \alpha' \log \beta' + a' \log b' + \log z.$$

Substituting a', b', α' and β' into this equation, and defining $Z = \log z$, we finally obtain the cost function in Eq. 2.

References

1. Sanfilipo, M.P., Benedict, R.H., Zivadinov, R., Bakshi, R.: Correction for intracranial volume in analysis of whole brain atrophy in multiple sclerosis: the proportion vs. residual method. Neuroimage **22**(4), 1732–1743 (2004)
2. Lemieux, L., Hagemann, G., Krakow, K., Woermann, F.G.: Fast, accurate, and reproducible automatic segmentation of the brain in T1-weighted volume MRI data. Magn. Reson. Med. **42**(1), 127–135 (1999)
3. Smith, S.M., Zhang, Y., Jenkinson, M., Chen, J., Matthews, P., Federico, A., De Stefano, N.: Accurate, robust, and automated longitudinal and cross-sectional brain change analysis. Neuroimage **17**(1), 479–489 (2002)
4. Buckner, R.L., Head, D., Parker, J., Fotenos, A.F., Marcus, D., Morris, J.C., Snyder, A.Z.: A unified approach for morphometric and functional data analysis in young, old, and demented adults using automated atlas-based head size normalization: reliability and validation against manual measurement of total intracranial volume. Neuroimage **23**(2), 724–738 (2004)
5. Fischl, B.: Freesurfer. Neuroimage **62**(2), 774–781 (2012)
6. Smith, S.M., Jenkinson, M., Woolrich, M.W., Beckmann, C.F., Behrens, T.E., et al.: Advances in functional and structural MR image analysis and implementation as FSL. Neuroimage **23**, S208–S219 (2004)
7. Ashburner, J., Friston, K.J.: Unified segmentation. Neuroimage **26**(3), 839–851 (2005)
8. Penny, W.D., Friston, K.J., Ashburner, J.T., Kiebel, S.J., Nichols, T.E.: Statistical Parametric Mapping: The Analysis of Functional Brain Images. Academic Press, New York (2011)
9. Keihaninejad, S., Heckemann, R.A., Fagiolo, G., Symms, M.R., Hajnal, J.V., Hammers, A.: A robust method to estimate the intracranial volume across MRI field strengths (1.5T and 3T). Neuroimage **50**(4), 1427–1437 (2010)
10. Huo, Y., Asman, A.J., Plassard, A.J., Landman, B.A.: Simultaneous total intracranial volume and posterior fossa volume estimation using multi-atlas label fusion. Hum. Brain Mapp. **2**, 599–616 (2017)
11. Manjón, J.V., Eskildsen, S.F., Coupé, P., Romero, J.E., Collins, D.L., Robles, M.: Nonlocal intracranial cavity extraction. Int. J. Biomed. Imaging **2014**, 11 p. (2014). Article ID 820205. doi:10.1155/2014/820205
12. Kuklisova-Murgasova, M., Aljabar, P., Srinivasan, L., Counsell, S.J., Doria, V., Serag, A., Gousias, I.S., Boardman, J.P., Rutherford, M.A., Edwards, A.D., et al.: A dynamic 4D probabilistic atlas of the developing brain. NeuroImage **54**(4), 2750–2763 (2011)
13. Licandro, R., Langs, G., Kasprian, G., Sablatnig, R., Prayer, D., Schwartz, E.: Longitudinal diffeomorphic atlas learning for fetal brain tissue labeling using geodesic regression. In: Brain 2011 (2011)
14. Tyson, J.E., Parikh, N.A., Langer, J., Green, C., Higgins, R.D.: Intensive care for extreme prematurity moving beyond gestational age. N. Engl. J. Med. **358**(16), 1672–1681 (2008)
15. Blencowe, H., Cousens, S., Oestergaard, M.Z., Chou, D., Moller, A.B., Narwal, R., Adler, A., Garcia, C.V., Rohde, S., Say, L., et al.: National, regional, and worldwide estimates of preterm birth rates in the year 2010 with time trends since 1990 for selected countries: a systematic analysis and implications. Lancet **379**(9832), 2162–2172 (2012)

16. Liu, L., Johnson, H.L., Cousens, S., Perin, J., Scott, S., Lawn, J.E., Rudan, I., Campbell, H., Cibulskis, R., Li, M., et al.: Global, regional, and national causes of child mortality: an updated systematic analysis for 2010 with time trends since 2000. Lancet **379**(9832), 2151–2161 (2012)
17. Muñoz-Moreno, E., Arbat-Plana, A., Batalle, D., Soria, G., Illa, M., Prats-Galino, A., Eixarch, E., Gratacos, E.: A magnetic resonance image based atlas of the rabbit brain for automatic parcellation. PLoS ONE **8**(7), e67418 (2013)
18. Shewchuk, J.R.: An introduction to the conjugate gradient method without the agonizing pain (1994)
19. Modat, M., Cash, D.M., Daga, P., Winston, G.P., Duncan, J.S., Ourselin, S.: Global image registration using a symmetric block-matching approach. J. Med. Imaging **1**(2), 024003–024003 (2014)
20. Modat, M., Ridgway, G.R., Taylor, Z.A., Lehmann, M., Barnes, J., Hawkes, D.J., Fox, N.C., Ourselin, S.: Fast free-form deformation using graphics processing units. Comput. Methods Programs Biomed. **98**(3), 278–284 (2010)
21. Steiger, J.H.: Tests for comparing elements of a correlation matrix. Psychol. Bull. **87**(2), 245–251 (1980)
22. DeLong, E.R., DeLong, D.M., Clarke-Pearson, D.L.: Comparing the areas under two or more correlated receiver operating characteristic curves: a nonparametric approach. Biometrics **44**, 837–845 (1988)

Assessing Reorganisation of Functional Connectivity in the Infant Brain

Roxane Licandro[1,2]([✉]), Karl-Heinz Nenning[2], Ernst Schwartz[2],
Kathrin Kollndorfer[2], Lisa Bartha-Doering[3], Hesheng Liu[4], and Georg Langs[2]

[1] Institute of Computer Aided Automation - Computer Vision Lab,
Vienna University of Technology, Vienna, Austria
licandro@caa.tuwien.ac.at
[2] Department of Biomedical Imaging and Image-guided Therapy - Computational
Imaging Research Lab, Medical University of Vienna, Vienna, Austria
[3] Department of Pediatrics and Adolescent Medicine,
Medical University of Vienna, Vienna, Austria
[4] Department of Radiology, Martinos Center, MGH,
Harvard Medical School, Boston, USA

Abstract. As maturation of neural networks continues throughout childhood, brain lesions insulting immature networks have different impact on brain function than lesions obtained after full network maturation. Thus, longitudinal studies and analysis of spatial and temporal brain signal correlations are a key component to get a deeper understanding of individual maturation processes, their interaction and their link to cognition. Here, we assess the connectivity pattern deviation of developing resting state networks after ischaemic stroke of children between 7 and 17 years. We propose a method to derive a reorganisational score to detect target regions for overtaking affected functional regions within a stroke location. The evaluation is performed using rs-fMRI data of 16 control subjects and 16 stroke patients. The developing functional connectivity affected by ischaemic stroke exhibits significant differences to the control cohort. This suggests an influence of stroke location and developmental stage on regenerating processes and the reorganisational patterns.

1 Introduction

Human brain development starts during pregnancy and proceeds in building structural as well as functional trajectories through adulthood until senescence [17]. Morphological, functional, and cognitive maturation is shaped by genetic and environmental influence such as learning processes and experience after birth, and the resulting structure varies substantially across individuals [21]. While the functional and morphological organization of the adults' brain is known to a large extent, we are only starting to understand its emergence and maturation [17]. We know that we can observe distributed components similar to those in adults already in neonates [8], while substantial changes to the brain network structure occur during childhood, such as an increase in long-,

M.J. Cardoso et al. (Eds.): FIFI/OMIA 2017, LNCS 10554, pp. 14–24, 2017.
DOI: 10.1007/978-3-319-67561-9_2

and a decrease in short-distance connections from infants to adults [5]. However, these observations primarily focus on the comparison of age snapshots, and do not capture multivariate temporal change patterns of the connectome. There is a particularly critical gap in knowledge concerning normal development confronted with disease or adverse events such as stroke.

Paediatric Ischaemic Stroke (IS) is caused by a decreased blood flow in cerebral vessels (ischaemia), which in an irreversible case leads to the death of brain cells and forming of brain lesions [15]. Stroke in children is a rare event, with an international incidence of 1.2 to 13 per 100,000 children per year under 18 years of age [19]. Children, who survive an IS, suffer from lifelong motoric or cognitive disabilities as well as developing or learning problems. Their outcome varies over age, the stroke location or additional comorbidities [15]. Functional MRI techniques (fMRI) enable the measurement of functional organisation [4]. In comparison to task-based fMRI, pediatric resting state (rs)-fMRI aims to image neural activation and analyse brain signals due to their temporal correlation independent of a stimulus [1] in a non-invasive way.

Plasticity is the process which enables the central nervous system to dynamically adapt to external stimuli. Natural plasticity is induced by the age and developmental related changes of the brain and is triggered by learning and experience [2], where adaptive plasticity refers to pathology related modifications, e.g. functional and structural reorganisation of brain tissue after stroke [13]. Also genetic factors can drive these processes [12]. While we have gained some understanding in reorganization processes in adults [14], we have poor understanding of how reorganization interacts with development. Resting state fMRI enables the study of these processes driving the functional and structural organisation. Ultimately they can lead to improved functional outcome of children suffering from brain injuries, by developing novel interventional techniques or adapting therapy, dependent on the developmental stage of a disease [13].

Challenges. The challenges for studying reorganisation in children lies in capturing the dynamics of interactions between adaptive and developmental processes. After a damage, plasticity and vulnerability of the brain influence recovery together with the injuries severity, the age and the time since damage [2]. Functional recovery after brain injury depends on the ability of the brain to adapt to changes [9]. Recent studies suggest that cognitive abilities after brain injury are dependent on the plasticity of neural networks that control brain functions [10]. Thus, the impact of brain injury on cognition is best studied by investigating neuronal networks rather than circumscribed areas [3]. As maturation of neural networks continues throughout childhood [5], brain lesions insulting immature networks have a different impact on function than lesions acquired after full network maturation. A deeper understanding of individual continuous maturation processes, their interaction, and their link to cognition is essential for our understanding of the functional brain architecture, treatment and optimal promotion of children [12].

Contribution. The methodological contribution of this work is two-fold: (1) we propose a technique to quantify connectivity pattern deviation in the development of functional connectivity, and (2) a method to *track* regions which exhibit similar connectivity characteristics as *source* regions such as an area impacted by stroke after reorganization. We hypothesize that (1) stroke subjects exhibit higher deviation from a control population age specific mean than controls, and (2) reorganization causes new regions to adopt connectivity characteristics of areas impaired by stroke due to reorganization. We adapt an approach by [16] to extract connectivity pattern deviation over development and reorganisational patterns of functional connectivity in children induced by laesions forming after an ischaemic stroke. The methodologies proposed are summarised in Sect. 2. The evaluation setup and computed results are documented in Sect. 3 and a discussion and possibilities for future work are given in Sect. 4.

2   Methodology

In this section the methodology is introduced, by providing (1) a Connectivity Profile Deviation (CPD) score to analyse deviations between control and stroke subjects and (2) by tracking reorganization using the proposed prior. For the formulations we assume a graph based representation of the cortical surface, which is previously normalized to a standardized surface consisting of nodes $x = 1 \ldots N$. For every subject the Connectivity Matrix $CM \in \mathbb{R}^{N \times N}$ is computed and stroke masks are annotated (for more details regarding the preprocessing and dataset used cf. Sect. 3).

Age specific reference of connectivity profiles across the cortex. According to the size of the dataset and preliminary analysis we decided to perform element wise linear regression of correlation coefficient matrices of control subjects to derive the slope $B \in \mathbb{R}^{N \times N}$. An age matched correlation matrix $\overline{CM}$ is then computed using Eq. 1.

$$\overline{CM}^{age} = B * age + B_0 \tag{1}$$

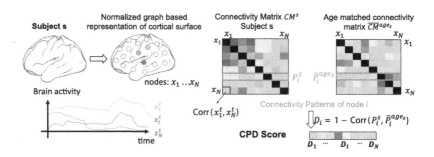

Fig. 1. Schematic illustration of the computation of the CPD score.

Identifying deviations of local connectivity characteristics. In a second step the CPD score $D \in \mathbb{R}^{1 \times N}$ is computed between every single subject's CM^s and the age matched $\overline{CM}^{age_s}$ using Pearson Correlation Coefficient (PCC) (cf. Eq. 2).

$$D_x^s = 1 - PCC(P_x^s, \overline{P}_x^{age_s}), x = 1 \dots N \tag{2}$$

Therefore, a connectivity pattern $P_x^s \in \mathbb{R}^{1 \times N}$ of a vertex x and the corresponding age matched connectivity pattern $\overline{P}_x^{age_s} \in \mathbb{R}^{1 \times N}$ of controls are computed, where $P_x^s = CM_{i=x,j}$, $\overline{P}_x^{age_s} = \overline{CM}_{i=x,j}^{age_s}$, $j = 1 \dots N$ (cf. Fig. 1). This CPD score is computed for every subject s in the dataset (control and stroke cases).

Finding target areas of reorganization. In this work we propose a *ReOrganisation Score (ROS)* for identifying possible regions, where functional networks of a stroke region transfer to. For clearer understanding its computation is schematically illustrated in Fig. 2. In a first step the corresponding stroke case's age matched $\overline{CM}^{age}$ is computed. In a second step for every stroke subject separately the stroke mask is used to determine the set $u, 1 \dots W, W \leq N$ of nodes corresponding to the stroke regions. In a third step we compute the Reorganisation Maps (RM) $RM_{u,z}^s$ and $RM_{u,z}^{age_s}$ between connectivity patterns using Eqs. 3 and 4. We define $z = x \setminus u$ as set of nodes not belonging to the stroke region. $\overline{P}_{u_l}^{age_s} = \overline{CM}_{i=u_l,j=z}^{age_s}$, $P_{z_k}^s = CM_{i=z_k,j=z}$, $\overline{P}_{z_k}^{age_s} = \overline{CM}_{i=z_k,j=z}$, $k = 1 \dots M, M = |x \setminus u|, l = 1 \dots W$.

$$RM_{u,z}^s = PCC(\overline{P}_u^{age_s}, P_{z_k}^s), s = 1 \dots S \tag{3}$$

$$RM_{u,z}^{age_s} = PCC(\overline{P}_u^{age_s}, \overline{P}_{z_k}^{age_s}), s = 1 \dots S \tag{4}$$

After the calculation of the RMs we extracted the vertex of set u with the maximum value. Since RM of the control model show higher values as RM of

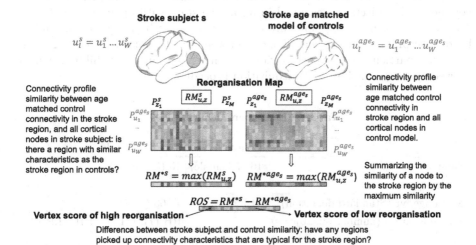

Fig. 2. Schematic illustration of the computation of the reorganisation score.

the stroke, we decided (for obtaining comparability for visualisation purposes) to perform histogram equalisation, resulting in two vectors $RM^{*s} \in \mathbb{R}^{1 \times M}$ and $RM^{*age_s} \in \mathbb{R}^{1 \times M}$. Subsequently, we estimate the ROS of a subject S as defined in Eq. 5.

$$ROS = RM^{*s} - RM^{*age_s}, \tag{5}$$

3 Results

The participants in this study are 32 children between 7 and 17 years consisting of 16 control cases and 16 ischaemic stroke cases (cf. participant demographics in Table 1). Subject No. 15 (control), No. 17 (stroke), and No. 21 (stroke) were excluded, due to technical issues during acquisition. During the preprocessing phase three stroke subjects (No. 3, 10 and 22) and control subjects (No. 26, 33 and 34) were excluded because of high motion artefacts (5 subjects) and severe stroke (more than the half of the size of a hemisphere was affected). The stroke events occurred at different spatial locations on the right (RH) or left hemisphere (LH). The children were right-, left- or mixed handed. The time frame between scan event and stroke event, as well as the range of the age at stroke of the children ranges from 0 to 15 years. All participants' guardians (parents) were informed about the aim of the study and gave their written, informed consent prior to inclusion. The protocol of this study was approved by the national ethics committee of the Medical University of Vienna and performed in accordance with the Declaration of Helsinki (1964), including current revisions and the EC-GCP guidelines. The scanning was performed on a 3T TIM Trio System (Siemens Medical Solution, Erlangen, Germany) Scanner and rs-fMRI measurements were performed using single-shot, gradient-recalled, echo-planar imaging with the following setup: TR = 2000 ms, TE = 42 ms, FOV = 210 × 210 mm, slices = 20, gap between slices = 1 mm, slice thickness = 4 mm, frames = 150 volumes. All subjects are scanned in an awake state with open eyes for 5 min. To restrict head motion, pillows are used as fixation on both sides of the child's head. The probands wore headphones to attenuate the noise level during scan. All study participants watched a video, explicitly designed for children, which showed and explained an MRI acquisition procedure.

Table 1. Participant demographics

	Control	Pediatric stroke
Sample size	16 (7 Female)	16 (5 Female)
Excluded	4	5
Mean age, yr (Standard deviation)	11.2 (3.19)	11.63 (3.14)
Stroke location (number of subjects)	-	RH (7), LH (7), RH + LH (2)

Anatomical and Functional Preprocessing. Anatomical and functional preprocessing is performed using Freesurfer[1][6] and FSL[2][11]. The functional preprocessing includes a registration to the anatomical data, head motion regression and bandpass temporal filtering (0.01–0.1 Hz) to remove constant offsets and linear trends. Cerebral signals of the stroke and control cases are resampled to common FreeSurfer fsaverage5 space [7]. After this alignment every subject's cortical surface is represented as a standardized mesh consisting of 20484 nodes. After resampling the data are spatially smoothed using a 4 mm FWHM Gaussian filter. For the identification of correlating regions, the PCC is computed between the time course of a node $x(t)_i$ in each subject's brain and every other node's $x(t)_j$ time course. This results in a correlation coefficient matrix $CM_{i,j} \in \mathbb{R}^{N \times N}$, where N is the number of nodes observed, $i = 1 \ldots N$ the ith row and $j = 1 \ldots N$ the jth column of the matrix [18]. For every subject in the stroke cohort masks of brain lesion are annotated by an expert and also preprocessed using the introduced preprocessing pipeline.

Deviation of local connectivity characteristics in the control cohort. Figure 3 illustrates the CPD score for control subjects of different age (left) and its change over increasing age (right). The intersubject deviation of controls is minimal in the visual, sensory and motor cortices and correlates with increasing age to the deviation estimates in [16] of adult controls. High deviation is observed in the temporal cortex including primary auditory cortex, Wernicke's area, in the prefrontal cortex and parietal lobe. Considering the age a decrease of deviation in the heteromodal regions is observable with increasing age also visible in the corresponding boxplot of CPD scores in Fig. 4 (left).

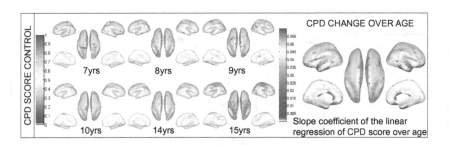

Fig. 3. Visualisation of the CPD score in control subjects during ageing: 6 control subjects and their deviation to the age matched average, and the visualisation of the change: red regions exhibit increased deviation/deviation change, while blue regions are more stable. (Color figure online)

---

[1] http://surfer.nmr.mgh.harvard.edu [accessed 16th May 2017].
[2] http://fsl.fmrib.ox.ac.uk/fsl/fslwiki/FSL [accessed 16th May 2017].

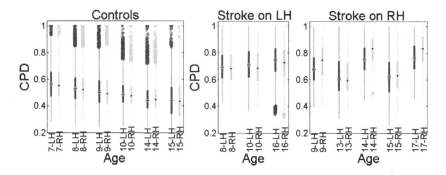

Fig. 4. Visualisation of CPD score of LH and RH within the stroke and control cohort (CPD scores of all subjects at same age are grouped here). Control cases show symmetric mean CPD between RH and LH and a decrease according to increasing age. The CPD scores of stroke subjects show higher means on the hemisphere of stroke location. (Color figure online)

Deviation of local connectivity characteristics in the stroke cohort. For the stroke subjects RH and LH stroke cases are grouped together for clearer visualisation in Fig. 5. The stroke cohort shows higher variabilities compared to the control cohort, which overlaps with the hypothesis that stroke affects the reorganisation of connectivity networks, resulting in higher CPD. It is observable that higher intersubject CPD over 0.8 are observable on the hemisphere of stroke location also visible in the corresponding boxplot of CPD scores in Fig. 4 (middle, right).

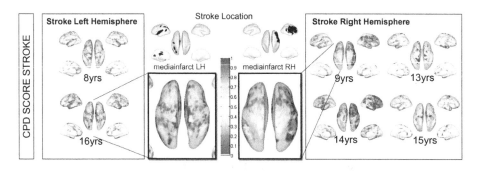

Fig. 5. Visualisation of CPD score of LH stroke subjects (left) and RH stroke subjects (right). (Color figure online)

Target regions of reorganisational processes. To evaluate the ability of the ROS to detect reorganisational regions we first divided the brain surface into 17 cortical networks using the parcellation proposed by Yeo et al. [20], which is computed based on rsfMRI acquisitions of 1000 subjects and additionally provides fsaverage 5 surface labels. For every region (total 36 - LH and RH are observed separately) the ratio of stroke voxels and the region's mean ROS and mean CPD are estimated. In Fig. 6 the first row illustrates correlation matrices $\in \mathbb{R}^{36 \times 36}$ based on correlations computed between the ratio of stroke voxels and mean CPD for all subjects (first column), for LH stroke subjects (second column) and RH stroke subjects (third column). In Fig. 6 second row the mean ROS score is used instead of the mean CPD to estimate the correlations. In Fig. 6 a deviation of correlation values between LH and RH stroke subjects is visible, since correlations only between a stroke voxel ratio (>0) on the ipsilateral side can be computed. In the first row of Fig. 6 positive correlations are observable, which can be interpreted as regions greater affected by a stroke lesion show a higher mean CPD and a lower mean CPD if they are less affected. Additionally, stronger blocks of correlation scores are observable in the default mode network regions (except the temporal component Default A) or somato motoric areas. In the second row of Fig. 6 especially for RH stroke subjects (right) a division of RH and LH correlation values according to their sign is visible, since the severity of stroke and number of subjects is higher in this cohort compared to LH stroke subjects. The voxel ratio positively correlates with the ROS of the contralateral side and negatively with the ROS of the ipsilateral side. This suggests a decrease of the ROS in ipsilateral and an increase of the ROS in contralateral regions with increased stroke voxel ratio in the stroke hemisphere. In Fig. 7 the target regions for possible reorganisational processes after stroke, computed using the ROS

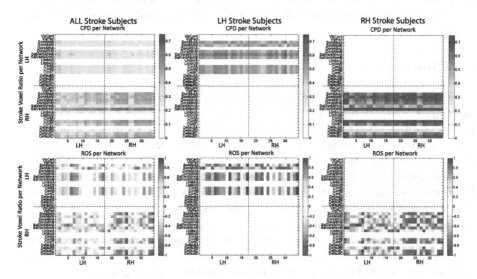

Fig. 6. Row one visualises the network wise correlations between the stroke voxel ratio and the CPD score using all stroke subjects (first column), LH stroke (second column) and RH stroke subjects (third column). Visualisation of network wise correlations between the stroke voxel ratio and the ROS are shown in row two. (Color figure online)

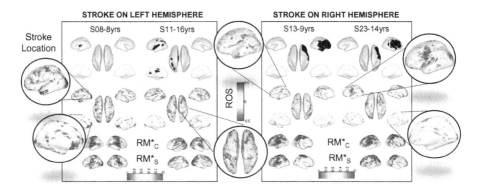

Fig. 7. Visualisation of regions that pick up connectivity patterns observed in the stroke region in age matched control average. Red ROS indicates regions that exhibit characteristics typical for the stroke regions if the subject is a control. (Color figure online)

proposed are visualised for LH stroke subjects (left) and RH stroke subjects (right). The first row visualises the stroke location, the second row the ROS and the third and fourth row the histogram equalized reorganisation vectors. Subject S08 shows possible target regions in its strokes neighbourhood on the ipsilateral side. S11 shows possible symmetric reorganisation targets. S13 and S23 with a severe mediainfarct on the RH show both on the contro and ipsilateral side of non-stroke region an increased ROS as well as on the contralateral side in the stroke region.

4   Conclusion

We present a methodology to assess connectivity pattern deviation in developing functional networks and to estimate possible target regions of reorganisational processes after ischaemic stroke. According to the results we can conclude that stroke subjects show a higher deviation compared to control subjects, especially more on the hemisphere of stroke location. Control subjects show decreasing deviation over age to age matched controls, with highest changes occuring in the prefrontal cortex and temporal lobe. We proposed a reorganisational score, which identifies ipsi-lateral and symmetric networks in neighbourhood of the stroke location as possible indicator for reorganisation in developing resting state networks. The limit of our approach lies in the size and heterogeneity of the dataset. For future work we will evaluate different stroke datasets with similar locations of the stroke lesions and a higher number of participants.

Acknowledgement. This work was co-funded by the Oesterreichische Nationalbank (Anniversary Fund, project number 15356), by the FWF under KLI 544-B27 and I 2714-B31, by the European Commision FP7-PEOPLE-2013-IAPP 610872 and by ZIT Life Sciences 2014 (1207843).

References

1. Altman, N.R., Bernal, B.: Clinical applications of functional magnetic resonance imaging. Pediatr. Radiol. **45**(3), 382–396 (2015)
2. Anderson, V., Spencer-Smith, M., Wood, A.: Do children really recover better? Neurobehavioural plasticity after early brain insult. Brain J. Neurol. **134**(Pt 8), 2197–221 (2011)
3. Bullmore, E., Sporns, O.: Complex brain networks: graph theoretical analysis of structural and functional systems. Nat. Rev. Neurosci. **10**(3), 186–198 (2009)
4. Casey, B., Tottenham, N., Liston, C., Durston, S.: Imaging the developing brain: what have we learned about cognitive development? TiCS **9**(3), 104–110 (2005)
5. Fair, D.A., Cohen, A.L., Power, J.D., Dosenbach, N.U.F., Church, J.A., Miezin, F.M., Schlaggar, B.L., Petersen, S.E.: Functional brain networks develop from a "local to distributed" organization. PLoS Comput. Biol. **5**(5), e1000381 (2009)
6. Fischl, B.: FreeSurfer. Neuroimage **62**(2), 774–781 (2012)
7. Fischl, B., Sereno, M.I., Tootell, R.B., Dale, A.M.: High-resolution intersubject averaging and a coordinate system for the cortical surface. Hum. Brain Mapp. **8**(4), 272–84 (1999)
8. Gao, W., Zhu, H., Giovanello, K.S., Smith, J.K., Shen, D., Gilmore, J.H., Lin, W.: Evidence on the emergence of the brain's default network from 2-week-old to 2-year-old healthy pediatric subjects. Proc. Natl. Acad. Sci. U.S.A. **106**(16), 6790–6795 (2009)
9. Huttenlocher, P.R.: Neural Plasticity: The Effects of Environment on the Development of the Cerebral Cortex. Harvard University Press, Cambridge (2002)
10. Ius, T., Angelini, E., Thiebaut de Schotten, M., Mandonnet, E., Duffau, H.: Evidence for potentials and limitations of brain plasticity using an atlas of functional resectability of WHO grade II gliomas: towards a minimal common brain. NeuroImage **56**(3), 992–1000 (2011)
11. Jenkinson, M., Beckmann, C.F., Behrens, T.E.J., Woolrich, M.W., Smith, S.M.: FSL. NeuroImage **62**(2), 782–90 (2012)
12. Johnston, M.V.: Plasticity in the developing brain: implications for rehabilitation. Dev. Disabil. Res. Rev. **15**(2), 94–101 (2009)
13. Kornfeld, S., Delgado Rodríguez, J.A., Everts, R., Kaelin-Lang, A., Wiest, R., Weisstanner, C., Mordasini, P., Steinlin, M., Grunt, S.: Cortical reorganisation of cerebral networks after childhood stroke: impact on outcome. BMC Neurol. **15**(1), 90 (2015)
14. La Corte, V., Sperduti, M., Malherbe, C., Vialatte, F., Lion, S., Gallarda, T., Oppenheim, C., Piolino, P.: Cognitive decline and reorganization of functional connectivity in healthy aging: the pivotal role of the salience network in the prediction of age and cognitive performances. Front. Aging Neurosci. **8**, 204 (2016)
15. Lynch, J.K., Han, C.J.: Pediatric stroke - what do we know and what do we need to know? Semin. Neurol. **25**(4), 410–423 (2005)
16. Mueller, S., Wang, D., Fox, M.D., Yeo, B.T.T., Sepulcre, J., Sabuncu, M.R., Shafee, R., Lu, J., Liu, H.: Individual variability in functional connectivity architecture of the human brain. Neuron **77**(3), 586–595 (2013)
17. Power, J.D., Fair, D.A., Schlaggar, B.L., Petersen, S.E.: The development of human functional brain networks. Neuron **67**(5), 735–48 (2010)
18. Sepulcre, J., Liu, H., Talukdar, T., Martincorena, I., Thomas Yeo, B.T., Buckner, R.L.: The organization of local and distant functional connectivity in the human brain. PLoS Comput. Biol. **6**(6), 1–15 (2010)

19. Tsze, D.S., Valente, J.H.: Pediatric stroke: a review. Emerg. Med. Int. **2011**, 734506 (2011)
20. Yeo, B.T.T., Krienen, F.M., Sepulcre, J., Sabuncu, M.R., Lashkari, D., Hollinshead, M., Roffman, J.L., Smoller, J.W., Zöllei, L., Polimeni, J.R., Fischl, B., Liu, H., Buckner, R.L.: The organization of the human cerebral cortex estimated by intrinsic functional connectivity. J. Neurophysiol. **106**(3), 1125–65 (2011)
21. Zilles, K., Palomero-Gallagher, N., Amunts, K.: Development of cortical folding during evolution and ontogeny. Trends Neurosci. **36**(5), 275–284 (2013)

Fetal Skull Segmentation in 3D Ultrasound via Structured Geodesic Random Forest

Juan J. Cerrolaza[1]([✉]), Ozan Oktay[1], Alberto Gomez[2], Jacqueline Matthew[2], Caroline Knight[2], Bernhard Kainz[1], and Daniel Rueckert[1]

[1] Biomedical Image Analysis Group, Imperial College London, London, UK
j.cerrolaza-martinez@imperial.ac.uk
[2] Division of Imaging Sciences and Biomedical Engineering,
King's College London, London, UK

Abstract. Ultrasound is the primary imaging method for prenatal screening and diagnosis of fetal anomalies. Thanks to its non-invasive and non-ionizing properties, ultrasound allows quick, safe and detailed evaluation of the unborn baby, including the estimation of the gestational age, brain and cranium development. However, the accuracy of traditional 2D fetal biometrics is dependent on operator expertise and subjectivity in 2D plane finding and manual marking. 3D ultrasound has the potential to reduce the operator dependence. In this paper, we propose a new random forest-based segmentation framework for fetal 3D ultrasound volumes, able to efficiently integrate semantic and structural information in the classification process. We introduce a new semantic features space able to encode spatial context via generalized geodesic distance transform. Unlike alternative auto-context approaches, this new set of features is efficiently integrated into the same forest using contextual trees. Finally, we use a new structured labels space as alternative to the traditional atomic class labels, able to capture morphological variability of the target organ. Here, we show the potential of this new general framework segmenting the skull in 3D fetal ultrasound volumes, significantly outperforming alternative random forest-based approaches.

Keywords: Random forest · Generalized geodesic distance · Structured class

1 Introduction

Ultrasound (US) imaging is the preferred screening modality for the diagnosis and monitoring of fetal anatomy during pregnancy. Its non-ionizing and non-invasive nature makes it possible to safely perform routine US-based examination of the unborn baby. In particular, an accurate gestational age (GA) estimation is essential. It defines the estimated date of delivery and may influence the success or safety of a clinical intervention. 2DUS-based biometrics, such as biparietal diameter, occipital-frontal diameter and head circumference, have been extensively used to establish the GA. However, these biometrics are prone to errors

© Springer International Publishing AG 2017
M.J. Cardoso et al. (Eds.): FIFI/OMIA 2017, LNCS 10554, pp. 25–32, 2017.
DOI: 10.1007/978-3-319-67561-9_3

due to the high intra- and inter-observer variability associated with manual measurements [15], and the subjectivity in 2D diagnostic plane selection. Moreover, the early detection of cranial malformations (e.g., craniosynostosis) requires the detailed analysis of the curvilinear cranial bones and their boundaries, which may be difficult to visualize in a single 2D plane. Despite 2DUS remains the gold standard of prenatal care [3], studies [1] have reported on the superiority of 3DUS in the evaluation of fetal anatomy and anomaly. The possibility to scan and store volumetric data offers a significant advantage over 2DUS, not only overcoming limitations associated with plane selection subjectivity, but also allowing a better understanding of fetal cranial structure [1], and the definition of new volumetric biometrics. In this context, the development of accurate automatic segmentation methods in 3DUS is paramount to alleviate the tedious and subjective manual delineation process. In recent years, there has been increasing interest in developing new segmentation strategies for sonographic images [2]. However, to the best of our knowledge, the automatic segmentation of the skull in prenatal 3DUS has not yet been satisfactorily addressed. In the early works of Lue et al. [4] and Shen et al. [5], the authors use the Hough transform to approximate the head contour to an ellipsoid in 2DUS. While the use of a predefined parametric curve can be useful to deal with fuzzy, or even incomplete skull boundaries, it cannot capture the local shape variations of skulls that are not perfectly elliptically shaped, or showing cranial malformations. Similarly, Foi et al. [7] proposed a fully automatic segmentation method of the fetal skull in 2DUS images, modeling the skull intensity as a difference of Gaussians revolved along predefined elliptical contours. More recently, Namburete and Noble [6] presented a simple random forest classifier to identify cranial pixels in 2DUS, using superpixels-based statistics as feature space. Chen et al. [8] proposed a first segmentation framework for 3DUS. However, despite acceptable results, the authors use a fetal phantom to impose shape priors, which limits the generality and applicability of this registration-based method.

In this paper, we introduce a new fully automatic framework for the segmentation of the skull in fetal 3DUS. We term this framework structured geodesic random forest (SGeo-RF). The integration of structural information in RF [9] was recently exploited by Oktay et al. [12] for the registration of cardiac images. However, its potential for the segmentation of medical images remains unexplored. The use of structured labels and semantic features is particularly relevant in the context of US image segmentation, where the low signal-to-noise ratio, signal attenuation, and missing boundaries often lead to noisy and inaccurate segmentation results which do not follow object boundaries, and anatomically inconsistent. SGeo-RF is a general framework that efficiently integrates semantic and structural information in the segmentation process, thanks to a new super-class label space introduced here.

2   Method

Traditional RF formulations suffer some important limitations. Typically, each observation is considered as a separate unit of information, making predictions for each sample independently, and preventing the classifier from enforcing dependencies between variables (i.e., predicting features), or in the label space. While the independence assumption enables efficient training and fast predictions, it also limits the capability of RF to incorporate valuable contextual and structural information into the framework. This is of particular relevance in challenging contexts such as fetal 3DUS.

Suppose $\mathbf{S}$ represents the set of data points extracted from all training images, $\mathbf{S} = \{\mathbf{p}_i, l_i\}_1^N$. Typically, each observation is defined by the corresponding voxel position, $\mathbf{p}_i$, the feature vector, $\mathbf{v}(\mathbf{p}_i) = (v_1, \ldots, v_m) \in \mathcal{X}$, and its associated class label, $l_i \in \mathcal{Y} = \{0, \ldots, K\}$ where $K \in \mathbb{N}$ is the number of organ classes we are trying to segment. RF are composed of multiple independently learnt random decision trees, tree-structured classifiers expressed as a recursive partition of the feature space $\mathcal{X}$. For a given node within the tree, $\mathcal{N}_j$, and the corresponding training subset, $\mathbf{S}_j \subset \mathcal{X} \times \mathcal{Y}$, the goal is to find a semi-optimal binary test function, $\Psi_j : \mathcal{X} \to \{0, 1\}$ that provides a good split of the data $\mathbf{S}_j = \{\mathbf{S}_{jL}, \mathbf{S}_{jR} | \Psi_j(\mathbf{S}_{jL}) = 0, \Psi_j(\mathbf{S}_{jL}) = 1\}$, according to an information gain criterion (e.g., maximizing the Shannon entropy-based information gain). The training process continues recursively on the left and right nodes with data $\mathbf{S}_{j,L}$ and $\mathbf{S}_{j,R}$, respectively, until the information gain or the training set size fall below a minimum threshold. During testing, each new sample $\mathbf{v}(\mathbf{p})$ is classified using $\Psi_j(\mathbf{v}(\mathbf{p}))$ to successively branching left or right down the tree until a terminal node (leaf) is reached. At this point, the corresponding label, l is estimated by using the empirical class distribution associated with the leaf node.

2.1   Geodesic Contextual Information

Typically, the feature space $\mathcal{X}$ is characterized by a set of appearance-based features extracted directly from the original raw images (or from filtered versions of them). Recent works on auto-context, and deep learning [14] has shown how the use of learned contextual information directly in the classification can lead to a significant improvement of the results, although at the cost of a significant computational over-head. Here, we use the GGD formulation presented by Kontschieder et al. [11], to efficiently compute the geodesic distance from each class and to incorporate additional contextual information within the same decision tree, without the need for additional heuristics and significant additional computing cost.

SGeo-RF trains trees in breadth-first order, and in sections, $\{s_0, s_1, \ldots, s_D\}$, as shown in Fig. 1(b). For each section of the tree, s_d, we use the class distribution associated with each node to generate new predictive contextual features for the next section, s_{d+1} (see Fig. 1(b) and (c)). Using the estimated class posterior $P_d^k(\mathbf{v})$ associated to each class $k \in \mathcal{Y}$, the GGD can be defined, for every data point $\mathbf{v}(p)$ in the image $\mathbf{I}$, as $G_d^k(\mathbf{p}) = \min_{\mathbf{p}' \in \mathbf{I}}(\delta(\mathbf{p}, \mathbf{p}') + \nu(1 - P_d^k(\mathbf{v}(\mathbf{p}'))))$, with $\delta(\mathbf{p}, \mathbf{q}) = \inf_\Gamma \int_0^{l(\Gamma)} \sqrt{1 + \gamma^2(\nabla \mathbf{I}(r) \cdot \Gamma_{\mathbf{p},\mathbf{q}}(r))^2} dr$, $(\nu, \gamma \in \mathbb{R})$, representing the geodesic distance between two points $\mathbf{p}$ and $\mathbf{q}$ (which can be efficiently computed in linear time [13]), and $\Gamma_{\mathbf{p},\mathbf{q}}$ being the path connecting these two points.

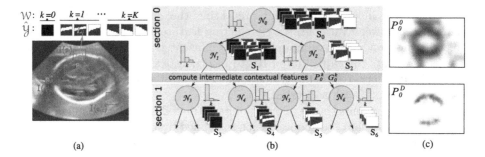

Fig. 1. SGeo-RF framework. (a) Image and labels patches extracted from the 3DUS images. The structured label space, $\hat{y}$, is used to define the super-class dictionary, $\mathcal{W}$. (b) Structured entangled tree. Intermediate super-class probabilities and GGD are used to as features for the lower sections. (c) Intermediate probability maps, P_d^k, for super-class $k = 0$ (background) computed at the first (s_0) and the last (s_D) section.

This new GGD-based connectivity features can be considered as a new set of features able to encode variable dependencies directly in the feature space the forests operate on. The intuition behind this is that these new features encode the edge-aware distance of any point in the image from the class k, thus enriching the feature space $\mathcal{X}$ with new long-range and soft connectivity features.

2.2   Structured Label Space

In traditional RF, the input data samples are processed independently, assuming independent output labels. However, for many applications, including the segmentation of anatomical organs, the label space does exhibit an inherently topological structure, thus rendering the class labels explicitly interdependent. For the particular case considered here, it is expected that the labels assigned to a certain patch of the image containing foreground information reflect the characteristic curved pattern of the skull. Here, we incorporate this structural information by defining a new structured label space $\hat{y}$, as alternative to the traditional space of independent atomic labels, y. In this new context, each training data is now associated to a $(N \times N \times N)$ structured label patch, $L_i \in \mathbb{R}^{N^3}$, centered at $\mathbf{p}_i$ (see Fig. 1(a)). During training, the set of structured labels reaching the node $\mathcal{N}_j$, $\{L_i\}$, is mapped to an intermediate continuous space, $\hat{y} \rightarrow \mathcal{Z}$, such that the dissimilarity between patches can be approximated by the Euclidean distance in $\mathcal{Z}$ (c.f., [10] for details). In order to apply the same information gain criterion when computing the corresponding splitting function Ψ_j, new cluster-based binary labels can be easily assigned to $\{L_i\}$, by applying k-means clusterization over $\mathcal{Z}$.

The dynamic assignment of labels provides an efficient strategy to work with a large and potentially heterogeneous set of patches. However, the computation of the new semantic GGD-based features requires a predefined set of atomic labels associated to each patch. In [9], the authors propose to use the original label of the patch central voxel defined over $\mathcal{Y}$ as label associated to the entire patch $\{L_i\}$. However, the new structured split functions are now defined over $\hat{\mathcal{Y}}$, thus leading to inaccurate or uninformative estimations of P_d^k and G_d^k (see Sect. 2.1). Alternatively, we also could use the original labels initially assigned to each of the voxels that constitute the new structured patches,$\{L_i\}$, to estimate P_d^k and G_d^k over the original space of atomic labels, $\mathcal{Y}$. However, none of these alternatives integrates the structural information provided by $\hat{\mathcal{Y}}$ when computing the new contextual features. Here, we define a new super-class label space $\mathcal{W}$ by clustering the entire set of training patches into K clusters (i.e., P_d^k and G_d^k are now defined over $k \in \mathcal{W}$). Intuitively, this new space of super-classes can be considered as a dictionary of representative patches, specifically tailored to the particular geometry of the organs of interest (see Fig. 1(a)). Moreover, $\mathcal{W}$ allows us to define new re-balancing factors to compensate the class imbalance, particularly important in segmentation problems where voxels in the background class are dominant. The global and node-based re-balancing factors are defined as $w_k = (\sum_{k \in K} n(k, \mathbf{S}_0))/n(k, \mathbf{S}_0)$, and $w_{k,j} = \sum_{k \in K} w_k n(k, \mathbf{S}_j)$, respectively, with $n(k, \mathbf{S}_j)$ denoting the number of training patches of super-class k in the training subset $\mathbf{S}_j$ reaching the node $\mathcal{N}_j$. The Shannon entropy used to define the splitting function Ψ_j is now defined as $E(\mathbf{S}_j) = -\sum_{l \in \{L,R\}} \sum_{k \in K} w_k n(k, \mathbf{S}_{jl}) \log(w_k n(k, \mathbf{S}_{jl}))/w_{k,jl}$.

2.3   Contextual Feature Space

In the proposed method, the original feature vector $\mathbf{v}(\mathbf{p}_i)$ is defined as set of appearance-based features extracted from images patches of fixed size ($M \times M \times M$) centered at $\mathbf{p}_i$. In particular, these features correspond to statistics extracted from different information channels, including the raw intensity, gradient magnitudes, six HoG-like channels, and the monogenic signal. Additionally, we extend $\mathcal{X}$ by generating new contextual-based features at the end of each section, s_d as described in Sect. 2.1. For each observation, $\{\mathbf{p}_i, L_i\}$, we define a set of T randomly located probe patches pairs, $\{\mathbf{q}_{i,t}^1, \mathbf{q}_{i,t}^2\}_{t=1}^T$ offset from $\mathbf{p}_i$. The new features are defined as the sum, difference and absolute difference between these two patches in different feature channels: the raw image intensities $(\mathbf{I}(\mathbf{q}_{i,t}^1), \mathbf{I}(\mathbf{q}_{i,t}^2))$, the intermediate class posteriors $(P_d^k(\mathbf{q}_{i,t}^1), P_d^k(\mathbf{q}_{i,t}^2))$, and the GGD $(G_d^k(\mathbf{q}_{i,t}^1), G_d^k(\mathbf{q}_{i,t}^2))$.

3   Results and Discussion

The new SGeo-RF segmentation framework is evaluated on a dataset of 59 fetal 3DUS images acquired under an IRB approved protocol during the routine second trimester obstetrical ultrasound examination (23.4 weeks average GA, range from 20 to 30). The images were acquired from the axial plane with transfrontal 3D acquisition, using a Philips iU22 system with an X6-1 xMATRIX array transducer. The ground truth was delineated manually under the supervision of an expert radiologist. All the images were denoised using non-local means filtering

and resampled to isotropic voxel size of 0.50 mm per dimension. The performance of SGeo-RF is compared with two alternative segmentation methods, a
classic non-structured RF classifier without any contextual information, and a
convolutional neural network (CNN) for image segmentation based on the U-net
architecture [14]. A total of 16 independent decision trees were used for both,
SGeo-RF and RF, with a maximum tree depth of 64 levels. For the rest of the
configuration parameters the selected values were: $M = 24$, $N = 12$, $D = 16$,
$K = 7$, $T = 20$, $\nu = 15$ and $\gamma = 30$.

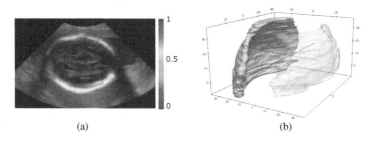

(a)   (b)

Fig. 2. Segmentation results obtained with SGeo-RF. (a) Output probability map for
the skull after merging all trees. SGeo-RF correctly identifies the skull region despite
the presence of highly echogenic regions with similar intensity pattern. (b) 3D render
of the segmented skull resulting from SGeo-RF inference, including the orthogonal
semiaxis used to estimate GA.

Table 1 shows the segmentation error for the three methods, using 49 images
for training and 10 images for testing. It can be observed that SGeo-RF provides better segmentation results than the classic RF for most of the metrics:
Dice's coefficient (DC), Jaccard index (JI), sensitivity, specificity, and accuracy.
In particular, the new method provides an average DC of 0.80 ± 0.03, a statistically significant improvement over the 0.65 ± 0.04 of RF (p-value < 0.05 using
Wilcoxon paired signed non-parametric test). CNN-based methods have become
very popular in recent years, providing some of the most accurate methods for
organ segmentation. However, in spite of the superior average DC obtained by
the CNN (0.84 ± 0.12), no statistically significant difference was found between
CNN and SGeo-RF (p-value > 0.16). However, we observed that both RF and
CNN provided a significantly higher number of false positives than SGeo-RF
(p-value < 0.05), obtaining specificities of 0.97 ± 0.01, 0.95 ± 0.02 and 0.99 ± 0.01,
respectively. While SGeo-RF provided more conservative results (0.80 ± 0.07 sensitivity), the calculation of 3D-based biometrics was more severely affected by
the presence of false positives far from the target organ observed in RF and CNN,
which required additional post-processing of the segmentation results. Figure 2
shows the resulting segmentation for one case using SGeo-RF.

The CNN required about 45 h of training on a GPU-accelerated system,
with an estimated testing time of 1.6 s. per 3D volume. SGeo-RF represents a
computationally more efficient option than CNN, requiring only 3 h of training

(no GPU used). However, the average execution time was 60 s. per volume. Even though this still represents a more efficient option than manual marking process, it represents a considerable increase over CNN. In the future, we plan to optimize the execution time of our new method by implementing a parallelized version of the code.

Finally, a linear regression model was used to automatically estimate the fetal GA, using the three orthogonal semiaxis of the segmented skull as predictive variables (see Fig. 2(b)). This simple predictive model provided a GA estimation error of 0.5 ± 0.3 weeks (statistically similar results were obtained with SGeo-RF and CNN), which is within the reported 7 to 12 days margin when using manually defined 2D biometrics parameters, such as the biparietal diameter or head circumference [15].

Table 1. Segmentation accuracy evaluation of the fetal skull segmentation using SGeo-RF, a classic non-structured RF method (RF), and CNN. The table present the average and standard deviation for the Dice's coefficient (DC), Jaccard index (JI), sensitivity, specificity and accuracy.

	DC	JI	Sensitivity	Specificity	Accuracy
SGeo-RF	0.80 ± 0.03	0.65 ± 0.04	0.80 ± 0.07	0.99 ± 0.01	0.98 ± 0.01
RF	0.65 ± 0.15	0.50 ± 0.17	0.97 ± 0.02	0.95 ± 0.02	0.93 ± 0.02
CNN	0.84 ± 0.12	0.70 ± 0.17	0.97 ± 0.02	0.97 ± 0.01	0.94 ± 0.01

4   Conclusions

In this paper, we present the first automatic framework for the segmentation and quantification of the skull in fetal 3DUS. In particular, we propose a new general RF-based method able to efficiently integrate semantic and structural information in the same decision forest. First, new contextual information and potential variable dependencies are encoded in a new extended feature space via GGD. Second, structural information of the target organs are also integrated in the system defining a structural label space. Both semantic and structural information are finally integrated into an intermediate super-class space introduced here. Moreover, the proposed RF-based framework represents an accurate and efficient alternative to the popular CNN-based methods, which are significantly more computationally demanding and less intuitive. The promising results obtained in the segmentation and characterization of the fetal skull demonstrate the potential utility of this general method for the automatic and objective analysis of the skull in fetal 3DUS. In the future, we plan to extend this framework in two directions. First, the study of more sophisticated predictive models based on 3DUS-based biometrics, able to provide even more accurate predictions of the GA and validated over a larger database. Second, we plan to incorporate a more detailed analysis of the skull, including the detection of sutures and fontanelles.

This would provide valuable anatomical information of the baby, enabling a more accurate structural analysis and the early and automatic assessment of congenital malformations, such as fetal craniosynostosis.

Acknowledgement. This research was supported in part by the Marie Sklodowska-Curie Actions of the EU Framework Programme for Research and Innovation, under REA grant agreement 706372.

References

1. Dikkeboom, C.M., et al.: The role of three-dimensional ultrasound in visualizing the fetal cranial sutures and fontanels during the second half of pregnancy. Ultrasound Obstet. Gynecol. **24**, 412–416 (2004)
2. Noble, J.A., Boukerroui, D.: Ultrasound image segmentation: A survey. IEEE Trans Med. Imag. **25**(8), 987–1010 (2006)
3. International Society of Ultrasound in Obstetrics and Gynecology: Sonographic examination of the fetal central nervous system: Guidelines for performing the basic examination and the fetal neurosonogram. Ultrasound Obstet. Gynecol. 29, 109–116(2007)
4. Lu, W., et al.: Automated fetal head detection and measurement in ultrasound images by iterative randomized hough transform. Ultrasound Med. Biol. **31**(7), 929–936 (2005)
5. Shen, Y., et al.: Fetal skull analysis in ultrasound images based on iterative randomized Hough transform. SPIE 7265 (2009)
6. Namburete, A.I.L., Noble, J.A.: Fetal cranial segmentation in 2D ultrasound images using shape properties of pixel clusters (2013). ISBI: 720–723
7. Foi, A., et al.: Difference of Gaussians revolved along elliptical paths for ultrasound fetal head segmentation. Comput. Med. Imaging Graph. **38**, 774–784 (2014)
8. Chen, H.C., et al.: Registration-based segmentation of three-dimensional ultrasound images for quantitative measurement of fetal craniofacial structure. Ultrasound Med. Biol. **38**(5), 811–823 (2012)
9. Kontschieder, P., et al.: Structured labels in random forests for semantic labelling and object detection. TPAMI **36**(10), 2104–2116 (2014)
10. Dollar, P., Zitnick, C.: Structured forests for fast edge detection. In: Proceedings of the ICCV, pp. 1841–1848 (2013)
11. Kontschieder, P., et al.: GeoF: Geodesic forests for learning coupled predictors. In: Proceedings of the CVPR (2013)
12. Oktay, O., et al.: Stratified decision forests for accurate anatomical landmark localization in cardiac images. TMI **36**(1), 332–342 (2017)
13. Toivanen, P.J.: New geodesic distance transforms for gray-scale images. Pattern Recogn. Lett. **17**, 437–450 (1996)
14. Ronneberger, O., Fischer, P., Brox, T.: U-Net: Convolutional networks for biomedical image segmentation. In: Navab, N., Hornegger, J., Wells, W.M., Frangi, A.F. (eds.) MICCAI 2015. LNCS, vol. 9351, pp. 234–241. Springer, Cham (2015). doi:10.1007/978-3-319-24574-4_28
15. Butt, K., Lim, K.: Determination of Gestational Age by Ultrasound. SOGC Clinical Practice Guidelines, 303 (2015)

Fast Registration of 3D Fetal Ultrasound Images Using Learned Corresponding Salient Points

Alberto Gomez[(✉)], Kanwal Bhatia, Sarjana Tharin, James Housden,
Nicolas Toussaint, and Julia A. Schnabel

Department of Biomedical Engineering, King's College London, London, UK
alberto.gomez@kcl.ac.uk

Abstract. We propose a fast feature-based rigid registration framework
with a novel feature saliency detection technique. The method works by
automatically classifying candidate image points as salient or non-salient
using a support vector machine trained on points which have previously
driven successful registrations. Resulting candidate salient points are
used for symmetric matching based on local descriptor similarity and
followed by RANSAC outlier rejection to obtain the final transform.
The proposed registration framework was applied to 3D real-time fetal
ultrasound images, thus covering the entire fetal anatomy for extended
FoV imaging. Our method was applied to data from 5 patients, and
compared to a conventional saliency point detection method (SIFT) in
terms of computational time, quality of the point detection and registration accuracy. Our method achieved similar accuracy and similar saliency
detection quality in < 5% the detection time, showing promising capa-
bilities towards real-time whole-body fetal ultrasound imaging.

1 Introduction

Ultrasound imaging is a fast, non-invasive and cost-effective modality that
enables real-time 3D imaging of soft tissues. Ultrasound imaging is widely used
in many clinical applications, and particularly in fetal imaging for screening purposes. The "anomaly scan" carried out at 20 weeks of gestational age (GA) provides detailed information of individual fetal organs. Inconveniently, the size of
the fetus at 20 weeks is such that the field-of-view (FoV) of a 3D ultrasound image
can only capture a small region of the fetal body. The lack of whole-body images
does not provide sufficient context for global interpretation of fetal anatomy, and
prevents researchers and clinicians from accurately estimating global parameters
such as fetal weight, which is an important biomarker of fetal growth [4].

Alberto Gomez — This work was supported by the Wellcome Trust IEH Award
[102431]. The authors acknowledge financial support from the Department of Health
via the National Institute for Health Research (NIHR) comprehensive Biomedical
Research Centre award to Guy's & St Thomas' NHS Foundation Trust in partnership
with King's College London and King's College Hospital NHS Foundation Trust.

M.J. Cardoso et al. (Eds.): FIFI/OMIA 2017, LNCS 10554, pp. 33–41, 2017.
DOI: 10.1007/978-3-319-67561-9_4

Extended FoV images can be achieved from multiple 3D ultrasound images using *mosaicing* [11] (or image stitching). Mosaicing involves at least two steps: first, the images must be spatially aligned; second, the aligned images must be stitched seamlessly to provide a single, extended FoV image. In this paper we focus on the first problem, that is, registering multiple 3D ultrasound images together. More precisely, we aim towards a fast registration method that can be used to register images in real time during acquisition. A simple max compounding fusion method [12] is used after registration to produce the mosaiced images for proof of principle.

1.1   Related Work

3D ultrasound image registration, particularly when aiming at real-time performance for fetal applications, presents a number of challenges for conventional registration techniques:

1. Fetal features will appear differently across images because of the different angle of insonation as the transducer or the fetus moves.
2. View-angle dependent artefacts, such as shadows, mirroring and reverberation will appear differently in different images, even if these images show the same object.
3. Surrounding maternal tissue and placenta can misguide the registration process when there is fetal motion.
4. Image quality varies from one image to another depending on other exogenous factors including applied force, as well as contact between the transducer surface and the skin.

For all the factors listed above, ultrasound-specific methods for pair-wise [3,6,7,11] and group-wise [10] *offline* 3D ultrasound image registration have been proposed. These methods mostly use intensity based registration using input images or feature images extracted from the input images. As a result, these techniques require the evaluation of computationally expensive cost functions over large voxel regions and are in general not well suited for fast image registration.

Recently, feature-based methods have been applied to fast and real-time 3D ultrasound image registration. Schneider et al. [9] proposed to use a simplified version of SIFT [5]. In their paper, point detection was followed by a symmetric matching of feature points, and from these matched points a rigid transform was estimated using RANSAC [2] for outlier rejection. Interestingly, they keep a database of feature points which allows a one-to-many registration of every newly arrived image. The proposed method is fast thanks to a GPU implementation, but is very sensitive to view changes and probe rotations, and it therefore is only able to capture relatively small displacements. As a result, their method is not suitable for applications where the target is moving and where sweeps are not linear.

A hybrid feature-intensity based registration scheme was proposed in [1]. This scheme uses block matching to find matching points between two sequences, and then to use a point correspondence method to remove outliers and find the true correspondence. Feature point selection is done using a regular grid. This feature extraction method is extremely fast since no image processing is involved; as a result, there is no guarantee that the selected points will have a distinct feature that can help to establish a correspondence. For this reason, the points are matched using normalized cross-correlation (NCC) in block matching [8], assuming small rotations and translations for the search window, and achieving volume registration at 8 Hz.

Both [1,9] focus on applications where the entire FoV contains the object of interest: an in-vitro, static heart model in [9] and a liver in [1]. However, both are unable to deal with moving objects or the combination of static and moving tissue that are typical in fetal ultrasound. In such cases, the ability to select relevant feature points to drive the registration is critical.

The novelty of this paper is two-fold: we introduce (i) a fast candidate point detection method and (ii) a salient point classification step to discard points that are not likely to contribute to the registration process. These two novelties allow us to maintain a fast registration rate while achieving an accurate registration by improving the selection of salient points. An overview of the method is covered in Sect. 2.1 and specific details are given for (i) in Sect. 2.2 and for (ii) in Sects. 2.3 and 2.4. Results in terms of efficiency, execution time and registration accuracy for 5 fetal patients are given in Sect. 4.

2   Method

2.1   Image Registration Framework

The feature-based registration framework between a fixed and a moving image is represented in Fig. 1. Salient points are extracted from each image **(1)**. This is achieved in a two step process where first candidate points are selected (Sect. 2.2) and then from those the points that are not salient are discarded (Sect. 2.3). Local feature descriptors are extracted at the salient point locations **(2)**. As in [9], we use a sparse sampling feature, which provides a good balance between complexity and accuracy for small rotations. Correspondence between points is found by symmetric matching of the two point sets **(3)** followed by RANSAC outlier rejection **(4)** to fit the matched points using a rigid transform **(5)** similar to [1,9]. The choice of parameters for each block is detailed in Sect. 3.

2.2   Extraction of Candidate Points

As in [1] we start from a uniform grid of points, but then search for the local maximum within a local neighbourhood. The size of this neighbourhood is fixed so that the entire image is covered. This approach ensures to have points that are local maxima, allows to control the number of candidate points and the distance between them. In our experiments we used a grid of 1000 points.

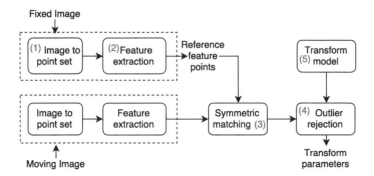

Fig. 1. Registration framework. Featured points are extracted from the fixed and the moving images using a point extractor (1) followed by a feature extraction (2) at the points location. Correspondences between fixed and moving points are found using symmetric matching (3) and the transform (5) between matched points is found through outlier rejection (4).

2.3   SVM Saliency Detector

The key to finding corresponding points in the method proposed in [9] (and, by extension, in our method) is the assumption that salient points can be found at corresponding locations in two different images. However this approach relies on the ability of the method to detect salient points and distinguish them from other feature points in the image that capture artefacts (e.g. edges generated by shadows) or points which belong to maternal tissue or other non-interesting structures which might mislead the registration. Schneider et al. [9] proposed a simple saliency model: a point was considered salient if the intensity value was in the range 150 to 200. We observed (as reported in our results) that this strategy admits too many points which in turn yields computationally expensive point matching and outlier rejection processes.

Instead we propose to learn a model for salient points by using a simple Support Vector Machine (SVM) classifier. Each candidate point is classified using a feature descriptor calculated on a N-voxel neighbourhood (i.e. a total of $(2N+1)^3$ values) around the point. The feature descriptor was designed to represent whether the central point is salient with respect to its environment and to capture texture and image patterns, while being rotation and translation invariant. For that reason we use a 2D histogram $H(i,j)$ with the distance to the centre on one axis and voxel intensity on the other as a descriptor:

$$H(i,j) = \#\{\mathbf{x} \in \mathcal{N}(\mathbf{c})|r_i \leq \|\mathbf{x} - \mathbf{c}\| \leq R_i, l_j \leq I(\mathbf{x}) \leq L_j\} \qquad (1)$$

where r_i, R_i are the minimum and maximum distances from a voxel $\mathbf{x}$ in the patch to the central voxel $\mathbf{c}$ for the i-th bin in the radial direction, l_j, L_j are the minimum and maximum intensities for the j-th bin along the intensity direction, and $\mathcal{N}(\mathbf{c})$ is the set of all voxels in the neighbourhood of $\mathbf{c}$.

2.4   Generation of Training Data

Each sample of the training data was an image patch where the centre point was either salient or non-salient. To reliably identify salient and non-salient points to generate the training data, pairwise registrations of every two consecutive images in each sequence were carried out. These registrations were manually intialized and artefacts and maternal tissue were manually masked out. The result of these registrations was verified by experts to ensure that they were successful. Each of these registrations defined a set of inlier points (i.e., points which were used after matching and RANSAC to define the parameters of the rigid transform) and outlier points (non-inlier points that were detected as salient following the method in [9]). Then a sliding temporal window of T consecutive volumes was defined. Points which were inliers in all registrations within the window were labelled as salient, and points which were outliers in all registrations were labelled as non-salient. Only points in the overlapping FoV of volumes within the window were considered. In this paper, inliers and outliers were generated with windows $T = 3$ and $T = 7$ respectively. This process produced 6813 ± 2820 samples per patient (790 ± 350 salient and 6023 ± 2465 non-salient).

3   Materials and Experiments

We used sequences of 3D images from five healthy fetuses, acquired with institutional ethical approval and informed consent of the mother. Details on GA, volumes per sequence, etc. are shown in Table 1. Data were acquired using a Philips EPIQ V7G and X6-1 matrix array transducer in 4D mode, by sweeping from the fetal head to the lower body. Experiments were carried out using 5-fold cross-validation: for each trial, images from four patients were used for training the SVM and the remaining patient was used for testing. Average and standard deviation values over these five trials are reported in the results section. The SVM classifier was trained twice, first with all support vectors and then restricting the maximum number of support vectors to 100 (approximately 10% of the total number of support vectors). The SVM parameters $\gamma = 10^{-3}$ (for the Gaussian kernel) and $C = 10^4$ (penalisation) were found by 3 fold cross-validation.

In addition to our proposed SVM saliency detector (Sect. 2.3), we carried out experiments using the image to point set filter (block 1 in Fig. 1) proposed by Schneider in [9], based on SIFT, which used using a single scale Laplacian of Gaussian (LoG, $\sigma = 3mm$). Note that, apart from the salient point extraction step, our proposed method is identical to that in [9], and unless otherwise stated the same parameters are used. The implementation of both methods was our own in C++, except for the use of ITK filters and dlib (CPU) for SVM. Each volume in each sequence was registered to the previous in a pair-wise fashion to prevent bias in the execution time measurements introduced by accumulated target points when using multiple images as in [1,9].

For the LoG and the proposed SVM methods we measured (1) the proportion of points classified as salient that were matched and, of those, the proportion

Table 1. Details on patient data, including the number of inlier and outlier points obtained from correctly registered volumes.

	GA	# volumes	volume rate	# inliers	# outliers
Pat 1	22w + 2	94	3 Hz	894	6855
Pat 2	23w + 5	90	3 Hz	739	4625
Pat 3	23w + 4	139	5 Hz	1311	9897
Pat 4	20w + 2	69	3 Hz	345	3529
Pat 5	22w + 3	101	4 Hz	661	5212

that turned out to be inliers, (2) the average time to register every new image including the breakdown into the different registration steps detailed above, and (3) the target registration error (TRE) for 25 manually picked landmarks distributed over the entire fetus.

4   Results

Figure 2 shows the results related to registration efficiency. Three salient point detection schemes are compared in this graph: local extrema of the LoG [9], and our SVM proposed method with all support vectors, and with 100 support vectors and different patch radius $N = 3, 4, 5$. The graph on Fig. 2a shows the average fraction of the salient points that are true inliers, matched but then resulting outliers, and not matched. In average the fraction of detected points that are inliers is comparable to the reference method (LoG). In all our experiments the value is actually higher with our method (by approximately 2% with 100 support vectors and $N = 4$), however this improvement is not supported by statistical evidence. The graph on Fig. 2b shows the total computation time, broken down into point detection, point matching and outlier rejection. Our method reduces execution time by two mechanisms: first, using a reduced number of support vectors makes salient point detection very fast (less that 100ms

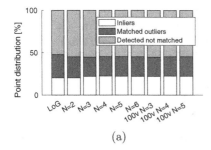
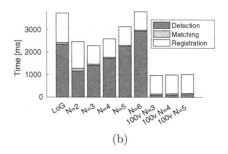

(a)   (b)

Fig. 2. Relation of points that determine the registration efficiency (a), for the different saliency detection methods and different values of the patch size N used by the SVM classifier. Computation time breakdown for image registration (b).

Table 2. Registration error in mm (average $\pm$ std.), from 5 patients. N = neighbourhood size, LoG = Laplacian of Gaussian, SVM 100v = SVM with only 100 vectors.

$N =$	LoG	SVM			SVM 100v		
		3	4	5	3	4	5
Pat 1	2.60 ± 1.87	2.58 ± 1.87	2.57 ± 1.87	2.57 ± 1.86	2.58 ± 1.87	2.57 ± 1.87	2.57 ± 1.87
Pat 2	2.65 ± 1.59	2.64 ± 1.54	2.65 ± 1.51	2.66 ± 1.55	2.65 ± 1.55	2.66 ± 1.56	2.68 ± 1.56
Pat 3	3.01 ± 1.93	2.97 ± 1.90	2.98 ± 1.90	3.01 ± 1.96	2.97 ± 1.90	2.98 ± 1.90	2.97 ± 1.90
Pat 4	3.62 ± 2.82	3.57 ± 2.75	3.78 ± 2.84	3.79 ± 2.84	3.58 ± 2.73	3.69 ± 2.81	3.83 ± 2.87
Pat 5	1.67 ± 1.61	1.71 ± 1.63	1.68 ± 1.63	1.69 ± 1.62	1.70 ± 1.63	1.69 ± 1.62	1.69 ± 1.62
Average	2.71 ± 1.97	2.69 ± 1.94	2.73 ± 1.95	2.75 ± 1.97	2.70 ± 1.94	2.72 ± 1.95	2.75 ± 1.96

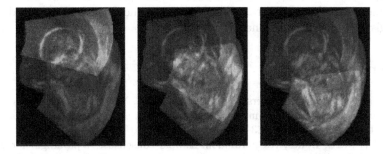

Fig. 3. Example slice of compounded volumes. The compounded image is represented in the background and three individual volumes are overlaid in green.

when using 100 support vectors and $N = 4$). We show later that this does not have a negative impact in accuracy. Second, the SVM picks salient points that are more likely to be inliers, hence less detected points are needed to achieve the same accuracy and the matching and registration (outlier rejection) processes can be done more rapidly.

Table 2 shows the average TRE calculated using 25 manually picked corresponding landmarks on each patient. Accuracy is comparable across methods (around 2.7 ± 1.9mm).

Figure 3 shows three example slices of registered and fused fetal volumes from patient 1[1] (using SVM with 100 vectors and $N = 4$). The compounded image is shown in grayscale in the background with three different images transformed to their location within the volume and overlaid in semi-transparent green.

5   Discussion and Conclusions

We have proposed a new method for fast extraction of salient points as part of a fast registration framework towards real-time 3D ultrasound image mosaicing.

---

[1] Additional figures with slices from all other patiens are available as supplementary material.

Our method aims to increase the chance that the salient points will be inliers in the feature matching process. An SVM classifier was trained using salient points that drove successful registrations, and used to classify candidate points into salient and non-salient. Our results indicate an improvement in the number of inliers out of the number of salient points with a substantial reduction of the point extraction time.

In the future, computational time can be further reduced by using more efficient point-matching algorithms and a parallel implementation. Future work will also include the use of non-rigid transformation models to deal with deformable types of fetal motion.

In summary, we have presented a new fast method to extract salient points from 3D ultrasound images to drive successful registrations. The method has been demonstrated on five fetal patients and has shown potential towards real-time registration in a real scenario.

References

1. Banerjee, J., Klink, C., Peters, E.D., Niessen, W.J., Moelker, A., van Walsum, T.: Fast and robust 3D ultrasound registration - Block and game theoretic matching. Med. Image Anal. **20**(1), 173–183 (2015)
2. Fischler, M.A., Bolles, R.C.: Random sample consensus: A paradigm for model fitting with applications to image analysis and automated cartography. Commun. ACM **24**(6), 381–395 (1981)
3. Grau, V., Becher, H., Noble, J.A.: Registration of multiview real-time 3-D echocardiographic sequences. IEEE Trans. Med. Imaging **26**(9), 1154–1165 (2007)
4. Kacem, Y., Cannie, M.M., Kadji, C., Dobrescu, O., Lo Zito, L., Ziane, S., Strizek, B., Evrard, A.-S., Gubana, F., Gucciardo, L., Staelens, R., Jani, J.C.: Fetal weight estimation: Comparison of two-dimensional US and MR imaging assessments. Radiology **267**(3), 902–910 (2013)
5. Lowe, D.G.: Distinctive image features from scale-invariant keypoints. Int. J. Comput. Vis. **60**(2), 91–110 (2004)
6. Ni, D., Qu, Y., Yang, X., Chui, Y.P., Wong, T.-T., Ho, S.S.M., Heng, P.A.: Volumetric ultrasound panorama based on 3D SIFT. In: Metaxas, D., Axel, L., Fichtinger, G., Székely, G. (eds.) MICCAI 2008. LNCS, vol. 5242, pp. 52–60. Springer, Heidelberg (2008). doi:10.1007/978-3-540-85990-1_7
7. Oktay, O., Schuh, A., Rajchl, M., Keraudren, K., Gomez, A., Heinrich, M.P., Penney, G., Rueckert, D.: Structured decision forests for multi-modal ultrasound image registration. In: Navab, N., Hornegger, J., Wells, W.M., Frangi, A.F. (eds.) MICCAI 2015. LNCS, vol. 9350, pp. 363–371. Springer, Cham (2015). doi:10.1007/978-3-319-24571-3_44
8. Ourselin, S., Roche, A., Prima, S., Ayache, N.: Block matching: A general framework to improve robustness of rigid registration of medical images. In: Delp, S.L., DiGoia, A.M., Jaramaz, B. (eds.) MICCAI 2000. LNCS, vol. 1935, pp. 557–566. Springer, Heidelberg (2000). doi:10.1007/978-3-540-40899-4_57
9. Schneider, R.J., Perrin, D.P., Vasilyev, N.V., Marx, G.R., Del Nido, P.J., Howe, R.D.: Real-time image-based rigid registration of three-dimensional ultrasound. Med. Image Anal. **16**(2), 402–414 (2012)

10. Wachinger, C., Navab, N.: Simultaneous registration of multiple images: similarity metrics and efficient optimization. IEEE Trans. Pattern Anal. Mach. Intell. **35**(5), 1221–1233 (2013)
11. Wachinger, C., Wein, W., Navab, N.: Three-dimensional ultrasound mosaicing. In: Ayache, N., Ourselin, S., Maeder, A. (eds.) MICCAI 2007. LNCS, vol. 4792, pp. 327–335. Springer, Heidelberg (2007). doi:10.1007/978-3-540-75759-7_40
12. Yao, C., Simpson, J.M., Schaeffter, T., Penney, G.P.: Multi-view 3D echocardiography compounding based on feature consistency. Phys. Med. Biol. **56**(18), 6109–6128 (2011)

Automatic Segmentation of the Intracranial Volume in Fetal MR Images

N. Khalili[1]([✉]), P. Moeskops[2], N.H.P. Claessens[3], S. Scherpenzeel[3], E. Turk[3],
R. de Heus[4], M.J.N.L. Benders[3,5], M.A. Viergever[1,5], J.P.W. Pluim[1,2],
and I. Išgum[1,5]

[1] Image Sciences Institute, University Medical Center Utrecht,
Utrecht, The Netherlands
nadieh@isi.uu.nl
[2] Medical Image Analysis Group, Department of Biomedical Engineering,
Eindhoven University of Technology, Eindhoven, The Netherlands
[3] Department of Neonatology, Wilhelmina Childrens Hospital,
University Medical Center Utrecht, Utrecht, The Netherlands
[4] Department of Obstetrics, University Medical Center Utrecht,
Utrecht, The Netherlands
[5] Brain Center Rudolf Magnus, University Medical Center Utrecht,
Utrecht, The Netherlands

Abstract. MR images of the fetus allow non-invasive analysis of the
fetal brain. Quantitative analysis of fetal brain development requires
automatic brain tissue segmentation that is typically preceded by segmentation of the intracranial volume (ICV). This is challenging because
fetal MR images visualize the whole moving fetus and in addition partially visualize the maternal body. This paper presents an automatic
method for segmentation of the ICV in fetal MR images. The method
employs a multi-scale convolutional neural network in 2D slices to enable
learning spatial information from larger context as well as detailed local
information. The method is developed and evaluated with 30 fetal T2-
weighted MRI scans (average age 33.2 ± 1.2 weeks postmenstrual age).
The set contains 10 scans acquired in axial, 10 in coronal and 10 in
sagittal imaging planes. A reference standard was defined in all images
by manual annotation of the intracranial volume in 10 equidistantly distributed slices. The automatic analysis was performed by training and
testing the network using scans acquired in the representative imaging
plane as well as combining the training data from all imaging planes. On
average, the automatic method achieved Dice coefficients of 0.90 for the
axial images, 0.90 for the coronal images and 0.92 for the sagittal images.
Combining the training sets resulted in average Dice coefficients of 0.91
for the axial images, 0.95 for the coronal images, and 0.92 for the sagittal images. The results demonstrate that the evaluated method achieved
good performance in extracting ICV in fetal MR scans regardless of the
imaging plane.

© Springer International Publishing AG 2017
M.J. Cardoso et al. (Eds.): FIFI/OMIA 2017, LNCS 10554, pp. 42–51, 2017.
DOI: 10.1007/978-3-319-67561-9_5

1   Introduction

Fetal magnetic resonance imaging (MRI) is increasingly used as a non-invasive tool for monitoring the fetal brain development. A number of papers describing automatic quantitative analysis of brain in MR scans of fetuses have been published [2,3,18]. Compared to automatic analysis of the brain in adults and neonates, analysis of the fetal brain carries unique challenges. In contrast to brain MRI of adults and neonates that mostly visualize the head only, fetal MR images have a larger field of view that includes the entire fetus as well as part of the maternal body. In addition, because of fetal movement, the brain location and orientation in fetal MRI may vary considerably. Hence, prior to analysis of the brain tissue classes, automatic methods often determine a volume of interest containing the brain.

To identify a volume of interest, several methods performed brain segmentation. Anquez et al. [1] proposed a method for automatic segmentation of intracranial volume (ICV) in fetal MR scans. The method first localizes the eyes and exploits this information to segment ICV using a graph cut approach that is guided by shape, contrast and biometrical priors. The method was applied to scans with unknown fetal orientation and the results demonstrate that it is able to perform segmentation with high accuracy. Rajchl et al. [11] proposed a deep learning approach for brain and lung segmentation. Their method combines a convolutional neural network and iterative graphical optimization to obtain the final segmentation. The method is trained with weakly labeled data consisting of the brain bounding boxes. It was applied to data with large anatomical variation and achieved high segmentation accuracy. Recently, Salehi et al. [13] proposed a method for segmentation of the brain in adult and fetal MR scans. In this approach, the fetal brain is first localized by defining a bounding box around it with ITKSNAP [20]. Next, the segmentation was performed using a multi-scale CNN as proposed by Moeskops et al. [10] with an iterative approach that uses input from the posterior probabilities of the previous segmentation step to refine the segmentations. The authors reported high segmentation accuracy.

Unlike methods performing ICV segmentation, several methods perform brain localization in fetal MRI. Ison et al. [5] proposed a pipeline to detect a bounding box in several stages. The method first employs a two-stage random forest classifier. In the first stage, maternal tissue is separated from the fetal head, and in the second stage the fetal brain tissue is classified in several classes. Thereafter, a Markov random field appearance model is used to find the brain orientation using results of the brain tissue classification. Hence, the detected bounding box follows the orientation of the brain in the scan. The results show that the proposed approach is robust but with moderate accuracy. Only 28% of the coronal images and 53% of the axial and sagittal images contained whole brain in the detected bounding box. Keraudren et al. [8] proposed a method for brain localization that determines a bounding box in the orientation of the image axis. The method first fits an ellipse around the brain in every image slice. Thereafter, ellipses meeting criteria about expected brain size and knowledge about gestational age are analyzed using SIFT features in a bag-of-words model to identify brain voxels. Thereafter, a bounding box is fitted to the extracted feature cloud using a RANSAC algorithm. The method can be applied to scans of any orientation and it achieved good results with 85% of the cases containing the whole brain within the bounding box. Taimouri et al. [16] proposed a template matching approach to find slices containing the brain. This was applied to determine a bounding box around the brain. Unlike methods that encode prior knowledge about the gestational age and brain size in the features, this method uses prior information from an age-matched template. The results demonstrate high success rate in determination of the brain bounding boxes.

In this study, we investigated whether the method previously developed for brain tissue segmentation by Moeskops et al. [10] can be used for the challenging task of segmentation of the ICV in fetal MRI. Unlike other methods for fetal brain segmentation, the proposed method directly segments the ICV from MRI data without the need to crop the image to a region of interest first or using prior knowledge about the brain size or gestational age. We evaluated the method with MR scans acquired in axial, coronal and sagittal imaging planes.

2   Data

This study includes T2-weighted MR scans of 10 fetuses. The gestational age of fetuses ranged from 22.9 to 34.6 weeks. For every patient, 3 images were acquired on a Philips Achieva 3 T scanner using a turbo fast spin-echo sequence. The data set contains 30 images in total: 10 images acquired in the axial, 10 images in the coronal and 10 images in the sagittal imaging plane. The acquired voxel size is $1.25 \times 1.25 \times 2.5$ mm^3 and reconstructed voxel size is $0.7 \times 0.7 \times 2.5$ mm^3. The reconstruction matrix is $512 \times 512 \times 80$.

To define the reference standard, manual segmentation of the ICV was performed by a trained medical student in 10 slices for each of the 30 MR images. The slices were equidistantly distributed over the brain. Manual annotation was performed using in-house developed software. The process was done by painting brain voxels in each slice.

Images were divided into training and test set. The training set contained images of 7 patients and the test set contained images of the remaining 3 patients.

3   Method

To segment ICV a multi-scale convolutional neural network (CNN) as proposed by Moeskops et al. [10] is employed. This network has been developed for brain tissue segmentation in neonatal and adult brain MR scans. The network analyzes 2D patches of different sizes to allow exploiting information from the local and global context. Hence, the network takes three patch sizes that are each analyzed in a separate network branch and combined in the last layer. Each branch consists of three convolutional layers alternated with downsampling layers to reduce feature map sizes. Convolution layers of each network branch are followed by a fully connected layer. Outputs of the three branches are concatenated and input

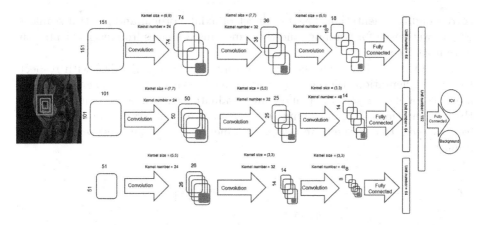

Fig. 1. CNN architecture: The network contains three branches which are fed by three different patch sizes extracted from the input image as illustrated by red squares in the input image. Each branch has three convolution layers and two fully connected layers. In the last layer, all three branches are concatenated in a single fully connected layer and classified as either ICV or background.

for a fully connected layer with a softmax function, which distinguishes between positive (ICV) and negative (mother and fetus excluding the brain) classes. As opposed to the network used for neonatal and adult images [10], the network in the current study uses larger input patches (51×51, 101×101 and 151×151 vs. 25×25, 51×51 and 75×75), and uses strided convolution instead of max-pooling. Detailed network parameters are shown in Fig. 1. To avoid bias towards the majority class, the network was trained with an equal number of positive (ICV) and negative (mother and fetus excluding the brain) samples randomly selected from each scan. In addition, training samples were randomly chosen in every epoch. In order to avoid overfitting, batch normalization [4] was used for the convolutional layers and dropout [15] was used for the fully connected layers. The CNN was trained by backpropagation using cross-entropy as loss function and Adam [9] for optimizing the weights and biases.

Pixel classification may result in isolated clusters of voxels that may locally resemble the brain. To prevent this, only the largest 3D connected component segmented by the CNN was retained.

4   Experiments and Results

Three sets of experiments were performed. In all experiments, segmentation performance was evaluated using Dice coefficients between manually and automatically segmented images.

First, to evaluate the performance of the network when training and testing with the representative data, the network was trained with images acquired in axial, coronal and sagittal planes separately and tested with images from the corresponding orientation. From each set of axial, coronal and sagittal scans, 7 images were used for training, and the remaining 3 images from each orientation were used for testing.

Second, to evaluate whether the network is able to generalize with respect to image orientation, the network was trained with a mix of images from the axial, coronal and sagittal planes, and evaluated with images acquired in all three orientations. Thus, training and test sets from the first set of experiments were merged. Hence, the training set contained 21 images and test set contained 9 images.

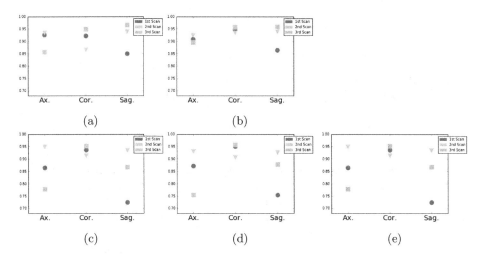

Fig. 2. Dice coefficients obtained between manual and automatic segmentation in different experimental settings for each test scan in axial (Ax.), coronal (Cor.) and sagittal (Sag.) imaging plane. Results were obtained when the CNN was trained with: (a) 7 scans from a single orientation and tested with scans acquired in the representative orientation; (b) a combination of 7 axial, 7 coronal, 7 sagittal scans; (c) 3 axial, 2 coronal and 2 sagittal; (d) 2 axial, 3 coronal and 2 sagittal scans; (e) 2 axial, 2 coronal and 3 sagittal scans.

Third, because the second experiment uses a much larger training set than the first experiment (21 vs. 7 training images), experiments with 7 training images acquired in axial, coronal and sagittal orientations were performed as well. For this purpose, experiments with three different training settings were performed: From a set of 3 axial, 3 coronal and 3 sagittal training scans, training was performed using 3 axial, 2 coronal and 2 sagittal images; 2 axial, 3 coronal and 2 sagittal images; and 2 axial, 2 coronal and 3 sagittal images.

Table 1 lists average of quantitative evaluation results of these experiments and Fig. 2 shows results obtained from each image. Figure 3 shows examples of the obtained segmentations.

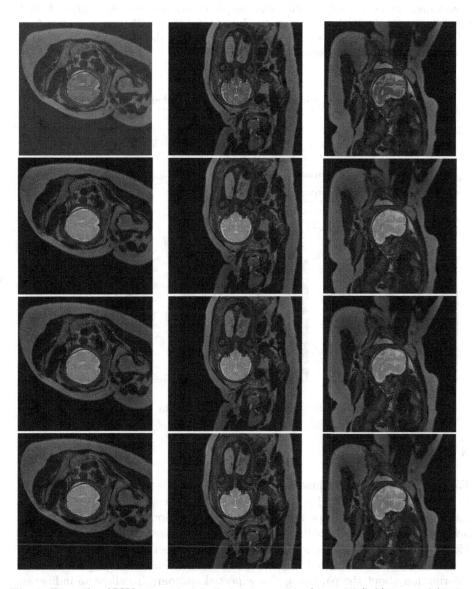

Fig. 3. Example of ICV segmentations in images acquired in axial (left), coronal (middle) and sagittal (right) planes. Top row: A slice from T2-weigted image; Second row: Automatic segmentations obtained using 7 training images from the representative imaging planes; Third row: Automatic segmentations obtained using all 21 training images from all 3 image orientations; Bottom row: Manual segmentation.

Table 1. Average Dice coefficients between manually and automatically obtained ICV segmentations: First three rows list results when network was trained with 7 images from a single plane and tested with images acquired in the corresponding plane. Fourth row lists results obtained when the network was trained with 21 training images from all three imaging planes. Last three rows list results of the network trained with 7 training images combined from all three imaging planes.

Training set composition	Test set		
	Axial	Coronal	Sagittal
7 axial	0.90	-	-
7 coronal	-	0.90	-
7 sagittal	-	-	0.92
7 axial, 7 coronal, 7 sagittal	0.91	0.95	0.92
3 axial, 2 coronal, 2 sagittal	0.86	0.93	0.84
2 axial, 3 coronal, 2 sagittal	0.85	0.94	0.85
2 axial, 2 coronal, 3 sagittal	0.89	0.93	0.84

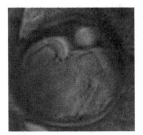 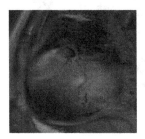 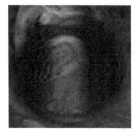

Fig. 4. Example of three slices strongly affected by imaging artifacts.

5   Discussion

We have presented an evaluation of a multi-scale CNN for segmentation of ICV in fetal MRI. The method was evaluated with images acquired in axial, coronal and sagittal imaging planes and the results demonstrate that the method achieves Dice coefficients of 0.91 regardless of the image orientation. Unlike previous fetal brain extraction methods, the proposed method segments ICV from fetal MRI without the need for bounding box localization or exploiting prior information about the patient age or expected anatomy. To allow an indication of the segmentation performance compared with other methods, the results from previous studies are summarized in Table 2. Note that these results are obtained on different data sets, and can therefore not be directly compared.

The segmentation performance appears similar when using representative training images and when using mixed training images with respect to imaging plane. This demonstrates that the method is robust with respect to image orientation. Results obtained in the experiment using a larger training set with

Table 2. Segmentation performance as reported in three previous studies. Note that these results are obtained on different data sets, and can therefore not be directly compared.

Previous studies	Dice coefficients	Hausdorff distance(mm)	Kappa
Salehi et al. [13]	0.98	-	-
Rajchl et al. [11]	0.94	-	-
Anquez et al. [1]	-	3.4	0.93

training images from all three imaging planes do not seem to lead to substantial improvement in performance, although they tend to be more consistent. Because a small test set of in total 9 test scans from 3 patients was available, statistical difference among the different experimental settings was not evaluated. In future research these results need to be confirmed in a larger set of images.

Because of the continuous fetal motion, fetal MR images contain motion artifacts that were most present in scans acquired in sagittal imaging plane. Slices that contained very strong artifacts were not segmented by the automatic method (Fig. 4). Because quantitative evaluation was performed only in slices with manual annotations, these did not affect the quantitative evaluation. Nevertheless, poor image quality in such slices prohibits manual expert as well as automatic brain segmentation. Hence, to solve this, motion correction, as e.g. proposed by Kainz et al. [6] could be applied prior to brain segmentation.

In this work, segmentation was performed using a multi-scale CNN as proposed by Moeskops et al. [10]. Similar multi-scale CNNs could likely also be used, such as the network proposed by Kamnitsas et al. [7]. In addition, other segmentation network architectures could be evaluated, such as the fully convolutional architectures as proposed by Shelhamer et al. [14] and Ronneberger et al. [12], which contain upsampling layers and skip-connections to acquire multi-scale information. Another approach used for segmentation are dilated CNNs [17,19], which can achieve large receptive fields with a limited number of trainable weights. Moreover, in future work, network architectures that use 3D information will be investigated.

The gestational age of fetuses included in this study was relatively narrow (range: 22.9 to 34.6). However, the method can likely be applicable to fetal MR scans made at other gestational ages. Our future work will investigate application of this method in a large set of fetal scans acquired in a broad range of gestational ages.

Acknowledgements. This study was sponsored by the Research Program Specialized Nutrition of the Utrecht Center for Food and Health, through a subsidy from the Dutch Ministry of Economic Affairs, the Utrecht Province and the Municipality of Utrecht.

References

1. Anquez, J., Angelini, E.D., Bloch, I.: Automatic segmentation of head structures on fetal MRI. In: 2009 IEEE International Symposium on Biomedical Imaging: From Nano to Macro. ISBI 2009, pp. 109–112 (2009)
2. Gholipour, A., Estroff, J.A., Barnewolt, C.E., Connolly, S.A., Warfield, S.K.: Fetal brain volumetry through MRI volumetric reconstruction and segmentation. Int. J. Comput. Assist. Radiol. Surg. **6**(3), 329–339 (2011)
3. Gholipour, A., Rollins, C.K., Velasco-Annis, C., Ouaalam, A., Akhondi-Asl, A., Afacan, O., Ortinau, C.M., Clancy, S., Limperopoulos, C., Yang, E., et al.: A normative spatiotemporal MRI atlas of the fetal brain for automatic segmentation and analysis of early brain growth. Scientific Reports 7 (2017)
4. Ioffe, S., Szegedy, C.: Batch normalization: Accelerating deep network training by reducing internal covariate shift. In: Proceedings of the 32nd International Conference on Machine Learning (ICML-15), pp. 448–456 (2015)
5. Ison, M., Donner, R., Dittrich, E., Kasprian, G., Prayer, D., Langs, G.: Fully automated brain extraction and orientation in raw fetal MRI. In: Workshop on Paediatric and Perinatal Imaging, MICCAI, pp. 17–24 (2012)
6. Kainz, B., Steinberger, M., Wein, W., Kuklisova-Murgasova, M., Malamateniou, C., Keraudren, K., Torsney-Weir, T., Rutherford, M., Aljabar, P., Hajnal, J.V., et al.: Fast volume reconstruction from motion corrupted stacks of 2D slices. IEEE Trans. Med. Imaging **34**(9), 1901–1913 (2015)
7. Kamnitsas, K., Ledig, C., Newcombe, V.F., Simpson, J.P., Kane, A.D., Menon, D.K., Rueckert, D., Glocker, B.: Efficient multi-scale 3D CNN with fully connected CRF for accurate brain lesion segmentation. Med. Image Anal. **36**, 61–78 (2017)
8. Keraudren, K., Kyriakopoulou, V., Rutherford, M., Hajnal, J.V., Rueckert, D.: Localisation of the brain in fetal MRI using bundled SIFT features. In: Mori, K., Sakuma, I., Sato, Y., Barillot, C., Navab, N. (eds.) MICCAI 2013. LNCS, vol. 8149, pp. 582–589. Springer, Heidelberg (2013). doi:10.1007/978-3-642-40811-3_73
9. Kingma, D., Adam, J.B.: A method for stochastic optimisation (2015)
10. Moeskops, P., Viergever, M.A., Mendrik, A.M., de Vries, L.S., Benders, M.J., Išgum, I.: Automatic segmentation of mr brain images with a convolutional neural network. IEEE Trans. Med. Imaging **35**(5), 1252–1261 (2016)
11. Rajchl, M., Lee, M.C., Oktay, O., Kamnitsas, K., Passerat-Palmbach, J., Bai, W., Damodaram, M., Rutherford, M.A., Hajnal, J.V., Kainz, B., et al.: Deepcut: Object segmentation from bounding box annotations using convolutional neural networks. IEEE Trans. Med. Imaging **36**(2), 674–683 (2017)
12. Ronneberger, O., Fischer, P., Brox, T.: U-Net: Convolutional networks for biomedical image segmentation. In: Navab, N., Hornegger, J., Wells, W.M., Frangi, A.F. (eds.) MICCAI 2015. LNCS, vol. 9351, pp. 234–241. Springer, Cham (2015). doi:10.1007/978-3-319-24574-4_28
13. Salehi, S.S.M., Erdogmus, D., Gholipour, A.: Auto-context convolutional neural network (auto-net) for brain extraction in magnetic resonance imaging. IEEE Trans. Med. Imaging **PP**(99), 1 (2017)
14. Shelhamer, E., Long, J., Darrell, T.: Fully convolutional networks for semantic segmentation. IEEE Trans. Pattern Anal. Mach. Intell. **39**(4), 640–651 (2017)
15. Srivastava, N., Hinton, G.E., Krizhevsky, A., Sutskever, I., Salakhutdinov, R.: Dropout: a simple way to prevent neural networks from overfitting. J. Mach. Learn. Res. **15**(1), 1929–1958 (2014)

16. Taimouri, V., Gholipour, A., Velasco-Annis, C., Estroff, J.A., Warfield, S.K.: A template-to-slice block matching approach for automatic localization of brain in fetal MRI. In: 2015 IEEE 12th International Symposium on Biomedical Imaging (ISBI), pp. 144–147. IEEE (2015)
17. Wolterink, J.M., Leiner, T., Viergever, M.A., Išgum, I.: Dilated convolutional neural networks for cardiovascular MR segmentation in congenital heart disease. In: Zuluaga, M.A., Bhatia, K., Kainz, B., Moghari, M.H., Pace, D.F. (eds.) RAMBO/HVSMR -2016. LNCS, vol. 10129, pp. 95–102. Springer, Cham (2017). doi:10.1007/978-3-319-52280-7_9
18. Wright, R., Kyriakopoulou, V., Ledig, C., Rutherford, M.A., Hajnal, J.V., Rueckert, D., Aljabar, P.: Automatic quantification of normal cortical folding patterns from fetal brain MRI. Neuroimage **91**, 21–32 (2014)
19. Yu, F., Koltun, V.: Multi-scale context aggregation by dilated convolutions. In: ICLR (2016)
20. Yushkevich, P.A., Piven, J., Hazlett, H.C., Smith, R.G., Ho, S., Gee, J.C., Gerig, G.: User-guided 3D active contour segmentation of anatomical structures significantly improved efficiency and reliability. Neuroimage **31**(3), 1116–1128 (2006)

Abdomen Segmentation in 3D Fetal Ultrasound Using CNN-powered Deformable Models

Alexander Schmidt-Richberg[1]([⊠]), Tom Brosch[1], Nicole Schadewaldt[1],
Tobias Klinder[1], Angelo Cavallaro[3], Ibtisam Salim[3], David Roundhill[2],
Aris Papageorghiou[3], and Cristian Lorenz[1]

[1] Philips Research Laboratories Hamburg, Hamburg, Germany
alexander.schmidt-richberg@philips.com
[2] Philips Ultrasound, Bothell, USA
[3] Nuffield Department of Obstetrics and Gynaecology,
Univerity of Oxford, Oxford, UK

Abstract. In this paper, voxel probability maps generated by a novel fovea fully convolutional network architecture (FovFCN) are used as additional feature images in the context of a segmentation approach based on deformable shape models. The method is applied to fetal 3D ultrasound image data aiming at a segmentation of the abdominal outline of the fetal torso. This is of interest, e.g., for measuring the fetal abdominal circumference, a standard biometric measure in prenatal screening. The method is trained on 126 3D ultrasound images and tested on 30 additional scans. The results show that the approach can successfully combine the advantages of FovFCNs and deformable shape models in the context of challenging image data, such as given by fetal ultrasound. With a mean error of 2.24 mm, the combination of model-based segmentation and neural networks outperforms the separate approaches.

1 Introduction

Ultrasound (US) is the modality of choice for fetal imaging. The advantages are above all that it is a widely available modality of limited cost, with no known adverse effects, being able to render fetal anatomy in sufficient detail to enable diagnostic decisions. At the same time, ultrasound is recognized as being a very operator-dependent modality, demanding high skill of the clinician to provide meaningful imaging material and being the contrary of a push-button modality. Historically, Ultrasound has been predominantly a 2D modality, showing the patient's anatomy in a fan-like portion of a plane and demanding high skills of anatomical orientation and recognition just to be able to find the right view-plane to answer a given clinical question.

In light of the above mentioned challenges, fetal imaging is an extreme case. Since a patient within a patient is examined, the anatomy and pose of the

C. Lorenz—We thank the authors of [9] for providing the automatic landmark detection.

M.J. Cardoso et al. (Eds.): FIFI/OMIA 2017, LNCS 10554, pp. 52–61, 2017.
DOI: 10.1007/978-3-319-67561-9_6

"outer patient". In addition, anatomical structures of the fetus are very small, sometimes just at the resolution level of the device. Since maternal tissue has to be penetrated before reaching the fetus, ultrasound frequencies cannot be chosen as high as the need for spatial resolution would demand. In this context, 3D ultrasound (3D US) may be of benefit. Since a whole volume is captured at once, the field of view needs to be defined with considerably less accuracy, only requiring that the anatomy of interest is included.

Fetal screening is routinely performed in two examinations at 18 to 22 weeks GA, covering a variety of fetal growth measures and the detection of fetal abnormalities. A third examination at 28 to 36 weeks GA is offered (depending on the setting) to all women or to those with specific risk factors, and is mainly devoted to assessment of growth control and fetal presentation.

Advanced image analysis tools can support the screening workflow in several ways. First of all, data navigation can be facilitated by automatic recognition of fetal anatomy and display of anatomy correlated views. Secondly, automatic delineation of anatomical structures enables automatic biometrical measurements. Thirdly, biometrical measurements and other image processing results may be used to support a diagnosis. One way to cope with the difficult image properties of fetal US image data is to introduce domain knowledge using a deformable shape model [13]. It can very well deal with noise, incomplete field of views, and drop-outs due to shadowing, and was successfully applied to 3D US fetal head screening [12]. In order to increase the capture range or the adaptation accuracy, the adaptation procedure can be extended to use not just one input image but several ones, e.g., in the case of MRI image data, where different sequences may be available [3,6].

As a first step in the direction of automatic assessment of fetal body measurements, we aim at automatically segmenting the fetal torso in 3D US data. This could be used to automatically determine the abdominal circumference, which is a critical measure of second trimester screening that suffers from high inter-observer variability [8]. To the best of our knowledge, this has not yet been addressed in the literature. We propose to improve accuracy of a model-based segmentation (MBS) by considering the output of a convolutional neural network (CNN) applied to the original 3D US as an additional input. On this behalf, a resource-friendly multi-scale convolutional network architecture is presented. Similar to [6], the network output is then integrated into the segmentation approach. We show that the combination of CNN and MBS considerably enhances robustness of the segmentation and outperforms both separate approaches.

2   Methods

2.1   Model-Based Segmentation

The approach for model based segmentation (MBS) used in this work was originally introduced for heart segmentation in 3D CT images [13] and since successfully applied to a variety of applications, e.g., for head segmentation in fetal ultrasound [12]. Here, the boundary of the structure to be segmented is represented by a triangulated mesh, which is propagated towards boundaries in the images. The segmentation task is formulated as an energy minimization, in which the energy functional consists of two parts: On the one hand, an external energy that attracts the triangle center points of the mesh c_i towards detected boundaries points x_i^{target} in an image (with a weight w_i):

$$E_{\text{external}} := \sum_{i=1}^{T} w_i \left(\frac{\nabla I(x_i^{\text{target}})}{||\nabla I(x_i^{\text{target}})||} \cdot (x_i^{\text{target}} - c_i) \right)^2 . \tag{1}$$

On the other hand, an internal energy that penalizes deviations of the mesh vertices v_k from a learned typical shape μ_k (mean shape plus eigenmodes):

$$E_{\text{internal}} := \sum_{k=1}^{V} \sum_{j \in N(k)} ((v_k - v_j) - (\mathcal{T}(\mu_k) - \mathcal{T}(\mu_j))^2 + E_{\text{eigenmodes}} . \tag{2}$$

Here, $\mathcal{T}$ is a global transformation that registers the model mesh on the target mesh and $E_{eigenmodes}$ weighs the eigenmode configuration. For details, please refer to [13]. The energy is minimized using gradient descent until a maximum number of deformations is reached.

The boundary detection function in the core of the algorithm looks for x_i^{target} by maximizing the feature response F_i along a search ray orthogonal to each triangle center. It considers gradient direction, strength, gray value range inside and outside and other distinctive features for each triangle individually. Thus, the resulting deformable model is locally specific for the organ or organ set to be segmented and highly discriminative. In this work, the limited projected gradient feature following [13] is used:

$$F_i(x) = (n \cdot \nabla I(x)) \frac{g_{max}(g_{max} + ||\nabla I(x)||)}{g_{max}^2 + ||\nabla I(x)||^2} , \tag{3}$$

where $I(x)$ is the gray value image at position x. The gradient norm $||\nabla I(x)||$ is limited by g_{max} and projected onto the triangle normal vector n. Additionally, if neighboring gray values violate learned intervals, the feature response is rejected and – if no other valid target point is found for that triangle – it is adapted only based on the internal energy. The optimal parameter g_{max} and the intensity intervals are learned specifically for each triangle using simulated search [13].

2.2   Model Initialization

Since deformable models only have a local capture range, a robust model initialization is of crucial importance. Well-established approaches like the Generalized Hough Transformation [1] are less suited for the given application, because they are generally not invariant to scale and rotation, while the fetus is growing rapidly and can be of arbitrary orientation in the womb.

In this work, the model is therefore initialized based on three characteristic landmarks in the fetus: heart, stomach, and bladder. Here, two sets of landmarks are compared: On the one hand, manual landmarks defined by a clinical expert. On the other hand, landmarks automatically detected using random forests (RF) [9]. Once these landmarks are determined, they define a transformation (rotation plus uniform scaling) from the model domain to the image domain, which is applied on the learned mean shape model [13] for initialization.

2.3 Fovea Fully Convolutional Networks (FovFCN)

Since the recent rejuvenation of neural networks, object segmentation – often referred to as semantic segmentation [11] – has gained a lot of attention. This task was originally approached by classifying center pixels of patches using neural networks consisting of convolutional, pooling and dense layers [4]. Larger images were then processed in a sliding window fashion, which leads to many redundant calculations in the network where patches overlap. To address this, fully convolutional networks (FCNs) were proposed [11]. By replacing dense layers with 1×1 convolutions, multiple voxels can be classified simultaneously by feeding whole images through the FCN. However, the resulting classification output is of a lower resolution than the original image. Several publications address this issue by combining convolution and pooling with convolution transpose and unpooling layers (with potential shortcut paths) [2,7,10]. Using such a succession of contraction and upsampling layers allows feature extraction on different abstraction levels and yields an output of original image resolution.

In particular for large patch sizes in 3D images, these approaches can lead to a significant memory footprint. If the network size exceeds the memory of the GPU– e.g., in ultrasound devices with strict hardware constraints – segmentation performance can be affected considerably. If the patch size is chosen too small, however, image context is lost by only considering local regions at a time. In particular in fetal ultrasound, it can be difficult even for a human observer to tell if a local patch is part of the fetus or the background (i.e., the placenta, cf. Fig. 2) without considering the "big picture".

To address this issue, we propose a fully convolutional network architecture that feeds in patches at different resolutions, which allows the network to take large context into consideration while reducing the amount of required memory compared to previously proposed architectures [2,7,10]. In contrast to the multi-resolution approach proposed in [5], our network successively integrates the information from an arbitrary number of resolutions instead of only two. To maintain image context, the patch to be segmented is regarded in conjunction with larger, but down-sampled patches at the same position. This approach is loosely inspired by the distribution of photoreceptor cells in the human eye, which have the highest resolution at the *fovea centralis*. As illustrated in Fig. 1, features are extracted on each resolution level. Then, feature maps of coarser resolutions are up-sampled using average unpooling and additively joined with finer levels. The network is trained using the cross-entropy between the output layer and the known labels as the cost function.

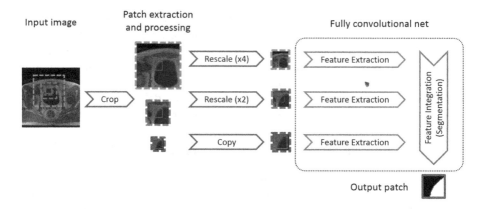

Fig. 1. Sketch of the Fovea CNN with three levels. To segment a patch of a given size (here: 74×74×74 voxels, red box), three input patches of different sizes are cropped from the input image. The larger "context" patches are then rescaled to a lower resolution. For each level, features are extracted (convolutional layers with ReLU activation) using cross entropy loss function. Feature maps at rescaled levels are up-sampled to original resolution using mean unpooling and then added to integrate features of all levels.

2.4   FovFCN-Powered Model-Based Segmentation

When segmenting the fetal torso in US images, the true boundary is often barely visible, e.g. due to shadow artifacts. Instead, other nearby boundaries of maternal tissue may attract the model searching for gradients. By considering a larger image context, techniques like FovFCN are superior to a local feature point search at distinguishing the true boundary of the torso in such regions. However, the resulting torso probability map does not directly provide a valid mesh. To combine advantages of shape models with the selective strengths of neural networks, probability maps are regarded as additional input to deformable models in this work. A similar idea was previously described for vertebra segmentation in MR images [6].

On this behalf, the ground truth torso segmentations are used for training features on torso-probability maps created by the FovFCN described in Sect. 2.3. Then, the model is used on the probability map instead of the original US image. An additional step is to combine the proposed target point search on probability maps and trained features for the original US image: For each triangle, both features search for target points and the external energy is a weighted average between both target point distances [3]. Thus, in contrast to [6], both the actual image information and the computed probability maps are part of the energy formulation for the optimization procedure.

3   Experiments and Results

3.1   Image Data

Experiments presented in this paper are based on 168 3D US datasets acquired with a Philips EPIQ 7 Ultrasound system using a V6-2 3D transducer. The imaged field of view covers the abdomen and parts of the thorax of the fetus. Typically, bladder, stomach, (internal) umbilical vein, and the heart are contained in the images. The gestational age ranges from 15 to 38 weeks. Depending on the gestational age and size of the fetus, the image matrix (x,y,z) contains $(256 \cdots 512) \times (263 \cdots 510) \times (143 \cdots 256)$ voxels with a voxel size of $(0.1 \cdots 0.5) \times (0.06 \cdots 0.4) \times (0.18 \cdots 0.8) \, \text{mm}^3$. For training, a subset of 126 cases was used, for testing the remaining 42 cases, aiming for equal age distributions. Figure 2 shows a random selection of case examples (only an abdominal slice of the 3D volume is shown). The variable image appearance and the influence of noise (especially for the smaller gestational ages) and of shadow artifacts caused by bone structures (especially for higher gestational ages) can be appreciated.

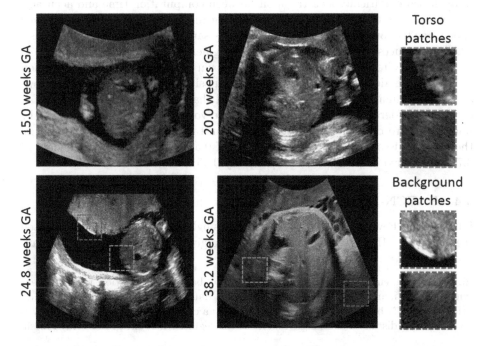

Fig. 2. Some exemplary cases of different gestational ages (GA). The selected slices (of the 3D data sets) show an abdominal region containing the bladder. Differentiating between torso and fetus can be impossible when only looking at small patches.

3.2   Intensity-Only MBS

In Table 1, quantitative results for the model-based segmentation MBS^I using only the ultrasound image I are given for both initialization approaches (manual and RF with mean landmark localization error of 16.5 mm). Exemplary results are shown in Fig. 3. In these experiments, deformable models are often attracted by wrong contours in the image. For example, the mother's tissue may exhibit stronger edges then the boundary of the fetus and therefore distract the model. Further, the impairing effect of false positive edges increases with the distance of the initial model to the correct boundaries. Therefore, the segmentation accuracy is considerably worse for RF-based initialization.

3.3   FovFCN

For segmenting the fetal torso, a FovFCN with three levels and a patch size of $74 \times 74 \times 74$ voxels and $7 \times 7 \times 7$ convolution kernels was employed. This implied input patches of sizes $86 \times 86 \times 86$ (level 0, original resolution), $52 \times 52 \times 52$ (level 1, after rescaling with factor 2) and $35 \times 35 \times 35$ (level 2, factor 4). Parameters were chosen empirically as a trade-off between computation time and accuracy. The network is trained using all 126 training images for 1000 epochs. In each epoch, one training patch per scan is randomly sampled (for all resolution levels), which introduces a certain degree of data augmentation.

Exemplary results of the FovFCN are shown in Fig. 3. The general position of the torso is detected well, with few false positives in the background. However, typical image artifacts like drop-off and shadows by the mother's ribs can entail a considerable amount of false negative voxels inside the torso. Also, the boundaries are often quite fuzzy. For a quantitative evaluation, the output of the FovFCN is binarized with a threshold of 0.5. In total, a Dice coefficient of 0.76 is obtained (sensitivity 0.89, specificity 0.95).

3.4   FovFCN-Powered MBS

Further, the FovFCN output P is used as single modality for a model-based segmentation MBS^P. Quantitative results are given in Table 1, with exemplary

Table 1. Segmentation results comparing model-based segmentation with different initialization (manual and RF-based) and input data (MBS^I: ultrasound intensities, MBS^P: FovFCN-based probabilities, and MBS^{IP}: a combination of both). Accuracy is given in mean distances of triangle centers of the segmented to the ground truth mesh.

	Metric	Init	MBS^I	MBS^P	MBS^{IP}
Manual initialization	Mean distance (mm)	4.01	2.23	**2.00**	2.06
	Max distance (mm)	6.28	4.43	**3.77**	4.17
Manual initialization	Mean distance (mm)	5.47	3.75	2.39	**2.24**
	Max distance (mm)	9.05	7.22	5.12	**4.97**

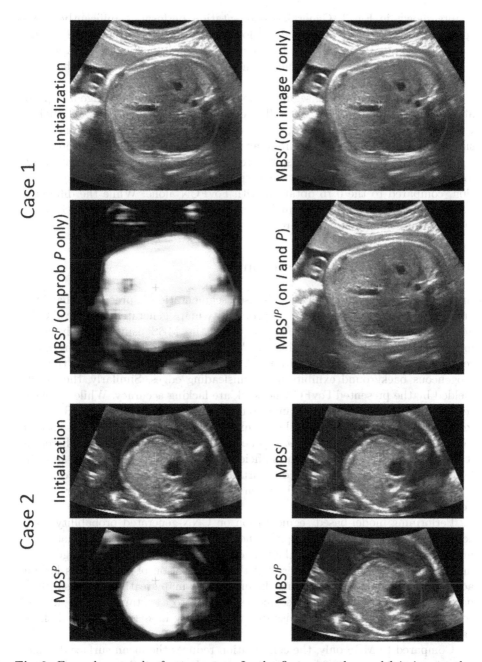

Fig. 3. Exemplary results for two cases. In the first case, the model is incorrectly attracted by a strong edge by from the mother's tissue. In the second example, a shadow artifact leads to a intensity drop-off at one side of the fetus, impairing the segmentation. In both cases, integrating the probability map yielded by the FovFCN considerably improves the result.

results shown in Fig. 3. Generally, segmentation performs significantly better (paired ttest, $p \leq 10^{-4}$ and $p \leq 10^{-12}$ for manual and RF initialization) on the probability maps P than on the ultrasound images I. In particular, the approach is much more robust against initialization errors because fewer edges in the image distract the model adaptation.

In the final experiments, segmentation was performed with image and probability map as input (MBS^{IP}, see Table 1 and Fig. 3). The results are slightly worse for well-initialized models, for RF-based initialization the combined consideration of images and probability maps is better than the separate approaches.

Dice values of the MBS^{IP} result were 0.87 (sensitivity 0.99, specificity 0.82) for manual and 0.86 (sensitivity 0.99, specificity 0.82) for RF-based initialization, compared to the 0.76 obtained with FovFCN alone. While the difference between MBS^{P} and MBS^{IP} is small, the use of both FovFCN and MBS clearly outperformes the individual approaches.

4 Discussion and Conclusion

In this work, an approach for model-based segmentation is presented that integrates image information with voxel probability maps generated by a novel CNN architecture. For segmenting the fetal torso, the MBS using solely intensity images is lacking robustness. This can be attributed to the challenging ultrasound data, which is impaired by noise and image artifacts. Further, the heterogeneous background exhibits many misleading edges. Similarly, the results yielded by the presented FovFCN network are lacking accuracy. While excellent results are obtained with the same architecture when segmenting MR or CT images, it can be assumed that the training set is too small to be representative for the wide range of (highly heterogeneous) fetal ultrasound scans. Therefore, it fails to learn the image content sufficiently well to be able to extrapolate the fetal anatomy in regions impaired by artifacts. This is further supported by the observation that the difference between training and test set is larger for the FovFCN than for the MBS.

Performing model-based segmentation on CNN-generated probability maps combines advantages of both approaches. The neural network eliminates the majority of distracting edges in the image and increases the capture range of the model. This is of particular interest if the initialization of the mesh is lacking accuracy, in which case considering the probability map greatly improves robustness. Further, the model-based segmentation is – to a certain degree – able to compensate for artifacts and noise due to explicitly modeled shape and shape variations.

Compared to MBS only, the combination reduces the mean surface distance error from 3.75 mm to 2.24 mm. Compared to FovFCN only, the combination increases the Dice coefficient from 0.76 to 0.86. Thus, FovFCN-powered MBS clearly outperforms either separate approach.

References

1. Ballard, D.H.: Generalizing the hough transform to detect arbitrary shapes. Pattern Recogn. **13**(2), 111–122 (1981)
2. Brosch, T., Tang, L.Y.W., Yoo, Y., Li, D.K.B., Traboulsee, A., Tam, R.: Deep 3D convolutional encoder networks with shortcuts for multiscale feature integration applied to multiple sclerosis lesion segmentation. IEEE Trans. Med. Imaging **35**(5), 1229–1239 (2016)
3. Buerger, C., Peters, J., Waechter-Stehle, I., Weber, F.M., Klinder, T., Renisch, S.: Multi-modal vertebra segmentation from MR dixon for hybrid whole-body PET/MR. In: Yao, J., Klinder, T., Li, S. (eds.) Computational Methods and Clinical Applications for Spine Imaging. LNCVB, vol. 17, pp. 159–171. Springer, Cham (2014). doi:10.1007/978-3-319-07269-2_14
4. Ciresan, D., Giusti, A., Gambardella, L.M., Schmidhuber, J.: Deep neural networks segment neuronal membranes in electron microscopy images. In: Pereira, F., Burges, C.J.C., Bottou, L., Weinberger, K.Q. (eds.) Advances in Neural Information Processing Systems, vol. 25, pp. 2843–2851 (2012)
5. Kamnitsas, K., Ledig, C., Newcombe, V.F., Simpson, J.P., Kane, A.D., Menon, D.K., Rueckert, D., Glocker, B.: Efficient multi-scale 3D CNN with fully connected CRF for accurate brain lesion segmentation. Med. Image Anal. **36**, 61–78 (2017)
6. Korez, R., Likar, B., Pernuš, F., Vrtovec, T.: Model-based segmentation of vertebral bodies from mr images with 3D CNNs. In: Ourselin, S., Joskowicz, L., Sabuncu, M.R., Unal, G., Wells, W. (eds.) MICCAI 2016. LNCS, vol. 9901, pp. 433–441. Springer, Cham (2016). doi:10.1007/978-3-319-46723-8_50
7. Noh, H., Hong, S., Han, B.: Learning deconvolution network for semantic segmentation. In: IEEE International Conference on Computer Vision (ICCV), pp. 1520–1528 (2015)
8. Papageorghiou, A.T., et al.: International standards for fetal growth based on serial ultrasound measurements: The Fetal Growth Longitudinal Study of the INTERGROWTH-21st Project. Lancet **384**, 869–879 (2014)
9. Raynaud, C., Ciofolo-Veit, C., Lefèvre, T., Ardon, R., Cavallaro, A., Salim, I., Papageorghiou, A., Rouet, L.: Multi-organ detection in 3D fetal ultrasound with machine learning. In: MICCAI Workshop on Fetal and InFant Image Analysis (FIFI 2017) (2017)
10. Ronneberger, O., Fischer, P., Brox, T.: U-Net: Convolutional networks for biomedical image segmentation. In: Navab, N., Hornegger, J., Wells, W.M., Frangi, A.F. (eds.) MICCAI 2015. LNCS, vol. 9351, pp. 234–241. Springer, Cham (2015). doi:10.1007/978-3-319-24574-4_28
11. Shelhamer, E., Long, J., Darrell, T.: Fully convolutional networks for semantic segmentation. IEEE Trans. Pattern Anal. Mach. Intell. **39**(4), 640–651 (2017)
12. Waechter-Stehle, I., Klinder, T., Rouet, J.M., Roundhill, D., Andrews, G., Cavallaro, A., Molloholli, M., Norris, T., Napolitano, R., Papageorghiou, A., et al.: Learning from redundant but inconsistent reference data: anatomical views and measurements for fetal brain screening. In: SPIE Medical Imaging, p. 97841A (2016)
13. Weese, J., Kaus, M., Lorenz, C., Lobregt, S., Truyen, R., Pekar, V.: Shape constrained deformable models for 3-D medical image segmentation. In: Information Processing in Medical Imaging (IPMI), vol. 2082, pp. 380–387 (2001)

Multi-organ Detection in 3D Fetal Ultrasound with Machine Learning

Caroline Raynaud[1](✉), Cybèle Ciofolo-Veit[1](✉), Thierry Lefèvre[1],
Roberto Ardon[1], Angelo Cavallaro[2], Ibtisam Salim[2], Aris Papageorghiou[2],
and Laurence Rouet[1]

[1] Philips Research MediSys, Paris, France
{caroline.raynaud,cybele.ciofolo-veit}@philips.com
[2] Nuffield Department of Obstetrics and Gynaecology,
University of Oxford, Oxford, England

Abstract. 3D ultrasound (US) is a promising technique to perform automatic extraction of standard planes for fetal anatomy assessment. This requires prior organ localization, which is difficult to obtain with direct learning approaches because of the high variability in fetus size and orientation in US volumes. In this paper, we propose a methodology to overcome this spatial variability issue by scaling and automatically aligning volumes in a common 3D reference coordinate system. This preprocessing allows the organ detection algorithm to learn features that only encodes the anatomical variability while discarding the fetus pose. All steps of the approach are evaluated on 126 manually annotated volumes, with an overall mean localization error of $11.9\,mm$, showing the feasibility of multi-organ detection in 3D fetal US with machine learning.

Keywords: 3D ultrasound · Volume alignment · Landmark localization

1 Introduction

In clinical routine, 2D Ultrasound (US) is the preferred scanning protocol for biometry measurements, growth monitoring and anatomy assessment during pregnancy. Obtaining reproducible and accurate values requires to follow strict guidelines, especially regarding the selection of the standard 2D viewing planes which are used to search for abnormalities or perform biometry measurements such as head and abdomen circumference or femur length. This task can be very difficult because of multiple factors: the mother morphology, the unknown and highly variable orientation of the fetus as well as well-known US artefacts, in particular the shadowing effect. 3D US is a more recent imaging technique that has the potential to overcome some of the above mentioned difficulties. In particular, the acquisition of a single 3D volume makes it possible to automatically select the required viewing planes, even for less experienced users. In addition, the clinicians can perform offline reading and, if necessary, adjust the position of the extracted planes prior to standard measurements.

© Springer International Publishing AG 2017
M.J. Cardoso et al. (Eds.): FIFI/OMIA 2017, LNCS 10554, pp. 62–72, 2017.
DOI: 10.1007/978-3-319-67561-9_7

Various strategies have been proposed for automatic viewing planes extraction in 2D. Views of interest can be selected from 2D US sequences by classifying the content of each frame to determine if it corresponds to a standard plane using a radial component model [1] or a pre-trained recurrent neural network [2]. Another 2D approach consists in fitting geometrical templates built at multiple resolutions and orientations in order to label the anatomical content [3].

In this study, we propose a new approach using 3D US to localize fetal abdominal organs which will be used as landmarks for subsequent standard planes extraction. Because 3D fetal US imaging is a relatively new field and only limited datasets are available, we chose the random forests method [4–6] among others possible learning techniques. However, the size, position and orientation of the fetuses in acquired volumes are highly variable due to fetal presentation, gestational age or probe position. To overcome this difficulty, our method first aligns and scales all fetuses in a common normalized reference coordinate system, so that the learning algorithm focuses only on analyzing fetal anatomy, without including variations due to spatial misalignments and pregnancy stages.

Overall, the proposed approach consists in tackling the successive difficulties step by step, by focusing on well identified problems to ensure the robustness of the whole processing pipeline. An initial volume alignment based on spine and torso detection is performed, followed by the disambiguation of head-toe orientation. Additional scaling normalizes the organ and fetus sizes. Once all volumes are aligned, a random forest is trained in order to regress the position of the main fetal abdominal organs. Finally, we evaluate both the pre-processing steps and the complete pipeline by using manually annotated landmark positions.

2   Method

To localize fetal organs from 3D US abdominal acquisitions with a learning-based approach, the input material is a database of 3D volumes associated to expert annotations of the main abdominal structures. Figure 1 (Left) illustrates, for each case, the position of the spine (lines) and main organ centers (dots) in the original acquisition coordinate system. The graph reflects the high variability of

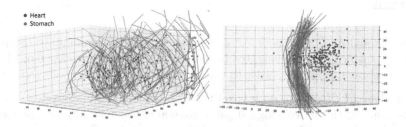

Fig. 1. Expert annotations of fetal spine (lines) and organs (dots). (Left) illustration of orientation variability of fetal volumes before alignement of fetus coordinate systems. (Right) Organs positions after volume alignement.

fetus positions and orientations and confirms that learning on such a database will include variability due to spatial positioning instead of focusing on real anatomical variations.

As explained above, this section describes how to solve this issue with a complete workflow, including a specific alignment and scaling preprocessing (Sect. 2.1) followed with a multi-organ localization method with random forests (Sect. 2.2).

2.1   Fetus Reference Coordinate System Definition

To align the whole database of N volumes, a local, fetus-based coordinate system noted $R_i = (O_i, x_i, y_i, z_i)$ is defined in each volume $i, i \in \{1 \dots N\}$ (see Fig. 2). An affine transformation is then applied to the volumes so that the fetus coordinate systems are scaled and aligned with a common arbitrary reference coordinate system $R = (O, x, y, z)$.

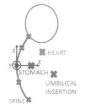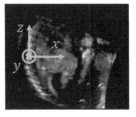

Fig. 2. Definition of a fetus-based coordinate system

Among all anatomical structures, the fetal spine is unique, clearly visible and specific enough to provide some basic orientation information, which makes it a good starting point for coordinate system definition. The first step of the alignment processing is thus to detect the spine of the fetus, which leads to the definition of the local origin O_i and a first axis z_i. A second, transverse axis x_i is then found by locating the fetus abdomen and the head-toe orientation is finally determined.

Spine Detection. The spine is automatically detected by combining a morphological filter which detects elongated bright structures and a deep learning (DL)-based vertebrae detector, in order to take advantage of both methods strengths.

Morphological filter. For each voxel **x** in the US volume, in a given spherical neighbourhood, the morphological filter compares the intensity of the voxels along a direction **u** with the intensity of the other voxels. The filter responses are computed for various neighbourhood radii and orientations **u** and combined to obtain a global response. The global responses of neighbouring voxels are aggregated to define connected components which correspond to the best filter responses (red overlay in Fig. 3 (Left)). Although some of the responses are accurately positioned on the spine, others are outliers that may be located on ribs or other elongated structures such as long bones.

Deep learning-based vertebrae detector. The DL-based vertebrae detector consists in a 2D fully convolutional network. The input of the network consists in 2D slices, extracted orthogonally to the original z-axis. The network architecture is as follows: a succession of three convolution blocks (each composed of 32 filters of two 3×3 convolutional layers with relu activation and one pooling layer), followed by two dense-equivalent blocks (each composed of 512 filters of 1×1 convolutions) and a final 1×1 convolution. The volume slicing produces a large amount of data with similar features, which is appropriate for deep learning methods. The network output is a downsampled probability map, with values closer to one where the spine might be located. A 3D DL-based vertebrae detector is built by stacking all the obtained 2D probability maps for one volume. This output heatmap is coarser than the morphological filter output, but more robustly located around the vertebrae (Fig. 3 (Center)).

Combined spine detector. By selecting the intersection between the DL vertebrae detector and the morphological filter responses, the network output is refined and the filter responses that are outside the spine are rejected, so that a more robust spine binary mask is finally obtained (Fig. 3 (Right)).

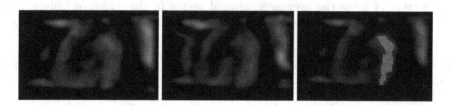

Fig. 3. Spine detection with: (Left) morphological filtering, Center: DL approach, (Right) combination of both approaches.

Origin and Vertical Axis. The center of mass of the spine binary mask is used as the center of the fetus coordinate system O_i. If the detected spine is highly curved, its center of mass might not belong to the binary mask. In this case, the binary mask point that is the closest to the center of mass is used. Then the extremities of the spine binary mask are used to define the z_i axis, a vertical axis tangent to the spine (see Fig. 2).

Abdomen Detection and Transverse Axes Definition. The x_i and y_i axes are searched in the plane orthogonal to z_i at O_i, noted (O_i, x_i, y_i). To do so, the fetus abdomen is detected in various transverse planes, with the following steps:

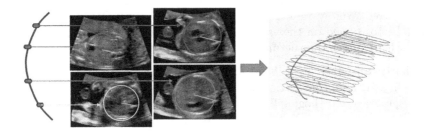

Fig. 4. (Left) Transverse planes extraction and abdomen detection. (Right) Torso volume of interest from transverse abdomen detections.

- Transverse planes extraction at evenly spaced points along the spine (Fig. 4).
- Abdomen detection in all transverse planes, by using a variant of the Hough transform tailored to the detection of circular shapes. In practice, the best convolution of the image with a radially-symmetric kernel modeling a disk with the desired border profile is searched among a range of radii (Fig. 4 (Left)).
- For each plane, computation of the vector going through the spine intersection with the plane and the center of the detected circle (orange segments in Fig. 4 (Left)).
- Projection of all vectors on the (O_i, x_i, y_i) transverse plane.
- Selection of x_i as the average projected vector in the (O_i, x_i, y_i) plane (see Fig. 2 (Left)). The y_i vector is chosen so that the coordinate system is orthogonal with right-handed orientation.

Additionally, the stack of abdomen detection results in transverse planes defines a mask of the abdomen, as shown in Fig. 4 (Right).

Head-Toe Orientation. At this stage, it is necessary to find the head-toe orientation of the volume and choose between the two possible directions of the z_i axis. This is done by training a classifier to distinguish between the two configurations in the 2D (O_i, x_i, z_i) slice of the volume (Fig. 5). In practice we use a convolutional neural network similar to AlexNet [7]. In order to be robust to possible inaccuracies during the spine detection step, random noise is added during the (O_i, x_i, z_i) slice extraction so that the network is fed with corrupted data during the training. Then random patches are selected in the slice to train the classifier, whose output is binary (1 when the fetus head is at the top of the image, O if it is at the bottom). The testing is done with a similar process, without the random noise addition.

Scaling. To reduce scale variability due to varying gestational ages (GA), a scaling factor is also applied to all volumes based on existing growth tables [8].

After this processing, the volumes are rotated and translated so that the associated fetus coordinate systems R_i are aligned with the common reference

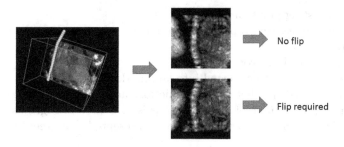

Fig. 5. Plane extraction along spine and patch extraction for classification.

coordinate system R. An illustration of the alignement is visible in Fig. 1 (Right), where the spine and various fetal organs have been annotated by experts.

2.2 Organ Detection

The detection of fetal organs is done with a random forest algorithm [4], with a similar approach as the one proposed in [5]. The principle is to learn, for a given point in a volume, the relative direction to the target organ landmarks. In the following description, such a relative direction is referred to as a voting vector.

Training. In order to train the random forest algorithm, it is necessary to set the values of a number of parameters. The most influential ones are the following: number of trees, depth of trees, number of training points per image and threshold on variance of voting vectors in a node, respectively noted N_T, D_T, N_P, α. The algorithm also depends on image-based features $F = \{f\}$. In the present study, the features are mostly derived from local gradients, such as locally normalized gradients and distance to gradients.

A splitting criterion is defined for all nodes. It aims at finding two subsets of training points so that the sum of the entropy of both subsets is minimal. To obtain the splitting criterion, a large set of random features is tested at each node. Within this set, the feature f that provides the optimal subset separation and the corresponding splitting threshold θ are selected and stored in the node. The entropy is defined as the variance of the voting vectors to each landmark.

Multiple stopping criteria are defined for all leaves: *(i)* a given depth D_T of the tree is reached, *(ii)* the intra-subset variance is below a given threshold α, *(iii)* the subset is too small. The mean of the voting vectors is stored in each leaf. This will be the voting vector of each point classified in this leaf.

Testing. Testing describes the actual landmark localization process, which is restricted to the volume area located inside the abdomen mask, as defined in Sect. 2.1. For a given input volume, the following steps are performed:

- P random testing points are selected.
- The testing points are propagated throughout the tree, using the (f, θ) splitting criteria, until they reach a leaf.
- Each point provides a voting vector.
- All voting vectors are converted into landmark predictions.
- To provide a single prediction, all predictions are combined through Gaussian estimation. An example of all predictions is presented in Fig. 6 as a coloured overlay. The extracted single prediction is presented as a green point.

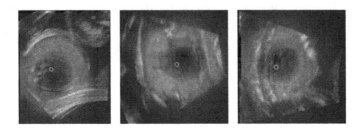

Fig. 6. Cross-section planes from a 3D ultrasound volume with overlay of all voting predictions and extracted single prediction (green point). (Color figure online)

3   Results and Discussion

3.1   Material and Experimental Setup

The database consists in 126 3D ultrasound abdominal volumes, acquired in 2015 at John Radcliffe Hospital, Nuffield Department of Obstetrics and Gynaecology. The acquisitions are performed on a EPIQ 7G system (Philips Ultrasound, Bothell, WA), using a mechanical V6-2 probe. The probe orientation is axial with respect to the fetal abdomen and the mechanical sweep spans the spine longitudinal axis. The database includes gestational ages ranging from 16 to 38 weeks. The volumes dimensions in voxels are $512 \times 512 \times 256$, with a spatial resolution around $0.25 \times 0.25 \times 0.5$ mm.

The whole approach uses learning algorithms at various steps. In order to perform validation, the data is split into 4-folds of about 32 volumes each. Each fold reflects the GA distribution in the database. For all validation experiments, the same folds are used. For each fold, the algorithm is trained on the three remaining folds. Parameters for random forests training are $N_T = 20$, $D_T = 20$, $N_P = 20.10^6$, $\alpha = 7$.

For each volume in the database, a spine annotation is provided as a point set, together with the landmarks corresponding to main organs (heart, stomach, umbilical vein and bladder) annotated as 3D points, when present in the volume.

3.2   Fetus Reference Coordinate System Validation

Spine Orientation Validation. The spine orientation is validated through comparison with manual annotations. Two metrics are used: *(i)* the distance d between the point set center of the annotated spine and the point set center of the automatically detected spine, *(ii)* the angle ϕ between the tangents to the spine of annotated and detected points sets.

Results show a mean distance $d = 12$ mm [±6.3]. The measured mean angle $\phi = 12°[\pm 7]$. These errors seem low enough to use the spine detection as a first step for volume alignment.

Torso orientation and x_i axis validation. In order to evaluate the accuracy of the abdomen detection and the transverse x_i axis, the spatial variances of different structures in two different coordinate systems are compared. Both coordinate systems use the spine direction as z_i axis. The first one (R_{curv}) is defined using the curvature of the spine in order to define the x_{curv} axis. Indeed, if the spine is curved, its center and both extremities define a plane. The x_{curv} axis is the orthogonal vector to z_i that points towards the convex side of the curve. The second coordinate system (R_i) is obtained as described in Sect. 2.1: the x_i axis is obtained through abdomen detection, being the average vector pointing from the spine to the center of the abdomen. The variance in the spatial distribution of two given organs, heart and stomach, are compared. Regarding the heart, the variance is 13.9 mm in the R_{curv} and 5.6 mm in R_i. For the stomach it goes from 10.4 mm to 4.3 mm, which shows that the use of the method described in Sect. 2.1 makes the x_i axis definition more accurate (Fig. 7).

Head-Toe Orientation Validation. As in the previous sections, we have validated the training of our network in a 4-fold scheme using images patches of size 128×128. On the 126 volumes the successful classification rate is 86%.

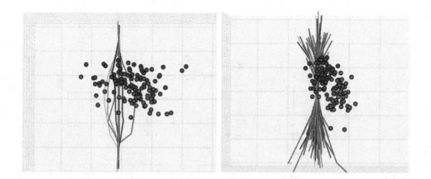

Fig. 7. (Left) Landmarks of heart (blue) and stomach (red) using alignment deduced from spine curvature (R_{curv}). (Right) Heart and stomach landmarks in aligned coord. system after torso detection combined with spine detection (R_i). (Color figure online)

Processing Time. With a standard CPU architecture (Intel Core i7, 8 GB RAM), the alignment process takes between 10 and 15 s per image.

3.3   Landmarks/Organs Detection Validation

The validation of organ detection consists in processing all volumes with the full pipeline. The output of the processing is a set of landmarks corresponding to fetal organs. In the present study, the localization of heart, stomach, umbilical vein and bladder is evaluated.

In order to separate localization errors due to both automatic coordinate system definition and the random forest algorithm itself, two series of evaluations are performed. The first series consists in using the manually annotated spine as input to define the fetus coordinate system R_i, thus removing errors due to its automatic detection. In the second evaluation series, the landmark localization follows the automatic fetus coordinate system definition. Errors are defined, for each landmark, as the distance between the annotated landmark and its predicted position. Results for the whole database are presented in Fig. 8. The localization error using the fully automatic pipeline is $\{10.2; 11.1; 11.1; 15.4\}$ mm respectively for umbilical vein, heart, stomach and bladder, which is close to $\{10.0; 10.8; 11.0; 15.3\}$ mm for same organs using manually annotated spine to initialize volume alignment.

Such results assert the quality of the fetus coordinate system automatic detection, which is a key in the whole processing. The variance of error using the automatic pipeline varies depending on the organ of interest. For the bladder, the error variance is higher. These results may be explained by factors such as its varying spatial extent, which depends on its filling state, and its location,

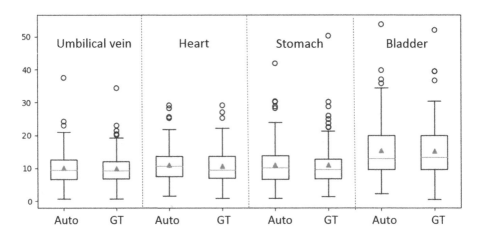

Fig. 8. Comparison of distances in mm from prediction to ground truth, per organ. Errors are measured for detection following automatic volume alignment (Auto), and also for detection based on spine annotations (GT).

most often at the edge of the volume, which limits the amount on information carried by features in its surroundings.

4   Conclusion

The overall performance of the presented approach depends on acquisition related characteristics, such as limited US field-of-view, especially for late pregnancy stages, and fetus orientation and size variations. The number of available volumes for training is another factor that limits the learning of anatomical variability. Finally, the successive processing steps also generate errors accumulation. Taking all these aspects into account, a mean error of 11.9 mm on landmarks detection appears acceptable for use in later processing, such as automatic viewing plane extraction.

This study shows that machine learning approaches can be used to detect fetal organs in 3D US, even when the dataset is relatively small and presents a high spatial variability. To do so, it is necessary to pre-process the US volumes by scaling and aligning them in a common spatial reference coordinate system, so that the learning algorithm focuses on anatomical variability rather than on spatial discrepancies. In order to increase the detection performance, directions such as the use of more volumes, data augmentation, image resolution refinement or separation of learning according to pregnancy stages are foreseen.

Acknowledgements. This work was done in Philips Research Paris (MediSys), with images acquired and manually annotated at the John Radcliffe Hospital, Oxford, in collaboration with the University of Oxford, with funding from Philips Ultrasound.

References

1. Dong, N., Xin, Y., Xin, C., Chien-Ting, C., Siping, C., Pheng Ann, H., Shengli, L., Jing, Q., Tianfu, W.: Standard plane localization in ultrasound by radial component model and selective search. Ultrasound Med. Biol. **40**, 2728–2742 (2014)
2. Chen, H., Dou, Q., Ni, D., Cheng, J.-Z., Qin, J., Li, S., Heng, P.-A.: Automatic fetal ultrasound standard plane detection using knowledge transferred recurrent neural networks. In: Navab, N., Hornegger, J., Wells, W.M., Frangi, A.F. (eds.) MICCAI 2015. LNCS, vol. 9349, pp. 507–514. Springer, Cham (2015). doi:10.1007/978-3-319-24553-9_62
3. Yaqub, M., Kelly, B., Papageorghiou, A.T., Noble, J.A.: Guided random forests for identification of key fetal anatomy and image categorization in ultrasound scans. In: Navab, N., Hornegger, J., Wells, W.M., Frangi, A.F. (eds.) MICCAI 2015. LNCS, vol. 9351, pp. 687–694. Springer, Cham (2015). doi:10.1007/978-3-319-24574-4_82
4. Criminisi, A., Shotton, J., Konukoglu, E.: Decision forests: a unified framework for classification, regression, density estimation, manifold learning and semi-supervised learning. Foundations and Trends in Computer Graphics and Vision (2012)
5. Cuingnet, R., Prevost, R., Lesage, D., Cohen, L.D., Mory, B., Ardon, R.: Automatic detection and segmentation of kidneys in 3D CT images using random forests. In: Ayache, N., Delingette, H., Golland, P., Mori, K. (eds.) MICCAI 2012. LNCS, vol. 7512, pp. 66–74. Springer, Heidelberg (2012). doi:10.1007/978-3-642-33454-2_9

6. Gauriau, R., Cuingnet, R., Lesage, D., Bloch, I.: Multi-organ localization with cascaded global-to-local regression and shape prior. Med. Image Anal. **23**, 70–83 (2015)
7. Krizhevsky, A., Sutskever, I., Hinton, G.E.: Imagenet classification with deep convolutional neural networks. In: Advances in Neural International Proceedings Systems (NIPS) (2012)
8. Papageorghiou, A.T., et al.: for the Internat. Fetal, for the 21st Cent., N.G.C.: Internat. standards for fetal growth based on serial ultrasound measurements: the fetal growth longitudinal study of the INTERGROWTH-21st project. The Lancet (2014)

Robust Regression of Brain Maturation from 3D Fetal Neurosonography Using CRNs

Ana I.L. Namburete$^{(\boxtimes)}$, Weidi Xie, and J. Alison Noble

Department of Engineering Science, Institute of Biomedical Engineering,
University of Oxford, Oxford, UK
`ana.namburete@eng.ox.ac.uk`

Abstract. We propose a fully three-dimensional Convolutional Regression Network (CRN) for the task of predicting fetal brain maturation from 3D ultrasound (US) data. Anatomical development is modelled as the sonographic patterns visible in the brain at a given gestational age, which are aggregated by the model into a single value: the brain maturation (BM) score. These patterns are learned from 589 3D fetal volumes, and the model is applied to 3D US images of 146 fetal subjects acquired at multiple, ethnically diverse sites, spanning an age range of 18 to 36 gestational weeks. Achieving a mean error of 7.7 days between ground-truth and estimated maturational scores, our method outperforms the current state-of-art for automated BM estimation from 3D US images.

1 Introduction

Estimation of fetal growth and developmental progression is paramount in obstetric care. The fetal brain undergoes a predictable sequence of structural changes across gestation: from a smooth surface, to progressively bearing more folds [1]. This process follows such a precise schedule, that any delays are indicative of impaired brain maturation. Thus, the presence of a cerebral abnormality may cause the level of brain maturation (BM) to differ from the chronological gestational age (GA). This work present a tool to automatically estimate BM from 3D ultrasound (US) images of the fetal brain from as early as 18 weeks.

Routinely used clinical methods for assessment of brain maturation are largely qualitative [2] or based on the size of a single brain structure [3]. In these examinations, obstetricians exploit the changes in texture and the emergence and evolution of structures at a given gestational timepoint to inform on BM [4]. They have to mentally fuse information from different brain structures, each of which follows a non-linear developmental trajectory, to then determine a maturational score [4]. The goal of this work is to capitalise on all available brain biomarkers, both spatially and temporally, in 3D US images to estimate BM.

Automated models have been successful in exploiting neurodevelopmental biomakers to predict age and maturation from brain images of neonates [5,6] and fetuses [7]. In [7], random regression forests (RRFs) were used to predict GA and BM from fetal ultrasound images and clinical biometric data. That approach demonstrated the ability of RRFs to map sonographic patterns visible

© Springer International Publishing AG 2017
M.J. Cardoso et al. (Eds.): FIFI/OMIA 2017, LNCS 10554, pp. 73–80, 2017.
DOI: 10.1007/978-3-319-67561-9_8

in standard clinical US data to gestational age within ± 11 days[1]. By design, RRFs are non-linear predictors that disregard any image regions which are not encapsulated within the set of hand-crafted features. Deep convolutional neural networks (DCNNs), on the other hand, have demonstrated that by not imposing priors on the data (i.e. no feature hypothesis), they are able to automatically identify relevant features for the prediction task. During training, the cost function is optimised to generate a model of high-level abstractions described by a multi-layered graph which encapsulates both linear and non-linear encodings of the data. This property makes them well-suited to making predictions about an organ as complex as the developing brain, with data as challenging as US.

Regression tasks are performed by convolutional regression networks (CRNs), and success has been achieved in estimating biological age from medical image data [8]. In this work, we follow this novel direction to apply CRNs to estimate BM from complex 3D neurosonographic data. However, while most regression models are designed to minimize the difference between ground-truth and predicted values by optimising a least-squares function, this tends to be sensitive to outliers. Within the context of ultrasound-based estimations, outliers are typically represented by images with strong acoustic shadows, partial anatomical occlusions, or variations in intensity patterns (due to acquisition protocol). They may also be represented by developmentally advanced or delayed fetal subjects, or the rare cases of fetuses affected by cerebral malformations. The L_2-norm is unlikely to perform well in such cases. In this work, we also explore an objective function that reduces emphasis on such outliers.

2   Methods

In the fetal period, the bright echoes visible in US images change, marking the emergence of cerebral structures [1]. This work explores two different CRN architectures for estimating BM from sonographic image patterns. The objective is to capture the brain features informative of structural brain changes and, potentially, the process of cortical folding. This section summarises the data processing pipeline and describes the architecture design.

2.1   Image Pre-processing

Fetal neurosonography is challenged by the fact that scanning through bone attenuates the ultrasound energy, and the concave shape of the skull surface refracts the signal. As the skull calcifies over the course of gestation, the US signal is increasingly affected, thereby lowering the image contrast and the visibility of anatomical boundaries. These interactions result in only the cerebral hemisphere farthest from the US probe producing an image with discernible structures. To circumvent this, a 'complete' representation of the brain was generated in our dataset by mirroring the visible hemisphere across the midsagittal plane.

---

[1] This result refers to the RRF model which exclusively used brain features, and did not incorporate information about fetal size (i.e. head circumference).

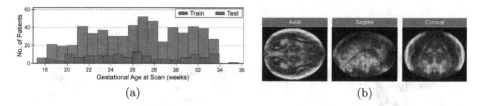

Fig. 1. (a) Gestational age distribution of the training ($N = 609$) and validation ($N = 120$) fetal datasets. (b) Example of preprocessed US brain image, following skull masking, alignment, and mirroring of visible hemisphere.

To exclude prior knowledge about the expected size of the brain, all ultrasound images were spatially normalized and aligned to a pre-defined coordinate frame prior to processing. Specifically, the skull was manually segmented, and the brain region was cropped and rigidly aligned to a predefined coordinate frame (Fig. 1b). To reduce the effect of intensity variations, the images were then individually normalised to have zero mean and unary standard deviation.

2.2 CRN Architectures

CRNs are sequential models consisting of layers which perform operations on the input data. The input to the network is an image $\mathbf{I} : \Omega \rightarrow \mathbb{R}^3$, and the output is a real-valued scalar $y \in \mathbb{R}$ corresponding to BM score. Given a training set $\{(\mathbf{I}_i, y_i)\}_{i=1}^{N}$ of N data samples, the goal of training a CRN is to learn a function $\varphi(\cdot; \theta)$ and its corresponding parameters θ to map an image to a prediction of BM: $\hat{y} = \varphi(\mathbf{I}; \theta)$. The function, $\varphi(\cdot; \theta)$ is minimized by a pre-defined loss function $\mathcal{L}(\mathbf{y}, \hat{\mathbf{y}} \mid \theta)$.

The input image is mapped to the output by a series of convolutional blocks (ConvBlocks). In each ConvBlock, feature extraction is performed by convolutional layers which convolve the images with a pre-defined number of filters (s) of kernel size k. In the first layer, we use a convolutional layer with filter of size $k \times k \times s$. All convolutional layers use kernels of fixed size ($k = 7$), with a sliding step of size $\delta_c = 1$. In order to improve feature generalizability, each convolution is followed by batch normalization. The batch-normalized filter outputs are then processed by a rectified linear unit (ReLU) as the non-linear activation function. Weight regularization of 10^{-4} is also used in each convolution to reduce the generalization error. In order to reduce computational burden, the image resolution is decreased by a Max-Pooling operation with a stride of $\delta_p = 2$. The last is the only layer of the network whose activation is not a ReLU; instead, it uses a linear activation to regress to GA as a proxy for BM.

We test two networks, each consisting of four pooling layers. The architecture of network CRN-2D consists of a ConvBlockA (Fig. 2b) before each pooling layer, for a total of eight two-dimensional (2D) convolutional layers between the input and output layers (Fig. 2a). Due to memory limitations associated with performing 3D convolutions, network CRN-3D was designed as a shallower network. It

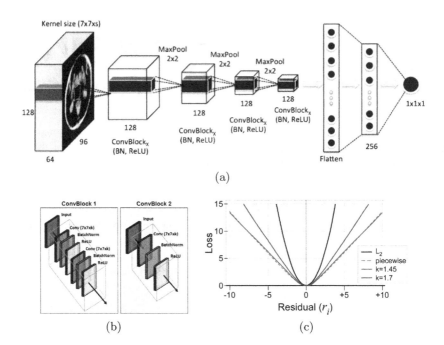

Fig. 2. (a) Basic architecture for the CRN-2D network. (b) Schematic of the components of ConvBlocks A and B. Each convolution (Conv) is followed by batch normalization (BN) and ReLU activation. (c) L_2 increases rapidly with increasing residual magnitude. We use a smooth approximation (red) of the piecewise (dashed green) Huber function. Higher values of k bias the curve towards L_2.

comprises of a ConvBlockB preceding each pooling operation, amounting to a total of four three-dimensional (3D) convolutions.

2.3   Loss Functions for Robust Maturation Regression

During the training process, the output of the CRN ($\hat{\mathbf{y}}$) is compared with the ground-truth labels $\mathbf{y}$ through a loss function $\mathcal{L}$, and the error is back-propagated to update the filter weights of all the layers. This process is repeated until convergence is reached. The goal of the loss function is to minimize the difference (or residuals, $\mathbf{r}$) between the known ($\mathbf{y}$) and estimated ($\hat{\mathbf{y}}$) values. Thus, the loss function ultimately dictates the speed of convergence, and the quality of the trained parameters.

In the back-propagation step, the magnitude of the gradient is proportional to the residual. As a result, the estimations that are close to the ground-truth (inliers) have a lower influence on the updated network parameters (θ), and the outliers yielding higher residuals have a greater influence and may thus bias the model to adapt itself to such examples. There are several options for objective functions. To achieve a robust BM estimator, we explored the effect of different loss functions on the CRN models. Namely, the familiar least-squares estimator ($\mathcal{L}_2$),

$$\mathcal{L}_2(\mathbf{r}) = \frac{1}{n} \sum_{i=1}^{n} r_i^2 \tag{1}$$

and the Huber estimator ($\mathcal{L}_{\text{hub}}$) which is less vulnerable to outliers [9],

$$\mathcal{L}_{\text{hub}}(\mathbf{r}) = \frac{1}{n} \sum_{i=1}^{n} k^2(\sqrt{1 + (r_i/k)^2} - 1). \tag{2}$$

where $r_i = \hat{y}_i - y_i$, and k is the tuning constant for the Huber estimator. As shown in Fig. 2c, both the L_2 and Huber functions increase without bound as the residual r_i departs from zero. The Huber estimator approximates the L_2-norm for small residuals, but the key difference is observed at high residuals when it approximates a linear model. While the L_2-norm assigns equal weight to all residuals, the weights of the Huber estimator decline when $|r_i| > k$, thus reducing the emphasis on outliers during training. Furthermore, a small value of k increases the resistance to outliers, at the cost of performance when errors follow a normal distribution. For our experiments, we set $k = 1.45$ for CRN-2D, and $k = 1.7$ for CRN-3D.

3 Experiments

In our experiments, we explore two network architectures for the task of predicting brain maturation from 3D ultrasound images. We explore the effect of either treating the 3D input image ($\mathbf{I} \in \mathbb{R}^{n_x \times n_y \times n_z}$) as a multi-channel image, or preserving its 3D nature during feature extraction. Specifically, Fig. 2a shows that in network CRN-2D, the depth of the feature extraction kernels in the first layer extends to encompass the third dimension of the image, such that the kernel dimensions are $k \times k \times n_z$. In network CRN-3D, the CRN performs 3D convolutions throughout the image space, and the kernel dimensions are $k \times k \times k$, where $k \ll n_z$. Furthermore, we investigate the effect of the choice of loss function on output predictions. In particular, we compare the L_2-norm and Huber loss functions.

Dataset: The dataset of volumetric US images used in this work comprised of the same 447 volumes ($247 \times 190 \times 179$ voxels at a resolution of $0.6 \times 0.6 \times 0.6\,\text{mm}^3$) used in [7], the results of which constitute the baseline for automated image-based BM estimation. The sonographic images of the fetal head were obtained from the INTERGROWTH-21st study database [10], which were collected using a Philips HD9 curvilinear probe at a 2–5 MHz wave frequency. Images were selected from fetuses with known gestational age ranging from 18 to 36 gestational weeks, spanning the second and third trimesters of pregnancy: an active period of spatiotemporal changes visible on the cortical surface. 'True age' was defined by the last menstrual period (LMP) and confirmed by first-trimester (≤ 14 weeks) crown-rump length measurement agreeing within 7 days.

Experimental setup: The performance of each of the five proposed models was evaluated in five-fold cross-validation rounds. In each round, the volumes of 121 subjects were reserved for testing, while the remaining 489 images were used in training. As shown in Fig. 1a, the age distribution in each dataset was uniform across the gestational age range. To reduce the number of parameters optimized by the CRNs, the input volumes were resized to $128 \times 96 \times 64$ or $96 \times 64 \times 48$ voxels for networks A and B, respectively. Each CRN was re-trained on a dataset of 584 volumes, and tested on an independent set of 146 US volumes from subjects whose scans were collected as part of a multi-site, ethnically diverse study.

Implementation details: The proposed framework was implemented using the Keras framework with a Tensorflow backend, using a parallel computing architecture (CUDA, NVIDIA Corp). All testing was performed on an Intel Xeon E5-2630 CPU (2.4 GHz, 16 cores) with a NVIDIA Titan X GPU. Optimization was achieved using the RMSprop algorithm over a maximum of 100 epochs to ensure convergence [11]. The initial learning rate was set to 10^{-2}, which was decreased by a factor of ten every 20 epochs. Due to memory limitations, the CRN-2D and CRN-3D networks were trained with batches of size 32 and 10, respectively, in each epoch.

4   Results and Discussion

We validated and tested five different models for automated BM prediction from US images for the fetal brain. The results for BM prediction are summarised in Table 1, where the first row shows the result of using the RRF baseline model. The RRF model yielded an accuracy of 10.65 ± 12.65 days on the test set, which was outperformed by all CRN networks with the exception of CRN-2D trained with L_2 loss. While we observed that both 2D and 3D CRN models were able to automatically generate filters that extract and characterise patterns of brain development, notable performance gains were achieved with the 3D CRNs (< 8 days). This may be attributed to the fact that the 3D models preserve the appearance statistics and spatial distribution of structures in the dimension that is 'compressed' by the 2D models during feature extraction.

Comparing the performance of the loss function, we observed faster converge with Huber loss (i.e. 40 epochs versus 45 epochs with L_2 loss). In general, the models trained with Huber loss performed better and with reduced variance. However, the best-performing model was CRN-3D trained with L_2 loss. This may be due to the fact that our data contained few samples of subjects with brain abnormalities (i.e. outliers) and so the L_2-norm was able to model these data. Future work may explore whether the same is true when fetuses with cerebral abnormalities are included in the dataset. Figure 3 shows that when applied to the test dataset, the CRN-3D model had lower variance and fewer outliers than the RRF predictions.

It is important to note, however, that the BM predicted in this study is representative of the average level of structural development and brain appearance in fetal subjects of the same GA. Thus, it is expected that the biological variation

Table 1. Errors in predicting BM as a regression target using networks CRN-2D and CRN-3D. Mean absolute differences ($\pm$ standard deviation) between ground-truth GA and predicted BM score. Results shown for the five-fold cross-validation sets (each $N = 121$), and for the independent test set ($N = 120$). CRN-3D trained with an L_2 loss function (in bold) outperformed the others.

Network	Loss function	Training time (s/epoch)	Validation error (days)	Test error (days)	No. params
RRF (baseline)	L_2-norm	60 s/tree	11.62 ± 10.43	10.65 ± 12.65	0.36 M
CRN-2D	L_2-norm	13	12.33 ± 10.09	11.43 ± 9.35	7.60 M
	Huber		10.32 ± 8.48	10.15 ± 9.88	
CRN-3D	L_2-norm	105	$\mathbf{6.93 \pm 5.46}$	$\mathbf{7.72 \pm 6.01}$	6.13 M
	Huber		7.61 ± 6.15	7.81 ± 7.01	

within a given GA is captured within our dataset. GA was used as a proxy for the ground truth BM score in the knowledge that the INTERGROWTH-21st dataset comprises of optimally healthy fetuses, with confirmed absence of neurocognitive delays on post-birth follow-up. Furthermore, our 'true age' values were annotated with a confidence level of ± 7 days, so our potential accuracy is limited by this value. Therefore, our result of 7.72 ± 6.01 days is considered a successful prediction of brain maturation. Thus, our algorithm trained on healthy fetuses, is designed to identify fetuses at risk of maturational delays.

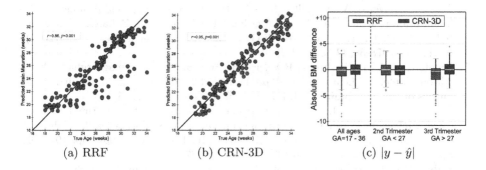

(a) RRF   (b) CRN-3D   (c) $|y - \hat{y}|$

Fig. 3. Chronological gestational age plotted against BM of the (a) RRF model and (b) the best-performing CRN-3D applied to the test dataset. (c) BM estimation results for the second and third trimesters of pregnancy, comparing the best performing CRN (red) and to the baseline RRF (blue) model. (Color figure online)

5   Conclusion

This paper presents and validates an automated method to predict brain maturation from 3D US scans of the fetal brain. Two proposed models were applied to an ethnically diverse fetal cohort, ranging from 18 to 34 weeks' gestation. We have demonstrated that without specifying a feature hypothesis or providing any information about fetal size, the CRN model is capable of identifying and characterizing neurodevelopment both spatially and temporally. The proposed CRN model is generalizable to different fetal cohorts, and capable of accurately estimating BM even in subjects where the state-of-art method fails.

References

1. Toi, A., Lister, W.S., Fong, K.W.: How early are fetal cerebral sulci visible at prenatal ultrasound and what is the normal pattern of early fetal sulcal development? Ultrasound Obstet. Gynecol. **24**(7), 706–715 (2004)
2. Monteagudo, A., Timor-Tritsch, I.E.: Normal sonographic development of the central nervous system from the second trimester onwards using 2D, 3D and transvaginal sonography. Prenat. Diagn. **29**(4), 326–339 (2009)
3. Vinkesteijn, A., Mulder, P., Wladimiroff, J.: Fetal transverse cerebellar diameter measurements in normal and reduced fetal growth. Ultrasound Obstet. Gynecol. **15**(1), 47–51 (2000)
4. Pistorius, L.R., Stoutenbeek, P., Groenendaal, F., de Vries, L., Manten, G., Mulder, E., Visser, G.: Grade and symmetry of normal fetal cortical development: a longitudinal two- and three-dimensional ultrasound study. Ultrasound Obstet. Gynecol. **36**(6), 700–708 (2010)
5. Franke, K., Luders, E., May, A., Wilke, M., Gaser, C.: Brain maturation: predicting individual BrainAGE in children and adolescents using structural MRI. NeuroImage **63**(3), 1305–1312 (2012)
6. Toews, M., Wells, W.M., Zöllei, L.: A feature-based developmental model of the infant brain in structural MRI. In: Ayache, N., Delingette, H., Golland, P., Mori, K. (eds.) MICCAI 2012. LNCS, vol. 7511, pp. 204–211. Springer, Heidelberg (2012). doi:10.1007/978-3-642-33418-4_26
7. Namburete, A.I.L., Stebbing, R.V., Kemp, B., Yaqub, M., Papageorghiou, A.T., Alison Noble, J.: Learning-based prediction of gestational age from ultrasound images of the fetal brain. Med. Image Anal. **21**(1), 72–86 (2015)
8. Štern, D., Payer, C., Lepetit, V., Urschler, M.: Automated age estimation from hand MRI volumes using deep learning. In: Ourselin, S., Joskowicz, L., Sabuncu, M.R., Unal, G., Wells, W. (eds.) MICCAI 2016. LNCS, vol. 9901, pp. 194–202. Springer, Cham (2016). doi:10.1007/978-3-319-46723-8_23
9. Huber, P.J.: Robust estimation of a location parameter. Ann. Math. Stat. **35**(1), 73–101 (1964)
10. Papageorghiou, A.T., Ohuma, E.O., Altman, D.G., Todros, T., Cheikh Ismail, L., Lambert, A., Jaffer, Y.A., Bertino, E., Gravett, M.G., Purwar, M., Noble, J.A., Pang, R., Victora, C.G., Barros, F.C., Carvalho, M., Salomon, L.J., Bhutta, Z.A., Kennedy, S.H., Villar, J.: International fetal and newborn growth consortium for the 21st century (INTERGROWTH-21st): international standards for fetal growth based on serial ultrasound measurements: the Fetal growth longitudinal study of the INTERGROWTH-21st project. Lancet **384**(9946), 869–79 (2014)
11. Tieleman, T., Hinton, G.: Lecture 6.5-RMSprop: divide the gradient by a running average of its recent magnitude. COURSERA Neural Networks Mach. Learn. **4**, 26–31 (2012)

4th International Workshop on Ophthalmic Medical Image Analysis, OMIA 2017

Segmentation of Retinal Blood Vessels Using Dictionary Learning Techniques

Taibou Birgui Sekou[1,3]([✉]), Moncef Hidane[1,3], Julien Olivier[1,3],
and Hubert Cardot[2,3]

[1] Institut National des Sciences Appliquées Centre Val de Loire, Blois, France
`taibou.birgui_sekou@insa-cvl.fr`
[2] Université de Tours, Tours, France
[3] LI EA 6300, Tours, France

Abstract. In this paper, we aim at proving the effectiveness of dictionary learning techniques on the task of retinal blood vessel segmentation. We present three different methods based on dictionary learning and sparse coding that reach state-of-the-art results. Our methods are tested on two, well-known, publicly available datasets: DRIVE and STARE. The methods are compared to many state-of-the-art approaches and turn out to be very promising.

Keywords: Retinal blood vessel segmentation · Medical image segmentation · Dictionary learning · Sparse coding · Linear classification · Random forests

1 Introduction

Retinal fundus images are now widely used for the diagnosis of various pathologies, including age-related macular degeneration, diabetic retinopathy and glaucoma. As a part of the central nervous system, the retina, and in particular its vasculature, is also used as a biomarker for early detection of neurodegenerative diseases.

Manual analysis of retinal images by ophthalmologists is a tedious task and, as for other manual delineation tasks, is subject to inter- and intra-operator variability. Thus, automatic and semi-automatic tools have been proposed, in particular, for retinal blood vessel segmentation (RBVS). While these tools are now starting to pervade clinical practice, the low image quality and the scale variation of the vessels still represent major challenges to most recent methods.

We examine in this paper a family of *supervised* RBVS methods based on *sparse representations* in *learned dictionaries*. These methods make use of the sparse representation of a patch around a pixel to determine its label. The differences between the proposed methods depend mainly on the number of learned dictionaries and the way the classifier is trained.

The general framework is composed of three stages: data preparation, segmentation, and post-processing. Data preparation consists in patches extraction

© Springer International Publishing AG 2017
M.J. Cardoso et al. (Eds.): FIFI/OMIA 2017, LNCS 10554, pp. 83–91, 2017.
DOI: 10.1007/978-3-319-67561-9_9

and normalization. Then, in the segmentation phase, a patch around each pixel is used by a dictionary learning method to assign its label. The output of the previous step leads to impulsive segmentation errors and we propose a robust regularization approach to tackle this problem. The remainder of this paper is outlined as follows. We review in Sect. 2 some recent state-of-the-art methods for RBVS. Section 3 reviews the supervised and unsupervised dictionary learning approaches and explains how both paradigms yield three different methods for RBVS. In Sect. 4, the experimental setup and the results are exposed. We conclude the paper in Sect. 5, pointing to possible directions for future work.

2 Related Work

RBVS has attracted a number of researchers for over two decades. Fraz et al. [1] presented a global review of the proposed methods in the field, up to 2012. They divided the methods into 6 classes: machine learning methods, matched filtering methods, morphological processing methods, vessel tracing/tracking methods, multi-scale methods, and model-based methods. It turns out that machine learning methods, especially the supervised ones, are in general the best. A more specific review focusing on computer-aided diagnosis for diabetic retinopathy is presented in [2].

In recent machine learning based approaches, a Lattice Neural Network with Dendritic Processing (LNNDP) framework is presented in [3]. Each pixel is classified using a $5-$dimensional feature vector extracted from an enhanced version of the green channel of the original RGB images. In [4], a discriminative dictionary learning technique is used. Image patches are extracted from an enhanced version of the green channel image to learn a specific dictionary per class. Two classes of patches are considered: patches containing a blood vessel and the others. Given a test image, overlapping patches are first extracted. The class of each patch is attributed according to the dictionary that best represents it. Then a segmentation map of each patch is obtained by thresholding the blood vessel patches and setting to zero the non-vessel ones.

The numerical results reported in [5,6] indicate that these works constitute the current state-of-the-art in RBVS. Wang et al. [5] proposed to follow two steps: a hierarchical feature extraction followed by an ensemble classification. The hierarchical features are obtained from different layers of a Convolutional Neural Network (CNN). Then Random Forest classifiers are trained on some levels of the CNN. The final class is obtained with a winner-take-all strategy. Liskowski et al. [6] used a CNN both as a feature extractor and a classifier.

3 RBVS Using Dictionary Learning

In what follows, we write patches as vectors. Let $\mathbf{X} = [\mathbf{x}_1, ..., \mathbf{x}_n] \in \mathbb{R}^{m \times n}$ be the input dataset consisting of n patches $\mathbf{x}_i \in \mathbb{R}^m$. In the supervised setting, one has also access to a vector of labels $\mathbf{y} \in \mathbb{R}^n$, with y_i denoting the label associated with the sample $\mathbf{x}_i$. This section first introduces a general view of dictionary learning, then, presents the methods proposed for RBVS.

3.1   Sparse Coding and Dictionary Learning

By choosing an overcomplete family $\{\mathbf{d}_k\}_{k=1}^{p}$ of vectors in $\mathbb{R}^m$ one can decompose an input patch $\mathbf{x} \in \mathbb{R}^m$ as a linear combination $\mathbf{x} = \sum_{k=1}^{p} a_k \mathbf{d}_k = \mathbf{Da}$, where $\mathbf{D} \in \mathbb{R}^{m \times p}$ is called a *dictionary*, and $\mathbf{a} \in \mathbb{R}^p$ is the vector of coefficients. Due to overcompleteness, the previous decomposition is not unique. In order to enforce sparsity, the following formulation has been widely adopted:

$$\mathbf{a}^* \leftarrow \min_{\mathbf{a} \in \mathbb{R}^p} \|\mathbf{x} - \mathbf{Da}\|_2^2 + \lambda \|\mathbf{a}\|_1, \tag{1}$$

where λ balances the trade-off between sparsity and reconstruction error, $\|.\|_q$ is the ℓ_q-norm[1]. The first term ensures a good reconstruction of the patch $\mathbf{x}$ from the dictionary, and the last term encourages the vector to be sparse. In general, increasing the value of λ yields sparser solutions.

The general idea of dictionary learning is to learn $\mathbf{D}$ from the dataset $\mathbf{X}$ by ensuring that each patch $\mathbf{x}_i$ is decomposed in a parsimonious manner (*see* [7] and references therein for more details). The formulation we retain for our present work is the following [8]

$$\mathbf{D}^*, \mathbf{A}^* \leftarrow \min_{\mathbf{D} \in \mathbb{R}^{m \times p}, \mathbf{A} \in \mathbb{R}^{p \times n}} \left[\mathcal{R}(\mathbf{X}, \mathbf{D}, \mathbf{A}) = \frac{1}{n} \sum_{i=1}^{n} \frac{1}{2} \|\mathbf{x}_i - \mathbf{Da}_i\|_2^2 + \lambda \|\mathbf{a}_i\|_1 \right], \tag{2}$$

where $\mathbf{A} = [\mathbf{a}_1, ..., \mathbf{a}_n]$ is the matrix of sparse coefficients. To resolve scale ambiguity, the columns of $\mathbf{D}$ are further constrained to be in the unit Euclidean ball. This constraint is applied to all subsequent dictionary learning variants.

3.2   RBVS by Sparse Coding Then Classifier (SCTC)

This method first learns a dictionary that best represents the entire training set (without class discrimination). Then, a random forest (RF) classifier is trained on the generated sparse codes. The method uses the dictionary learning phase as a high dimensional feature extractor. The training is done in the two following steps:

- Step 1: Solve a classical dictionary learning problem (Eq. (2)).
- Step 2: Train a random forest classifier of 50 trees using the matrix of sparse coefficients produced in Step 1 as input.

Given a patch query $\mathbf{z}$, its label l is computed by first solving a sparse coding problem using the learned dictionary. Then, the classifier is applied on the produced vector of coefficients to predict the label.

---

[1] The ℓ_q-norm ($q \geq 1$) of a vector $\mathbf{x}$ is: $\|\mathbf{x}\|_q = [\sum_i |x[i]|^q]^{1/q}$.

3.3   RBVS by Joint Dictionary and Classifier Learning (JDCL)

This method consists in learning jointly a dictionary and a linear classifier instead of separating them as done in SCTC. Introduced in [9], the method is formulated as follows

$$\mathbf{D}^*, \mathbf{A}^*, \mathbf{W}^* \leftarrow \min_{\mathbf{D}, \mathbf{A}, \mathbf{W}} \alpha \|\mathbf{L} - \mathbf{W}\mathbf{A}\|_F^2 + \beta \|\mathbf{W}\|_F^2 + \mathcal{R}(\mathbf{X}, \mathbf{D}, \mathbf{A}), \qquad (3)$$

where $\mathcal{R}$ is as defined in Eq. (2), $\mathbf{W} \in \mathbb{R}^{N \times p}$ contains the linear classifier's parameters, N is the number of classes, α and β are weight parameters, $\|.\|_F$ is the Frobenius norm[2], and $\mathbf{L} = [\mathbf{l}_1, ..., \mathbf{l}_n]$ is the label matrix where the vector $\mathbf{l}_i \in \mathbb{R}^N$ is 1 at the index corresponding to the class of the sample $\mathbf{x}_i$ and 0 elsewhere. Equation (3) can be solved efficiently using standard dictionary learning techniques (*see* [9] for more optimization details).

The label l of a query patch $\mathbf{z}$ is obtained using the following equation:

$$l = \arg\max_{i=1,...,N} [e_i = \mathbf{W}^* \mathbf{a}^*], \qquad (4)$$

where $\mathbf{W}^*$ is the previously learned classifier of Eq. (3) and $\mathbf{a}^*$ is obtained by applying Eq. (1) using the query patch $\mathbf{z}$ and the learned dictionary $\mathbf{D}^*$.

3.4   RBVS by One Dictionary per Class (DPC)

Let $\mathbf{X} = [\mathbf{X}_1, ..., \mathbf{X}_N]$ be the division of the dataset into sub-matrices, where each sub-matrix $\mathbf{X}_i \in \mathbb{R}^{m \times n_i}$ contains only the n_i samples that belong to the class i, and N is the number of classes ($N = 2$ in our setting).

In this method, we learn independently one dictionary on each sub-matrix. A query patch is classified by selecting the associated class of the dictionary that best reconstructs it, similarly to [10].

A dictionary $\mathbf{D}_i^*$ associated with the class i is learned using the corresponding sub-matrix by solving the problem in Eq. (2).

The label l of a query patch $\mathbf{z}$ is obtained by first computing the associated sparse coefficient $\mathbf{a}_i^*$ (using Eq. (1)) on each learned dictionary. Then, the following equation is used to predict the label:

$$l = \arg\min_{i=1,...,N} \left[e_i = \|\mathbf{z} - \mathbf{D}_i^* \mathbf{a}_i^*\|_2^2 + \lambda \|\mathbf{a}_i^*\|_1 \right]. \qquad (5)$$

3.5   Post-processing: Total Variation with ℓ_1 Fidelity Norm (TV$-\ell_1$)

The three proposed methods produce systematic errors in the form of *impulse noise*. This is a common issue encountered in most pixel classification methods. The image c in Fig. 1 shows a typical example, here obtained after applying the SCTC method. We formulate the post-processing as a denoising problem:

---

[2] The *Frobenius*-norm of a matrix $\mathbf{A} \in \mathbb{R}^{m \times n}$ is: $\|\mathbf{A}\|_F = \left[\sum_{i=1}^{m} \sum_{j=1}^{n} A[i,j]^2 \right]^{1/2}$.

we seek to recover a clean, *piecewise-constant* classification image from a noisy version. We adopt the TV-ℓ_1 model of [11] since it accounts both for our prior (piecewise constant solution) and for the likelihood (impulse noise). This leads to the following variational problem

$$I^* \leftarrow \min_I \|\nabla I\|_1 + \kappa \|I - I_0\|_1, \tag{6}$$

where I_0 is a noisy classification image. We note at this point that we do not impose any binary constraints in (6) but we simply threshold I^* after solving (6).

4   Experiments

The previously presented methods are tested on the following datasets:

- The DRIVE (Digital Retinal Images for Vessel Extraction) [12] dataset contains 40 expert annotated color retinal images taken with a fundus camera. It is divided into two sets of 20 images: the training and testing sets. Each image comes with a ground-truth segmentation (two for the test images and one for the training ones) and a mask image delineating the field of view (FOV). The first observer's ground-truth is considered in this paper.
- The STARE (STructured Analysis of the REtina) [13] is another well-known, publicly available database. The dataset is composed of 20 color fundus photographs. Half of the images presents pathological cases and contains abnormalities, which make the segmentation task even harder. Unlike the DRIVE dataset, the mask images are not provided. We construct them with a threshold on the grayscale images followed by a morphological filter with a structuring element of size 10 pixels.

4.1   Data Preparation

Given the contrast variation from one image to another, data preparation aims at normalizing the illumination beforehand. The grayscale versions of the original RGB images are considered throughout this experiment.

Pre-processing

- Image normalization and patch extraction: the first normalization consists in applying the Contrast Limited Adaptive Histogram Equalization (CLAHE) algorithm to the grayscale image. Then, all pixels outside the FOV are set to zero. For a given pixel, we extract the centered squared neighborhood patches of size 8×8. On both datasets, about 140 000 pixels are randomly selected to build our training set (*i.e.* around 70 000 patches per class). Patches with standard deviation less than 0.15 are not considered in the training set.
- Patch normalization: the squared neighborhood patches are then flattened into 64-dimensional vectors. Additional contrast normalization consists in normalizing each patch vector to have unit ℓ_2-norm.

Post-processings

After classifying each pixel of an image, we first multiply the resulting image with an eroded version of the mask image. This procedure aims at removing the pixels on the edges of the FOV. Then, we apply a TV-ℓ_1 regularization.

4.2   Experimental Setup and Measurements

The number of atoms p in the dictionary depends on the method: for SCTC $p = 1000$, for JDCL $p = 1000$, and finally $p = 500$ for DPC for each sub-dictionary. The online dictionary learning [14], available in the sparse modeling software[3] (SPAMS), is used in all our experiments as a dictionary learning algorithm. The primal-dual algorithm of Chambolle and Pock [15] is used for solving the TV-ℓ_1 problem (6). The parameters λ (Eq. (2)) and κ (Eq. (6)) are set, respectively, to 0.5 and 0.9. Note that, all these values are obtained using a grid-search and cross-validating on the training sets.

Let TP, TN, FN, and FP respectively denote the number of true positive, true negative, false negative, and false positive. We use the sensitivity

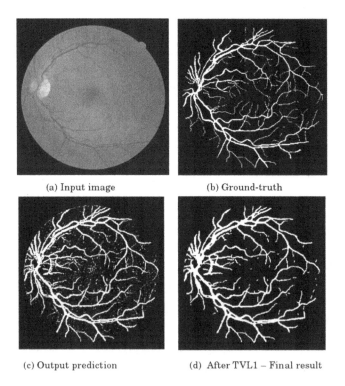

(a) Input image   (b) Ground-truth

(c) Output prediction   (d) After TVL1 – Final result

Fig. 1. Segmentation example using SCTC

---

[3] http://spams-devel.gforge.inria.fr/.

$\textbf{Sens} = \frac{TP}{TP+FN}$, the specificity $\textbf{Spec} = \frac{TN}{TN+FP}$ and the accuracy $\textbf{Acc} = \frac{TP+TN}{TP+FN+TN+FP}$ to quantify the performance of the RBVS methods.

4.3   Results and Discussions

Our results are depicted on Table 1 along with state-of-the-art results. Figure 1 illustrates a segmentation example.

Among the proposed methods, the SCTC approach seems to be the best only in terms of vessel detection (*i.e.* good sensitivity) while the DPC approach outputs good results with respect to all the performance measures.

The SCTC and JDCL methods tend to classify each patch with some line as vessel. This is due to the fact that these patches and the true vessel patches activate the same atoms, thus their sparse vectors are quite close. This problem is reduced when using the DPC model which uses the reconstruction error to classify a patch. Still, all the proposed methods reach the state-of-the-art results on the two datasets while being simple in terms of their architecture and number of parameters.

Other experiments, not reported in this paper, have been carried out with larger patches (*e.g.* 16×16). It turns out that the sensitivity can be improved but we are loosing on the specificity. This is due to the fact that, when using larger patches, more pixels near a blood vessel (but not belonging to it) tend to be classified as vessels.

Table 1. Our results on DRIVE and STARE versus the state-of-the-art.

Methods	Drive			Stare		
	Spec	Sens	Acc	Spec	Sens	Acc
This paper - SCTC	95.55	83.49	94.48	94.46	85.11	93.81
This paper - JDCL	96.32	80.60	94.93	95.78	77.24	94.45
This paper - DPC	97.05	77.88	95.36	96.75	75.58	95.23
Javidi et al. [4]	97.02	72.01	94.50	96.53	77.80	95.17
Singh et al. [16]	–	75.94	95.22	–	79.39	92.70
Orlando et al. [17]	96.84	78.97	–	97.38	76.80	–
Vega et al. [3]	96.00	74.44	94.12	96.71	70.19	94.83
Liskowski et al. [6]*	96.73	84.60	95.07	97.10	92.89	96.67
Wang et al. [5]*	97.33	81.73	97.67	97.91	81.04	98.13
Dasgupta et al. [18]*	98.01	76.91	95.33	–	–	–

* deep learning methods

5   Summary and Perspectives

In this paper, we presented three RBVS methods based on sparse representations in learned dictionaries. We showed that these methods can reach state-of-the-art results on the DRIVE and STARE datasets while remaining conceptually simple and computationally tractable. Future work will concentrate on taking patch correlations into account when learning the dictionary and on using more discriminative features.

References

1. Fraz, M., Remagnino, P., Hoppe, A., Uyyanonvara, B., Rudnicka, A., Owen, C., Barman, S.: Blood vessel segmentation methodologies in retinal images - a survey. Comput. Methods Programs Biomed. **108**(1), 407–433 (2012)
2. Mookiah, M.R.K., Acharya, U.R., Chua, C.K., Lim, C.M., Ng, E.Y.K., Laude, A.: Computer-aided diagnosis of diabetic retinopathy: a review. Comp. Bio. and Med. **43**(12), 2136–2155 (2013)
3. Vega, R., Sánchez-Ante, G., Falcón-Morales, L., Sossa, H., Guevara, E.: Retinal vessel extraction using lattice neural networks with dendritic processing. Comp. Bio. and Med. **58**, 20–30 (2015)
4. Javidi, M., Pourreza, H.R., Harati, A.: Vessel segmentation and microaneurysm detection using discriminative dictionary learning and sparse representation. Comput. Methods Programs Biomed. **139**, 93–108 (2017)
5. Wang, S., Yin, Y., Cao, G., Wei, B., Zheng, Y., Yang, G.: Hierarchical retinal blood vessel segmentation based on feature and ensemble learning. Neurocomputing **149**, 708–717 (2015)
6. Liskowski, P., Krawiec, K.: Segmenting retinal blood vessels with deep neural networks. IEEE Trans. Med. Imaging **35**(11), 2369–2380 (2016)
7. Mairal, J., Bach, F., Ponce, J.: Sparse modeling for image and vision processing. Found. Trends Comput. Graph. Vision **8**(2–3), 85–283 (2014)
8. Elad, M.: Sparse and Redundant Representation. Springer, New York, Dordrecht, Heidelberg, London (2010)
9. Zhang, Q., Li, B.: Discriminative K-SVD for dictionary learning in face recognition. In: IEEE Conference on Computer Vision and Pattern Recognition (CVPR), pp. 2691–2698 (2010)
10. Yang, A.Y., Wright, J., Ma, Y., Sastry, S.S.: Feature selection in face recognition: a sparse representation perspective. Technical Report UCB/EECS-2007-99, EECS Department, University of California, Berkeley (2007)
11. Nikolova, M.: A variational approach to remove outliers and impulse noise. J. Mathe. Imaging Vision **20**(1–2), 99–120 (2004)
12. Staal, J., Abrmoff, M.D., Niemeijer, M., Viergever, M.A., Ginneken, B.V.: Ridge-based vessel segmentation in color images of the retina. IEEE Trans. Med. Imaging **23**, 501–509 (2004)
13. Hoover, A., Kouznetsova, V., Goldbaum, M.: Locating blood vessels in retinal images by piecewise threshold probing of a matched filter response. IEEE Trans. Med. Imaging **19**, 203–210 (2000)
14. Mairal, J., Bach, F., Ponce, J., Sapiro, G.: Online learning for matrix factorization and sparse coding. J. Mach. Learn. Res. **11**, 19–60 (2010)
15. Chambolle, A., Pock, T.: A first-order primal-dual algorithm for convex problems with applications to imaging. J. Mathe. Imaging Vision **40**(1), 120–145 (2011)
16. Singh, N.P., Srivastava, R.: Retinal blood vessels segmentation by using Gumbel probability distribution function based matched filter. Comput. Methods Programs Biomed. **129**, 40–50 (2016)

17. Orlando, J.I., Prokofyeva, E., Blaschko, M.B.: A discriminatively trained fully connected conditional random field model for blood vessel segmentation in fundus images. IEEE Trans. Biomed. Eng. **64**(1), 16–27 (2017)

18. Dasgupta, A., Singh, S.: A fully convolutional neural network based structured prediction approach towards the retinal vessel segmentation. In: IEEE International Symposium on Biomedical Imaging (ISBI), pp. 248–251 (2017)

Detecting Early Choroidal Changes Using Piecewise Rigid Image Registration and Eye-Shape Adherent Regularization

Tiziano Ronchetti[1,3]([✉]), Peter Maloca[2], Christoph Jud[1], Christoph Meier[3], Selim Orgül[2], Hendrik P.N. Scholl[2], Boris Považay[3], and Philippe C. Cattin[1]

[1] Departments of Biomedical Engineering, University of Basel, Basel, Switzerland
Tiziano.Ronchetti@unibas.ch
[2] Ophthalmology, University of Basel, Basel, Switzerland
[3] HuCE-optoLab, Bern University of Applied Sciences, Bern, Switzerland

Abstract. Recognizing significant temporal changes in the thickness of the choroid and retina at an early stage is a crucial factor in the prevention and treatment of ocular diseases such as myopia or glaucoma. Such changes are expected to be among the first indicators of pathological manifestations and are commonly dealt using segmentation-based approaches. However, segmenting the choroid is challenging due to low contrast, loss of signal and presence of artifacts in optical coherence tomography (OCT) images. In this paper, we present a novel method for early detection of choroidal changes based on piecewise rigid image registration. In order to adhere to the eye's natural shape, the regularization enforces the local homogeneity of the transformations in nasal-temporal (x-) and superior-inferior (y-) direction by penalizing their radial differences. We restrict our transformation model to anterior-posterior (z-) direction, as we focus on juvenile myopia, which correlates to thickness changes in the choroid rather than to structural alterations. First, the precision of the method was tested on an OCT scan-rescan data set of 62 healthy Asian children, ages 7 to 13, from a population with a high prevalence of myopia. Furthermore, the accuracy of the method in recognizing synthetically induced changes in the data set was evaluated. Finally, the results were compared to those of manually annotated scans.

Keywords: Early choroidal changes · Piecewise rigid registration

1 Introduction

The choroid is a vascular tissue located between the rather rigid sclera and retina at the posterior pole of the eye. It provides oxygen and metabolites to the retinal structures [7]. The choroid shows a thickness between 50 and 300 μm with diurnal variations up to 29 μm. Several studies [2,6,7] argue that longitudinal changes of the choroidal thickness are related to the growth of the sclera and, therefore, to the elongation of the eye bulb. Monitoring choroidal thickness delivers insight into the pathogenesis and helps in the planning of treatment of various

© Springer International Publishing AG 2017
M.J. Cardoso et al. (Eds.): FIFI/OMIA 2017, LNCS 10554, pp. 92–100, 2017.
DOI: 10.1007/978-3-319-67561-9_10

ocular diseases such as myopia, glaucoma, diabetic retinopathy, choroidal tumors and macular degeneration [2]. The choroidal thickness is defined as the distance between the Choriocapillaris-Bruch's membrane-Retinal pigment epithelium complex (CBR) and the Choroid-Sclera Interface (CSI, see Fig. 1b). The common approach consists of localizing both CBR and CSI, using image segmentation [5,9]. To extract clinically relevant information, the distance CBR-CSI is visualized in a choroidal thickness map (see Fig. 1a). Due to the hyperreflectivity of the CBR in OCT imaging, its segmentation is relatively simple (e.g. using automatic graph-based segmentation methods [3]). In opposition, the CSI is difficult to segment because of the significantly lower image contrast, an increase of shadowing artifacts as well as unpredictable shape variations in the weakly scattering choroid [2]. The use of single frame segmentation as in [3,5,9] is difficult in longitudinal clinical studies where successive imaging sessions can strongly vary in signal quality.

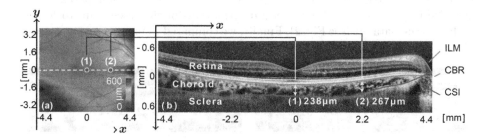

Fig. 1. (a) Choroidal (CBR-CSI) thickness map overlaid color-coded on fundus image. (b) OCT B-scan with segmented layers representing the section indicated by the white dotted line in (a). ILM is the Inner Limiting Membrane.

Due to the interleaved nature of the eye consisting of the soft choroid and surrounding more rigid tissues, the sclera and CBR, a piecewise rigid strategy [1] was used in recent developments to accurately model the deformation of the choroid. This approach allows to decompose the global non-rigid matching problem of the choroid into numerous local rigid registrations of the individual subregions. The results are embodied into a dense global non-rigid deformation field built such that it elastically deforms the soft choroid and preserves the rigid characteristics of the surrounding sclera and CBR.

In [8], the choroidal thickness changes were detected using atlas-based registration which could tackle the problem of low SNR. However, several challenges remain: (1) The method processes only scan-wise. (2) The regularization serves only as post-processing step and does not take the pixel spacing into account. (3) Due to the use of non-overlapping patches in the matching process the results become instable with increasing resolution.

In the proposed method, "Detecting early **C**horoidal changes using piecewise rigid image **R**egistration and eye-shape **A**dherent **R**egularization", as of now CRAR, we subdivide the volume around the CSI in partially overlapping cuboidal subregions, utilizing the rigid CBR as a reference surface. Using a multiresolution approach, a 3D regularized block-matching registration of the CSI is conducted. As the images are aligned to the rigid CBR, the displacement corresponds to shifts of the CSI. Thus, it is possible to determine the displacement field around the CSI and to use its outcome to quantify choroidal growth.

This paper's contribution is threefold: (1) By grouping two or more rectangular subregions around the CSI into cuboidal blocks, the matching is done fully in 3D (see Fig. 3). (2) We simultaneously regularized along the x- and y-axis taking different pixel spacing into account. This enforces uniform smoothness of the results matching the anatomic structure of the eye. (3) The regularization penalizes the radial differences of the transformations and favors similar displacements of patches within the same neighborhood (see Fig. 4). Mismatches are corrected during the gradient descent optimization.

In the pre-clinical experiment, we first analyzed the precision with scan-rescan data. Furthermore, we showed superior change-detection performance over the CSI using smooth synthetic deformations of the rescans up to $50\,\mu m$ built into the data set (see Fig. 2). Finally, we compared to manual segmentation.

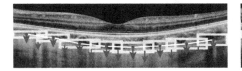 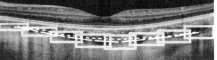

Fig. 2. Simulation of choroidal growth. Left: The white continuous line serves as reference for the deformation. Right: After blockwise transformation the reference line is shifted from the previous (white dotted line).

2   Material and Method

The eyes of 62 volunteers, aged 7 to 13, from Asian urban regions with a high prevalence of myopia were measured twice as scan-rescans within a few minutes, resulting in 124 OCT volume stacks. For half of them the left eye was measured, for the other the right one. For 36 of them a dual wavelength SD-OCT system prototype was used, which operated simultaneously at $800\,nm$ and $1075\,nm$ and was developed at the Bern University of Applied Sciences (see [8]). Each volume stack consisted of 25 slices of 768×496 pixels. The pixel spacing in nasal-temporal/x- and superior-inferior/y-direction were set to $11.47\,\mu m/pixel$ and to $245\,\mu m/pixel$, the one in anterior-posterior/z-direction was set to $3.87\,\mu m/pixel$. To examine the other 26 a Topcon SS-OCT system (DRI OCT Triton) was used, in which each volume stack consisted of 256 slices of 512×992 pixels. The pixel spacing in x-, y- and z-direction were set to 11.72, 23.44 and to $2.60\,\mu m/pixel$.

The preprocessing steps are the same as in [8]: the slices from the reference and template stack images are rigidly registered pair-wise at the CBR. Next,

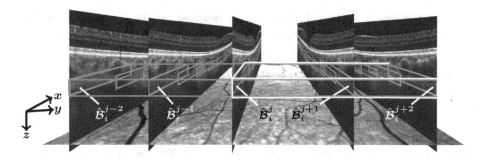

Fig. 3. The construction of the 3D cuboidal block $\mathcal{C}_i^s$ (green) by grouping five rectangular blocks $\hat{\mathcal{B}}_i^{j-2}$, $\hat{\mathcal{B}}_i^{j-1}$, $\hat{\mathcal{B}}_i^{j}$, $\hat{\mathcal{B}}_i^{j+1}$ and $\hat{\mathcal{B}}_i^{j+2}$ that have been normalized in height. The next block $\mathcal{C}_i^{s+1}$ (white) is created analogously.

using the algorithm presented in [3] based on graph search, the CBR is accurately segmented and becomes the shape-reference for the CSI.

Construction of the 3D Blocks: Let $\Omega_j \subset \mathbb{R}^2$ be the jth slice of size $m \times n$ pixels in a volume stack $\Omega = \bigcup_{j=1}^{S} \Omega_j \subset \mathbb{R}^3$ of S slices. In each slice Ω_j the area around the CSI is divided into N partially overlapping rectangular blocks $\mathcal{B}_i^j$. Each block has a variable height $h_i = (k_a + k_u) \cdot d_i$ and a center point x_i, where $i = 1, \ldots, N$. Here, d_i is the distance between the CBR and the roughly determined CSI at each location x_i, while k_a and k_u remain constant. The part of the block above the CSI is denoted by $k_a \cdot d_i$ and the part below by $k_u \cdot d_i$.

Since a high spatial resolution is needed to recognize small details, enough inner blocks are needed for a meaningful detection (the first and the last block are to be treated separately). Thus, the block matching is initialized with $N = 8$ blocks with a width $\omega = \frac{m}{7(1-\phi)+1}$, where ϕ is the lateral overlap (in percent) between two neighboring blocks at the resolution level $k = 1$. Using a multiresolution approach, the number N of blocks is doubled with increasing k (i.e. $N = 8 \cdot 2^{k-1} = 2^{k+2}$, $k \in \mathbb{N}$). To optimize the overlaps the values of $\phi, \beta \in \,]0, 1[$ are selected such that, at the level k, the block width $\omega_k = \omega \cdot \beta^{k-1}$ exponentially decreases, while the percentage overlap $\phi_k = 1 - (\frac{m}{\omega_k} - 1)/(2^{k+2} - 1)$ increases.

At each ith position on the x-axis, partially overlapping 3D cuboidal blocks $\{\mathcal{C}_i^s\}$ are formed in the y-direction by normalizing the height of the rectangular blocks of two or more successive slices, and then by grouping them as follows:

$$\mathcal{C}_i^1 = \bigcup_{j=1}^{G+1} \hat{\mathcal{B}}_i^j, \quad \mathcal{C}_i^s = \bigcup_{j=1+(s-2)G}^{1+sG} \hat{\mathcal{B}}_i^j \;\; (s = 2, \ldots, \bar{S} - 1), \quad \mathcal{C}_i^{\bar{S}} = \bigcup_{j=S-G}^{S} \hat{\mathcal{B}}_i^j,$$

where $\{\hat{\mathcal{B}}_i^j\}$ are the normalized blocks and $G+1$ indicates the number of slices of two successives cuboids C_i^s and C_i^{s+1} that overlap. For example, let $G = 2$ and $S = 25$ be given, then, at each position i on the x-axis $\bar{S} = 13$ cuboidal blocks are built: C_i^1 and C_i^{13} consist of 3 slices while $C_i^2 \ldots, C_i^{12}$ of 5 slices (see Fig. 3). Between the slices, cubic interpolation is used. As a result, $\bar{S} = \lceil \frac{S}{G} \rceil$ cuboidal blocks in the depth of the volume stack are obtained at the ith position on the x-axis. For each cuboid $\mathcal{C}_i^s$, the upper coordinate is defined as the minimum, the lower one as the maximum of all z values of the not yet normalized blocks $\mathcal{B}_i^j$.

3D Piecewise Registration: A reference I_R and a template image $I_T : \Omega \to \mathbb{R}$ mapping Ω to the corresponding intensities are given. Since this study focuses on quantitative choroidal thickness changes, only shifts in axial/z-direction are considered. The aim is to find a set $\mathcal{U} = \{u_i^s\}$ of blockwise constant transformations in z-direction $u_i^s : \mathcal{C}_i^s \to \mathbb{R}^3$ such that $I_T(p + u_i^s(p)) \approx I_R(p)$ for all $p \in \mathcal{C}_i^s$. Thus, the displacement vectors are $u_i^s(p) = u_i^s(p_i^s) \in \mathbb{R}^3$, for all $p \in \mathcal{C}_i^s$, in which $u_i^s(p_i^s)$ is the center displacement of the block $\mathcal{C}_i^s$. We consider image registration as a regularized minimization problem for the energy functional $\mathcal{J}$,

$$\arg\min_{\mathcal{U}} \mathcal{J}[\mathcal{U}], \quad \mathcal{J}[\mathcal{U}] := \mathcal{D}[I_R, I_T, \mathcal{U}] + \lambda \mathcal{R}[\mathcal{U}]. \tag{1}$$

$\mathcal{D}$ is a distance measure that quantifies the similarity between reference I_R and the transformed template image $I_T(p + u_i^s(p))$. The regularizer $\mathcal{R}$, with its corresponding trade-off parameter $\lambda > 0$, ensures certain properties of the transformation, which will be explained next. In order to indicate how well the transformed template image $I_T(p + u_i^s(p))$ matches the reference I_R, the similarity measure

$$\mathcal{D}[I_R, I_T, \mathcal{U}] := \sum_{s=1}^{\bar{S}} \sum_{i=1}^{N} \int_{p \in \mathcal{C}_i^s} ||I_T(p + u_i^s(p)) - I_R(p)||^2 \, dp$$

is defined, where p is the point position in block $\mathcal{C}_i^s \subset \Omega$. Using piecewise intensity-based locally rigid registration, an attempt is made to obtain the maximum correlation. This is done by matching blocks around the approximated CSI of the pre-registered image with the ones in the corresponding, slightly bigger search area $\hat{\mathcal{C}}_i^s \supset \mathcal{C}_i^s$ of the reference image.

Radial Differences Regularization: The regularizer $\mathcal{R}$ of Eq. (1) is defined by the fact that even in longitudinal studies of progressing diseases the shape of the CSI stays comparable to that of the CBR in small curvature and smoothness. Inspired by that, the regularization is defined as follows: (1) Neighboring displacements should be locally homogeneous. In other words, block centers within the same neighborhood should show a similar displacement. (2) To limit the influence of the displacement of a block to its own neighborhood, $\mathcal{R}$ ensures that the shifts of blocks further away converge to zero (see Fig. 4).

We therefore opted for a regularization based on radial differences [4] with a compactly supported radial kernel. Let $\mathcal{N} = N \cdot \bar{S}$ be the total number of cuboids, $p_i^s = (x_i^s, y_i^s, z_i^s)$ and $p_j^t = (x_j^t, y_j^t, z_j^t)$ the centers of the blocks $\mathcal{C}_i^s$ and $\mathcal{C}_j^t$ respectively. Then, the regularizer $\mathcal{R}$ is defined as follows:

$$\mathcal{R}[\mathcal{U}] = \frac{1}{\mathcal{N}} \sum_{s,t=1}^{\bar{S}} \sum_{i,j=1}^{N} ||u_i^s(p_i^s) - u_j^t(p_j^t)||^2 \, K(p_i^s, p_j^t), \tag{2}$$

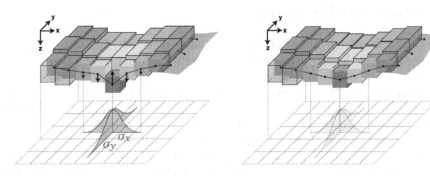

(a) The result after 3D block-matching   (b) The result after regularization

Fig. 4. (a) The position of the mismatched block (red) in the 3D registration is corrected by regularization. This has a smoothing effect, because the directly neighboring blocks (yellow) counteract this movement. Distant blocks (light green) have weaker influence. The blocks are drawn without overlap for better visualization. Both 1D B-spline kernels with their supports $2\sigma_x$ and $2\sigma_y$ are visualized underneath. (Color figure online)

where $u_i^s(p_i^s)$ and $u_j^t(p_j^t)$ are the corresponding displacement vectors of p_i^s and p_j^t as obtained from the 3D block-matching. Due to its smoothing properties and compact support, the radial cubic B-spline function $K : \Omega \times \Omega \to \mathbb{R}$ has been chosen as kernel. As the B-splines can be separated in single dimensions, the kernel K can be split into a product of two 1D cubic B-spline kernels

$$K(p_i^s, p_j^t) = \beta_3 \left(||x_i^s - x_j^t||/\sigma_x \right) \cdot \beta_3 \left(||y_i^s - y_j^t||/\sigma_y \right)$$

where σ_x, σ_y are the ratio of pixel spacing in x- and y-direction (Fig. 4a), and

$$\beta_3(r) = \begin{cases} 2/3 - ||r||^2 + ||r||^3/2 & \text{if} \quad 0 \le ||r|| < \sigma \\ (2 - ||r||)^3/6 & \text{if} \quad \sigma \le ||r|| < 2\sigma \\ 0 & \text{if} \quad 2\sigma \le ||r|| \end{cases}, \text{ where } r = \frac{||x_i^s - x_j^t||}{\sigma},$$

is the 1D radial cubic B-spline kernel in the corresponding axis and $\sigma \in \{\sigma_x, \sigma_y\}$. Here, 2σ describes the support in [mm] of the B-spline kernel in the x- and y-direction, respectively. The factor $||u_i^s(p_i^s) - u_j^t(p_j^t)||^2$ of Eq. (2) guarantees a local homogeneity of the transformations while the B-spline kernel takes care of a $(2\sigma_x \times 2\sigma_y)$-neighborhood. In other words, it makes sure that in case of two blocks being wide apart, displacements influence each other much less than if they are within the same neighborhood. The mismatched blocks of the registration process are not individually corrected. Instead, the entire neighborhood is moved until the block configuration with the least bending energy is reached (Fig. 4b).

3 Results and Discussion

The average displacements of all $\mathcal{N}$ blocks were detected using the proposed CRAR, a state-of-the-art method (ICR [8]) and the manual segmentation, each grouped by resolution level k. First, the methods were applied to the scan-rescan data set and then to the synthetically deformed data. In Fig. 5a the average displacements of the blocks from volume scan (reference) to its rescan (template) are shown. The average differences between the synthetically induced displacements (ground truth) and the measured ones are depicted in Fig. 5b.

CRAR shows, especially at higher resolution levels, a superior performance in comparison to ICR (see Fig. 5a). This is due to the fact that CRAR allows for the overlap of 3D blocks in both lateral, the x- as well as the y-direction, whereas in ICR only non-overlapping 2D rectangular patches are applied. With ICR a considerable deterioration of the scan-rescan results from level $k = 5$ occurs (see the trend in Fig. 5a), but with CRAR they remain precise.

This study aims at a precision in the detection of minute changes allowing clinical application: here it is set at $5\,\mu$m, i.e. in the range of the pixel scaling in z-direction. Hence, the ideal resolution level k for CRAR is found at $k = 7$, corresponding to the detected average displacements $|\Delta z| < 2\,\mu$m, which is a clear improvement to ICR ($k = 4, |\Delta z| > 4\,\mu$m) and manual segmentation ($k = 1, |\Delta z| > 7\,\mu$m). This is confirmed by applying CRAR to the synthetic deformations (see Fig. 5b): CRAR remains precise with only a slightly greater variance compared to the scan-rescans. Both graphs of Fig. 5 display an important, continuous deterioration of the results using manual segmentation with increasing k. To penalize lower resolutions in the evaluation, the displacements at each lower level are calculated by translating the corresponding blocks in the highest resolution level $k = 7$. Thus, at the sth position, the displacement of the first block $\mathcal{C}_1^s$ for $k = 1$ is the average of all the displacements of the centers $p_1^s, \ldots, p_{64}^s$ at $k = 7$. For the displacement of the second block $\mathcal{C}_2^s$ at $k = 1$, the average of the displacements of $p_{65}^s, \ldots, p_{128}^s$ at $k = 7$ is taken. The constants k_a and k_u are chosen in the range of $]0, \frac{2}{3}]$ and $]0, \frac{1}{3}]$. The higher blocks include rigid

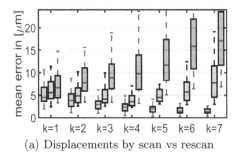

(a) Displacements by scan vs rescan

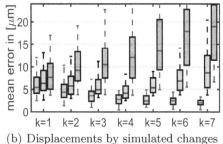

(b) Displacements by simulated changes

Fig. 5. Average displacements of the CSI obtained with CRAR (red), ICR (green), and manual expert segmentation (blue), applied on 62 OCT data set pairs (a) as scan-rescan and (b) after synthetic deformation for different k. (Color figure online)

tissue, thus detectability might be reduced and subtle changes could be missed. The ideal trade-off to define the blocks was found at $\phi = 0.3$ and $\beta = 0.55$. After analyzing the feature density of manually segmented interfaces, the minimal needed block width for the recognition of subtle thickness changes in the choroid was set at 5 pixels. Thus, only $k \leq 7$ is examined.

4   Conclusion

The advantages of our method are manifold: (1) The precision in the detection of choroidal thickness changes is achieved in the range of the pixel scaling in z-direction. Even for finer block sizes, such as $k = 5$, changes smaller than $5\,\mu m$ can be reliably recognized. By grouping the slices, the amount of information per patch increases, thereby reducing mismatches. (2) The regularization enforces uniform smoothness of the results matching the anatomic structure of the eye. (3) The simulated deformation proved that our method is able to detect long-term changes. (4) As the percentage overlap ϕ_k increases with k, the amount of information in the patches is still large, even at high resolution.

Our method, CRAR, enables unsupervised automated detection of choroidal and scleral changes and can be applied to large data sets to extract minute differences. It provides a sensitive objective progress indicator for several diseases and their respective treatments. The clinical results and interpretations of the ongoing longitudinal study of myopia development, utilizing CRAR, will be presented in an upcoming medical publication.

References

1. Čech, P., Andronache, A., Wang, L., Székely, G., Cattin, P.: Piecewise rigid multimodal spine registration. In: Handels, H., Ehrhardt, J., Horsch, A., Meinzer, H.P., Tolxdorff, T. (eds.) Bildverarbeitung für die Medizin 2006 Informatik aktuell. Springer, Heidelberg (2006). doi:10.1007/3-540-32137-3_43
2. Chhablani, J., Wong, I.Y., Kozak, I.: Choroidal imaging: a review. Saudi J. Ophthalmol. 28(2), 123–128 (2014)
3. Chiu, S.J., Li, X.T., Nicholas, P., Toth, C.A., Izatt, J.A., Farsiu, S.: Automatic segmentation of seven retinal layers in SDOCT images congruent with expert manual segmentation. Opt. Express 18(18), 19413–19428 (2010)
4. Jud, C., Möri, N., Bitterli, B., Cattin, P.C.: Bilateral regularization in reproducing kernel hilbert spaces for discontinuity preserving image registration. In: Wang, L., Adeli, E., Wang, Q., Shi, Y., Suk, H.-I. (eds.) MLMI 2016. LNCS, vol. 10019, pp. 10–17. Springer, Cham (2016). doi:10.1007/978-3-319-47157-0_2
5. Kajić, V., Esmaeelpour, M., Považay, B., Marshall, D., Rosin, P.L., Drexler, W.: Automated choroidal segmentation of 1060 nm OCT in healthy and pathologic eyes using a statistical model. Biomed. Opt. Express 3(1), 86–103 (2012)
6. Mutti, D.O., Gwiazda, J., Norton, T.T., Smith, E.L., Schaeffel, F., To, C.H.: Myopia yesterday, today, and tomorrow. Optom. Vis. Sci. 90(11), 1161–1164 (2013). Official publication of the American Academy of Optometry
7. Nickla, D.L., Wallman, J.: The multifunctional choroid. Prog. Retinal Eye Res. 29(2), 144–168 (2010)

8. Ronchetti, T., Maloca, P., Meier, C., Orgül, S., Jud, C., Hasler, P., Považay, B., Cattin, P.C.: Intensity-based choroidal registration using regularized block matching. In: Proceedings of the Ophthalmic Medical Image Analysis Third International Workshop (OMIA), pp. 33–40 (2016)
9. Tian, J., Marziliano, P., Baskaran, M., Tun, T.A., Aung, T.: Automatic segmentation of the choroid in enhanced depth imaging optical coherence tomography images. Biomed. Opt. Express **4**(3), 397–411 (2013)

Patch-Based Deep Convolutional Neural Network for Corneal Ulcer Area Segmentation

Qichao Sun[1(✉)], Lijie Deng[1,2], Jianwei Liu[1], Haixiang Huang[3], Jin Yuan[3], and Xiaoying Tang[1,2,4(✉)]

[1] Sun Yat-sen University Carnegie Mellon University (SYSU-CMU) Joint Institute of Engineering, Sun Yat-sen University, Guangzhou, Guangdong, China
tangxiaoy@mail.sysu.edu.cn
[2] Sun Yat-sen University Carnegie Mellon University (SYSU-CMU) SHUNDE International Joint Research Institute, Shunde, Guangdong, China
[3] State Key Laboratory of Ophthalmology, Zhongshan Ophthalmic Centre, Sun Yat-sen University, Guangzhou, Guangdong, China
[4] School of Electronics and Information Technology, Sun Yat-sen University, Guangzhou, Guangdong, China

Abstract. We present a novel approach to automatically identify the corneal ulcer areas using fluorescein staining images. The proposed method is based on a deep convolutional neural network that labels each pixel in the corneal image as either ulcer area or non-ulcer area, which is essentially a two-class classification problem. Patch-based approach was employed; for every image pixel, a surrounding patch of size 19×19 was used to extract the RGB intensities to be used as features for training and testing. For the architecture of our deep network, there were four convolutional layers followed by three fully connected layers with dropout. The final classification was inferred from the probabilistic output from the network. The proposed approach has been validated on a total of 48 images using 5-fold cross-validation, with high segmentation accuracy established; the proposed method was found to be superior to both a baseline method (active contour) and another representative network method (VGG net). Our automated segmentation method had a mean Dice overlap of 0.86 when compared to the manually delineated gold standard as well as a strong and significant manual-vs-automatic correlation in terms of the ulcer area size (correlation coefficient = 0.9934, p-value = 6.3e-45). To the best of our knowledge, this is one of the first few works that have accurately tackled the corneal ulcer area segmentation challenge using deep neural network techniques.

Keywords: Corneal ulcer · Deep learning · Convolutional neural network · Patch

1 Introduction

A corneal ulcer is an eye symptom that typically causes pain, red eye, mild or severe eye discharge, and reduced vision. There are a variety of reasons that might induce a corneal ulcer, including infection, physical and chemical trauma, corneal drying and

© Springer International Publishing AG 2017
M.J. Cardoso et al. (Eds.): FIFI/OMIA 2017, LNCS 10554, pp. 101–108, 2017.
DOI: 10.1007/978-3-319-67561-9_11

exposure, as well as over-wearing and misuse of contact lens. The corneal ulcers have been significantly affecting the eye health of human being.

Fluorescein staining is an important diagnostic tool for the detection of ocular surface diseases. The corneal staining pattern provides important information for characterizing corneal diseases, assessing severity, and monitoring clinical response to therapy [1]. Fluorescein staining has been effectively applied to characterizing the corneal ulcer abnormalities [2–4].

Relying on a fluorescein staining image, the severity of a corneal ulcer may be subjectively judged using two strategies. One is based on the chromaticity of the bright green color emitted from sodium fluorescein and the other is based on morphological characteristics such as the ulcer area size and the number of staining points. To objectively quantify the ulcer severity using the aforementioned strategies, an important prerequisite is to automatically segment the ulcer area. Usually, professional software packages such as the Photoshop (PS) are used to manually extract the corneal ulcer area, which is however time-consuming, labor-intensive, and subjective.

Regarding automated segmentation of the ulcer area, there have been methods relying on digital image analysis techniques. For example, some approaches applied a color extraction algorithm using RGB systems and edge detection algorithm [5, 6], whereas some others utilized thresholding techniques to detect conjunctival hyperemia and corneal staining collaterally [7]. However, these methods were mainly designed for fluorescein staining images with the ulcer pattern being a number of separate staining points but not for images with the ulcer pattern being flaky (a connected area of corneal ulcer).

Recently, deep neural network (DNN) has gained a substantial popularity due to its superior performance in many applications, especially in image-related fields (for a recent review please see LeCun et al. [8]). For example, Srivastava et al. [9] adopted a deep learning method for optic disc segmentation. An Inception-v3 architecture was employed for the detection of diabetic retinopathy in retinal fundus photographs [10]. DNN has also been successfully applied to image segmentation problems using patch-based methods [11–13]. To be specific, instead of predicting a segmentation label with features obtained from the entire image, this method uses features from small regions, known as patches, for training and testing in a DNN. In such cases, each image patch will become a training or testing object, and thus a single image will contain a large number of training or testing objects. In light of this, in this work, we propose a DNN based approach to automatically segment the corneal ulcer area from fluorescein staining images. We test the proposed algorithm on a dataset consisting of 48 fluorescein staining images with corneal ulcers. The proposed method is compared with a classic image segmentation approach (the active contour based segmentation) and another deep learning based method by replacing the network architecture with the VGG net. The performance of the proposed approach is evaluated using the Dice overlap score, sensitivity, and specificity, as compared to the manually delineated ulcer area segmentations. Correlations between the automatic segmentation results and the manual ones are statistically evaluated.

2   Materials and Methods

2.1   Dataset and Preprocessing

A total of 48 fluorescein staining images of size 2592 × 1728 were used in this study. To increase the computational efficiency, all images were down-sampled to be of size 648 × 432. The ulcer area was restricted to the cornea. To extract the cornea region, we manually labeled four key landmarks (the leftmost, rightmost, most top, and most bottom points of the cornea) on each image and then employed an ellipse shape model to fit those landmarks. After that, we constructed a pixel-specific patch of size 19 × 19 for all pixels in each corneal image. The RGB intensities of that patch (of size 19 × 19 × 3) for all pixels were used to be our features for classification. Pixels belonging to the ulcer area were assigned of label value 1 and those belonging to the non-ulcer area were assigned of label value 0. In Fig. 1, we demonstrate all preprocessing steps.

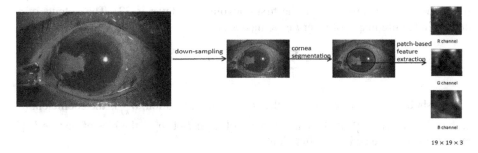

Fig. 1. The flow of prepossessing steps, including down-sampling, cornea segmentation, and patch-based feature extraction.

2.2   Deep Neural Network

During training, the inputs to our DNN are intensity patches of size 19 × 19 × 3. The intensity patches were passed through a stack of convolutional layers, for which we used different filters at different layers, followed by three fully connected (FC) layers. We

Table 1. The architecture of the deep convolutional neural network used in this study.

Layer	Parameter	Layer	Parameter
1. Convolution	7 × 7 × 3 × 32	9. Fully Connected	Neurons:128 × 128
2. ReLU		10. Dropout	Ratio: 0.5
3. Convolution	5 × 5 × 32 × 64	11. ReLU	
4. ReLU		12. Fully Connected	Neurons: 128 × 32
5. Convolution	3 × 3 × 64 × 96	13. ReLU	
6. ReLU		14. Fully Connected	Neurons: 32 × 2
7. Convolution	3 × 3 × 96 × 128	15. SoftmaxWithLoss	
8. ReLU			

used ReLU as the activation function for each layer. A dropout layer was used as a regularization technique to reduce overfitting in our DNN. Normalization layers were not utilized in our model because these layers did not improve the performance but largely increased the memory consumption and computation time. Table 1 lists details of our network architecture. We will now go through the detail of each type of layers.

Convolutional Layers. The $19 \times 19 \times 3$ intensity patches were processed with the convolutional layer [14] which was designed to detect local features at different positions of the patches. A neuron in a convolutional layer operates on a subset of the inputs which is called the receptive field. In our experiment, the size of our receptive field of the first convolutional layer was $7 \times 7 \times 3$. Therefore, each neuron in the first convolutional layer learned a local feature specific to its receptive field of size $7 \times 7 \times 3$. At the same layer, we desire to obtain image descriptors from a variety of angles. Therefore, a variety of kernels were used to process the same image intensity patches, obtaining multiple responses as different local characteristics, which collectively formed the feature maps (the number of feature maps in the first convolutional layer is 32). The outputs of a neuron in feature map k of layer l is defined as:

$$y_k^l = \sum_i W_{k,i}^l * y_i^{l-1} + b_k^l. \tag{1}$$

We should note that "$*$" denotes the convolution operation. $W_{k,i}^l$ is the coefficient of feature k of layer l, y_i^{l-1} is the feature map i of layer $l-1$, b_k^l is the bias of feature k of layer l, and α is the activation function.

Fully Connected Layers. The four convolutional layers were followed by three FC layers. The output of a fully connected layer l is given by:

$$y^l = \alpha(W^l * y^{l-1} + b^l). \tag{2}$$

We also used a dropout layer right after the first FC layer, which randomly disabled certain neurons in the network. This largely improved the robustness of the network by mitigating overfitting.

Activation Functions. During training, all layers except SoftMax layer were equipped with the same activation function (also named Rectified Linear Unit), which is defined as:

$$\alpha{:}x = max(0, x). \tag{3}$$

ReLU is less prone to the vanishing gradient problem when it compares to the sigmoid or tanh activation functions.

The probability for the input to be classified into each of the two categories (ulcer area versus non-ulcer area) can be found in the last FC layer followed by a softmax function. Suppose the output of the neuron i is z_i, and σ_i represents the probability of the input belonging to label i, then this probability can be computed as:

$$\sigma_i = \frac{e^{Z_i}}{\sum_{j=1}^{m} e^{Z_j}}. \tag{4}$$

2.3 Training

The training process used the mini-batch gradient descent approach based on back-propagation [15] with a momentum of 0.9. The batch size was set to be 64. Batch size defines number of samples that going to be propagated through the network in one forward or backward pass. The training was regularized by a weight decay (the L2 penalty multiplier was set to be 5×10^{-4}) and a dropout regularization for the first FC layer (drop out ratio was set to be 0.5). The learning rate was initially set to be 0.01. With the increase of the training steps, learning rate reduced gradually. Initialization of the network weights is important, since improper initialization may cause inappropriate result. The Xavier [16] initialization method is a very effective way of initializing neural network. And it works well with the ReLU activation function.

2.4 Implementation Details

Our network was constructed in the Caffe framework. Caffe is an open-source machine learning library specializing in deep learning algorithms. It also supports the use of GPUs, which can greatly accelerate the execution speed. Gradients were computed on batches, where each gradient update was the average of the individual gradients of the patches in the batch. A GTX Titan X was used for both training and testing.

3 Results

For the testing process, the Dice overlap coefficient is probably the most widely used measure for the comparison of two binary segmentations. The Dice coefficient takes values in the range [0.0, 1.0], where 1.0 is obtained for identical segmentations. In addition, Sensitivity and Specificity scores were also computed.

We also evaluated the correlation between the automatic segmentation results and the manual one in terms of the ulcer area size using the Pearson's correlation coefficient (PCC). All evaluation results are shown in Table 2.

Table 2. Results on dice, sensitivity, specificity, and PCC for the three automatic methods.

Method	Dice	Sensitivity	Specificity	PCC
Active contour	0.71 ± 0.206	0.74 ± 0.253	0.99 ± 0.009	0.970
VGG net	0.83 ± 0.114	0.78 ± 0.153	0.99 ± 0.002	0.987
Our DNN	$\mathbf{0.86 \pm 0.073}$	$\mathbf{0.82 \pm 0.112}$	$\mathbf{0.99 \pm 0.001}$	**0.993**

3.1 Baseline Method

Active contour is a classic approach for image segmentation. In this work, we applied Chan and Vese [17] region-based energy model to extract the boundary of ulcers and compared with results from the proposed method. For each image, we manually identified an initial contour and then iterated for 200 times to finalize. This method is semi-automatic since it requires users to manually provide an initial guess of the ulcer region.

3.2 VGG Net

In addition to the active contour segmentation, we also compared our network with another deep network called VGG net. A 5-fold cross-validation strategy was employed to evaluate the performance of the proposed approach and VGG net. For the training process, we can quantify their accuracy and loss. The loss function in our experiment is the SoftmaxWithLoss function, which is used to predict the label and calculate the loss during training phrase. The accuracy and loss of our DNN model and VGG net from one validation fold was illustrated in Fig. 2. Overall, we observe a fast convergence trend with a relatively high accuracy in both networks, wherein prolonged training yielded a small but steady improvement in terms of the accuracy.

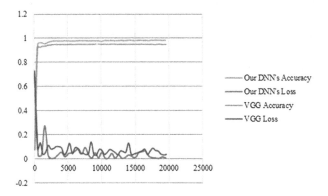

Fig. 2. Accuracy and loss of the training process during one validation fold for both networks.

As shown in Table 2, the proposed ulcer segmentation method has achieved a very high Dice score (0.86 on average) as well as high sensitivity and specificity. The Specificity was found to approach 1. This might be because that the main part of cornea is non-ulcer. In addition to the high overlap, we also observed a significantly positive correlation between the automatic ulcer area size and that of the manual delineations (PCC = 0.993, p-value = 6.3e–45). The proposed method was found to outperform both active contour and VGG net, especially in terms of Dice and sensitivity. Collectively, our results showed the superior performance of this proposed method in identifying ulcers from corneal staining images.

A comparison of results from the three automatic approaches (active contour, VGG net, and the proposed) and the manual ones for three representative cases is shown in

Fig. 3. The active contour method was generally not as precise as learning methods, indicating that deep learning methods are very promising when compared to conventional methods. Comparing VGG net and our DNN, we observed similar performance on some cases whereas the proposed network worked better for some other cases (see the 1st example). Despite its superior performance, two limitations of our method have been detected: firstly, it may mistakenly extract some tiny areas near the ulcer area (see the 2nd example); secondly, it may miss some pixels belonging to the ulcer area, such the 3rd example). The underlying reason is that the color intensity profiles for those missing spots are different from the major ulcer area. We conjecture that our DNN has not learned all characteristics of the ulcers, which will be a future direction to explore.

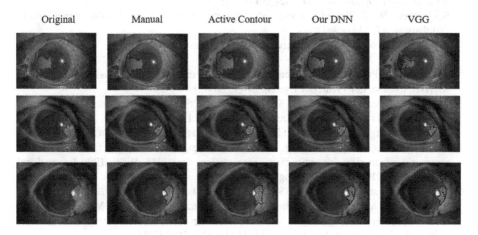

Original   Manual   Active Contour   Our DNN   VGG

Fig. 3. A comparison of the automatic ulcer segmentation results and the manual ones for three representative cases.

4   Conclusion

In this paper, we have proposed and validated an automatic segmentation method for corneal ulcers based on a deep convolutional neural network with the training and testing features obtained from image patches and compared the result with the active contour segmentation method and the VGG net based deep learning method. Utilizing a total of 48 images, we have demonstrated the superiority of the proposed method in terms of both segmentation accuracy and correlation to the manually delineated results. To the best of our knowledge, there have been very rare work on automatic ulcer segmentation even using traditional digital image analysis techniques. Methods relying on deep learning techniques have been even rarer. Our method is one of such kind. The proposed method can automatically extract corneal ulcers with very promising results. This will largely improve the diagnostic efficiency, especially in the big data era.

Acknowledgments. This study was supported by the National Key R&D Program of China (2017YFC0112400), the National Natural Science Foundation of China (NSFC 81501546), and the SYSU-CMU Shunde International Joint Research Institute Start-up Grant (20150306).

References

1. Joyce, P.: Corneal vital staining. Ir. J. Med. Sci. **42**, 359–367 (1967)
2. Kumar, A., Thirumalesh, M.: Use of dyes in ophthalmology. J. Clin. Ophthalmol. Res. **1**, 55 (2013)
3. Kaufman, H.: The diagnosis of corneal herpes simplex infection by fluorescent antibody staining. Arch. Ophthalmol. **64**, 382–384 (1960)
4. Schweitzer, N.: A fluorescein colored polygonal pattern in the human cornea. Arch. Ophthalmol. **77**, 548 (1967)
5. Peterson, R., Wolffsohn, J.: Objective grading of the anterior eye. Optom. Vis. Sci. **86**, 273–278 (2009)
6. Wolffsohn, J., Purslow, C.: Clinical monitoring of ocular physiology using digital image analysis. Contact Lens Anterior Eye **26**, 27–35 (2003)
7. Pritchard, N., Young, G., Coleman, S., Hunt, C.: Subjective and objective measures of corneal staining related to multipurpose care systems. Contact Lens Anterior Eye. **26**, 3–9 (2003)
8. LeCun, Y., Bengio, Y., Hinton, G.: Deep Learning. Nature **521**, 436–444 (2015)
9. Srivastava, R., Cheng, J., Wong, D., Liu, J.: Using deep learning for robustness to parapapillary atrophy in optic disc segmentation. In: 2015 IEEE 12th International Symposium on Biomedical Imaging (ISBI) (2015)
10. Gulshan, V., Peng, L., Coram, M., Stumpe, M., Wu, D., Narayanaswamy, A., Venugopalan, S., Widner, K., Madams, T., Cuadros, J., Kim, R., Raman, R., Nelson, P., Mega, J., Webster, D.: Development and validation of a deep learning algorithm for detection of diabetic retinopathy in retinal fundus photographs. JAMA **316**, 2402 (2016)
11. de Brebisson, A., Montana, G.: Deep neural networks for anatomical brain segmentation. In: 2015 IEEE Conference on Computer Vision and Pattern Recognition Workshops (CVPRW) (2015)
12. Wachinger, C., Reuter, M., Klein, T.: DeepNAT: deep convolutional neural network for segmenting neuroanatomy. NeuroImage (2017)
13. Havaei, M., Davy, A., Warde-Farley, D., Biard, A., Courville, A., Bengio, Y., Pal, C., Jodoin, P., Larochelle, H.: Brain tumor segmentation with deep neural networks. Med. Image Anal. **35**, 18–31 (2017)
14. Lecun, Y., Bottou, L., Bengio, Y., Haffner, P.: Gradient-based learning applied to document recognition. Proc. IEEE **86**, 2278–2324 (1998)
15. LeCun, Y., Boser, B., Denker, J., Henderson, D., Howard, R., Hubbard, W., Jackel, L.: Backpropagation applied to handwritten zip code recognition. Neural Comput. **1**, 541–551 (1989)
16. Glorot, X., Bengio, Y.: Understanding the difficulty of training deep feedforward neural networks. J. Mach. Learn. Res. **9**, 249–256 (2010)
17. Chan, T., Vese, L.: Active contours without edges. IEEE Trans. Image Process. **10**, 266–277 (2001)

Model-Driven 3-D Regularisation for Robust Segmentation of the Refractive Corneal Surfaces in Spiral OCT Scans

Joerg Wagner$^{(\boxtimes)}$, Simon Pezold, and Philippe C. Cattin

Department of Biomedical Engineering, University of Basel, Allschwil, Switzerland
joerg.wagner@unibas.ch

Abstract. Measuring the cornea's anterior and posterior refractive surface is essential for corneal topography, used for diagnostics and the planning of surgeries. Corneal topography by Optical Coherence Tomography (OCT) relies on proper segmentation. Common segmentation methods are limited to specific, B-scan-based scan patterns and fail when applied to data acquired by recently proposed spiral scan trajectories. We propose a novel method for the segmentation of the anterior and posterior refractive surface in scans acquired by 2-D scan trajectories – including but not limited to spirals. Key feature is a model-driven, three-dimensional regularisation of the region of interest, slope and curvature. The regularisation is integrated into a graph-based segmentation with feature-directed smoothing and incremental segmentation. We parameterise the segmentation based on test surface measurements and evaluate its performance by means of 18 *in vivo* measurements acquired by spiral and radial scanning. The comparison with expert segmentations shows successful segmentation of the refractive corneal surfaces.

Keywords: Optical Coherence Tomography · Segmentation · Cornea

1 Introduction

Optical Coherence Tomography (OCT) is an emerging modality in ophthalmology – including measurement of the cornea. Although the cornea consists of multiple layers, refraction mainly occurs at the anterior and posterior surface. Correct three-dimensional delineation of the anterior and posterior corneal surfaces is therefore crucial for determining the corneal refractive power and the generation of corneal topography maps, used for diagnostics and surgical planning. For corneal measurement by OCT, the cornea is usually scanned by scan patterns consisting of multiple straight scans (B-scans). Raster patterns consist of parallel B-scans. Radial scan patterns consist of meridional B-scans rotated around the apex of the eye and are commonly used for corneal topography [4]. Recently, Wagner *et al.* [5] proposed a spiral scan pattern for corneal topography with reduced susceptibility to disturbances caused by eye blinking or abrupt movements. However, the appearance of the cornea in spiral scans is different

© Springer International Publishing AG 2017
M.J. Cardoso et al. (Eds.): FIFI/OMIA 2017, LNCS 10554, pp. 109–117, 2017.
DOI: 10.1007/978-3-319-67561-9_12

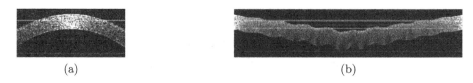

(a)   (b)

Fig. 1. (a) A typical radial B-scan. (b) One eighth (one cycle) of a spiral scan where the center of the scan pattern is aligned to the apex of the eye.

and more variable (*cf.* Fig. 1), e.g. it varies with the relative position of the eye. This asks for new, more versatile segmentation and regularisation methods.

Common methods are optimised for the segmentation of classical B-scans – using active contours or graph theory. To overcome the typically low signal-to-noise ratio (SNR) of OCT images, 2-D regularisation schemes are applied. Yazdanpanah *et al.* [8] add 2-D shape and smoothness terms to their active contour approach. Williams *et al.* [6] use graph cut with 2-D curvature and shape terms. LaRocca *et al.* [3] use a two step process for segmenting corneal layers in radial B-scans. They restrict the search region by parabolic extrapolation from the central high SNR area into the lateral low SNR areas. Recently, Williams *et al.* [7] added a 2-D shape prior to their shortest path method, resulting in more accurate segmentation compared to level set and graph cut methods. Fu *et al.* [2] used graph-search to find markers for a later segmentation by a fourth order.

These methods are by design inappropriate for the segmentation of images obtained by spiral scan patterns. We present a model-driven 3-D regularisation for robust graph-based segmentation of the anterior and posterior refractive surface in scans from 2-D scan trajectories – including but not limited to spirals. Apart from the novel regularisation, the graph-based segmentation features intrinsic, feature directed smoothing for enhanced robustness to noise. Further, we developed an incremental segmentation scheme that enables the processing of long scans (as obtained by spiral scanning) on systems with limited memory.

2 Methods

2.1 Graph-Based Segmentation

Although the regularisation is our main contribution, we first describe the basic segmentation method. Because graph-search methods performed best in recent work [7], we convert the segmentation into a shortest path problem on a weighted directed graph. The nodes represent individual image pixels. Contrary to the state of the art, we only assign nodes to every b^{th} A-scan and introduce edges that span the A-scans lying in between, where edge length b is an integer greater than one. We will refer to A-scans with assigned nodes as *nodal A-scans*. The edge weights are calculated from the intensities of pixels lying on a straight line between their start and end pixel, which is done by means of kernel convolution (see Fig. 2a). This leads to a piecewise linear segmentation with averaging in edge direction. The averaging results in feature-directed smoothing and enhances the

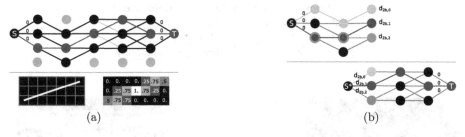

Fig. 2. (a) The graph structure (top) with source (S) and target (T) nodes and the shortest path (red), while gray colour indicates nodes and edges outside the ROI or slope limits. An ideal edge (bottom, left) and the resulting kernel for edge weight calculation (bottom, right). (b) Piecewise segmentation scheme. The shortest distances $(d_{2b,i})$ to the last nodal A-scan of the first frame graph (top) are used as weight to connect the start node (S*) for the next frame (bottom). (Color figure online)

robustness to noise. Because the intensity of a nodal pixel is used twice – for incoming and outgoing edge weights – these pixels are weighted half. To ensure an unrestricted start and end, we connect a source and a target node by zero weight edges with all the nodes from the first and last nodal A-scan, respectively.

Incremental Segmentation. We developed an incremental scheme to solve the global graph search problem. With this scheme, neither the complete scan nor the complete graph has to be in memory at once. We divide the scan image into frames containing $ab+1$ A-scans, where b is the edge length and a an integer greater than one. Therefore, each frame starts and ends with a nodal A-scan. Because the last A-scan of a frame is the first A-scan of the following frame, the frames overlap by one A-scan. Thus, the first frame contains the A-scan indices 0 up to ab and the second frame contains ab to $2ab$. The procedure consists of the following steps (*cf.* Fig. 2b): (1) Generate the graph for the first frame, (2) determine the shortest path $d_{ab,j}$ to all nodes in the last A-scan, (3) generate the graph for the next frame using the path distances $d_{ab,j}$ to connect the new start node, (4) repeat steps (2) and (3). The shortest path to the target is then put together from the shortest paths determined in step (2). To save memory, the single frames are read in and preprocessed on demand for steps (2) and (3).

Preprocessing. After applying the fast Fourier transform to the spectral OCT scans, subtracting the background scan and taking the logarithm (of base 10), a specific preprocessing is performed for each feature to segment (see Sect. 2.2). The given filter widths are specific for the used scan system (see Sect. 2.3). For the *stroma*, Gaussian smoothing ($\sigma = 7\,\text{px}$) and box filtering (width $= 28\,\text{px}$) in scan direction and 2D sub-scaling by the factor 7 is performed. For the *anterior surface* and *posterior surface*, filtering in scan direction with the negative and positive first derivative of a Gaussian ($\sigma = 4\,\text{px}$) is performed, respectively.

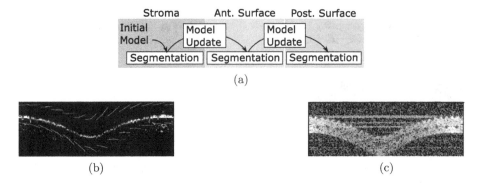

(a)

(b)   (c)

Fig. 3. (a) Segmentation procedure. (b) Section of a scan, preprocessed for the segmentation of the anterior surface, with the regularisation limits for ROI, slope and curvature (cyan). (c) Original scan section with the resulting segmentations. (Color figure online)

2.2   Regularisation

Based on a three-dimensional model, the region of interest (ROI), slope and curvature are selectively limited. To increase robustness, we perform a stroma segmentation prior to the segmentation of the anterior and posterior corneal surfaces (see Fig. 3). The regularisation model is updated between the segmentations. Figure 5 shows the positive effect of this regularisation scheme, especially for segmentation of the posterior corneal surface.

Regularisation Model. We used Zernike polynomials as the basis for our regularisation model because they are state of the art for the description of optical surfaces [5]. Our model consists of a 6th-order Zernike surface, defined by its radius and coefficients $c_{n,m}$, and tolerances $t_{n,m}$ assigned to the coefficients (all in millimeters), where n and m indicate the radial and azimuthal degree of the Zernike polynomials Z_n^m, respectively. For the initial model, we constructed a Zernike surface that approximates a sphere with radius of 7.8 mm – the shape and size of a typical cornea. A relative coefficients tolerance $t_{n,m} = 0.2 \cdot c_{n,m}$ was applied, except for the offset tolerance which was set to $t_{0,0} = 0.5$. Thus, the operator has to adjust the distance between OCT system and subject in advance with an accuracy of ± 0.5 mm. For the model updates, the Zernike surfaces are constructed based on the previous segmentation as described in [5]. We use the coefficients' standard errors $s_{n,m}$, measures for the confidence in the reconstruction [5], to calculate the tolerances of the coefficients by $t_{n,m} = 4 \cdot s_{n,m}$.

The reconstructed surface is shifted by redefining the offset coefficient $c_{0,0} := c_{0,0} + dz$, where dz is the estimated distance from the previous surface. The corresponding coefficient tolerance is modified as $t_{0,0} := t_{0,0} + \Delta dz$, where Δdz is the tolerance of the surface position. Assuming a corneal thickness of 0.8(5) mm and a corneal refractive index of $n_c = 1.38$, we use a distance shift for the anterior surface of $dz_{sa} = 0.4 \cdot 1.38$ with a tolerance of $\Delta dz_{sa} = 0.25 \cdot 1.38$ and a shift for the posterior surface of $dz_{ap} = 0.8 \cdot 1.38$ with a tolerance of $\Delta dz_{ap} = 0.5 \cdot 1.38$.

Implementation. To restrict the ROI, nodes are generated only for pixels lying in an estimation band for the depth $z_E(i) \pm z_M(i)$. The depth $z_E(i)$ is estimated by sampling the model surface at the scan position i. The margin $z_M(i)$ is determined based on the coefficients tolerances $t_{n,m}$. Because the Zernike polynomials Z_n^m are orthogonal, the margin from the individual tolerance Zernike polynomials $z_M^{n,m}(i) = \mathrm{abs}(t_{n,m} \cdot Z_n^m(x_i, y_i))$ are added to obtain the total margin $z_M(i) = \sum z_M^{n,m}$. To restrict the slope, two nodes at scan positions i_1 and i_2 are only connected when the slope $\Delta z(i_1, i_2)$ is in the slope estimation band $\Delta z_E(i_1, i_2) \pm \Delta z_M(i_1, i_2)$. The slope $\Delta z_E(i_1, i_2)$ is estimated by sampling the model surface at the scan positions and calculating the depth difference $\Delta z_E(i_1, i_2) = Z(x_{i2}, y_{i2}) - Z(x_{i1}, y_{i1})$. For calculating $\Delta z_M(i_1, i_2)$, the slope margins of the tolerance polynomials are determined and added analogously. The curvature is restricted while solving the shortest path problem with an adapted version of Dijkstra's algorithm: The curvature is restricted by considering only the nodes that result in a discrete curvature that is in the allowed range. The curvature at a certain scan point i is defined by $c_i = z(i-1) - 2z(i) + z(i+1)$. The estimated curvature is calculated from the model surface by $c_E = z_E(i-1) - 2z_E(i) + z_E(i-1)$. The margin c_M is determined in analogy with the position and slope margin.

2.3   Evaluation

Scan Patterns and Setup. For the evaluation of the method, we used two scan patterns with different 2-D scan trajectories: a spiral scan pattern (Fig. 4a) with 32768 points and a radial scan pattern 5920 points (Fig. 4b) that includes turning loops between B-scans. We implemented the segmentation in Python 2.7, using Numpy and NetworkX, and used a custom swept-source OCT system at

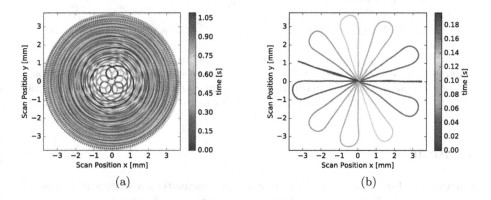

(a)   (b)

Fig. 4. (a) The spiral scan pattern and (b) the radial scan pattern.

1060 nm featuring telecentric scanning and a sweep rate of 30 kHz. Bandwidth-limited full-width at half maximum axial resolution of the system is 40 μm. Segmentation is based on data interpolated to 12 μm axial pixel dimension.

Parameter Optimisation. Edge length b is a crucial parameter. A short edge results in low averaging and high susceptibility to noise. On the other hand, a long edge is expected to bias the segmentation because the piecewise linear approximation is not adequate anymore. Thus, we optimised the edge length by means of test surface measurements with both scan patterns. We used three test surfaces with different shapes: a sphere with a radius of 6.4 mm, a sphere with a radius of 8.8 mm, and a torus with radii of 7.6 mm and 8.0 mm. We performed a torus fit on the points obtained by the individual segmentations and used the RMS of the fit error to find the trade-off between high robustness to noise and accuracy.

In Vivo Evaluation. For the *in vivo* evaluation, we used an edge length of 20 for the segmentation of the corneal surfaces and an edge length of 10 for the sub-scaled stroma segmentation. We used a edge length at the lower end of the optimal range (see parameter optimisation results) because the test surfaces only represent normal eyes and idealized astigmatism. The method was evaluated by comparing to expert segmentations. Nine different eyes from nine healthy volunteers were measured with both scan patterns. The expert manually marked the pixel-position of the anterior and posterior cornea surface in 10 randomly selected A-scans (*cf.* Fig. 5). This procedure was done a second time for the same A-scans, by the same expert. For each of the 180 A-scans, we calculated the differences between the piece-wise linear interpolated automatic segmentation z_S and the expert segmentation z_{E1} by $dz_{SE1} = z_S - z_{E1}$ as well as the differences between the two expert segmentations $dz_{E12} = z_{E1} - z_{E2}$.

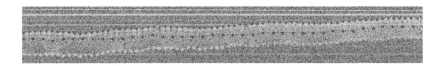

Fig. 5. Section of a spiral *in vivo* scan. The segmented cornea anterior (blue) and posterior (green) corneal surface. The stroma segmentation is shown in red. As comparison, the unregularised segmentation of the posterior surface is shown in magenta. Expert segmentations are shown in yellow. (Color figure online)

3   Results

Parameter Optimisation. The test surface measurements confirm the positive effect of the feature-directed smoothing introduced by the A-scan-spanning edges. Figure 6a shows minimal fitting error for an edge width between 16 and

28 for the radial scan pattern. For the spiral scan pattern, the error still seems to decrease when increasing the edge length above 24, albeit being close to convergence. This can be explained by the fact that the radial pattern scans along the maximal surface gradient whereas the spiral pattern scans nearly along the minimal surface gradient.

In-Vivo Evaluation. Figure 6b shows the comparison with expert segmentations. For the difference to the expert segmentation dz_{SE1} we removed two outliers (-72 px and -66 px), caused by exceptionally low SNR in one radial scan. This results in a mean difference $\bar{dz}_{SE1}$ of -0.73 ± 1.06 px (mean $\pm$ SD) for the anterior surface and -0.13 ± 2.91 px for the posterior surface, over both scan patterns. The mean difference between expert segmentations $\bar{dz}_{E12}$ is -0.31 ± 0.87 px for the anterior surface and -0.35 ± 2.85 px for the posterior surface.

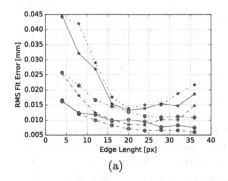 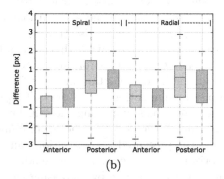

(a)   (b)

Fig. 6. (a) Optimisation curve of the edge width for the scan patterns (spiral: red, radial: blue) and test surfaces (small sphere: dashed, big sphere: dash-dot, torus: solid). (b) *In vivo* differences between automatic segmentation and expert segmentation d_{SE1} (blue) and between the expert segmentations d_{E12} (green). (Color figure online)

4 Discussion

Motivated by the recently proposed spiral scan pattern and the limitations of current segmentation methods, we introduce a novel 3-D regularised segmentation for the anterior and posterior corneal surface in scans acquired by 2-D scan trajectories like spirals. The *in vivo* comparison with expert segmentations shows successful segmentation of the anterior and posterior corneal surfaces. Both differences, between our method and expert segmentations and between the expert segmentations, are within ± 3 px. With the pixel resolution of 12 μm, this corresponds to a spatial range of $\pm 36\,\mu$m, which is less than the full-width at half maximum axial resolution (40 μm) of the OCT system. This indicates segmentation of the accurate surfaces. Because our method works for two contrary 2-D scan trajectories, one scanning along the maximal surface gradient and one scanning along the minimal surface gradient, we suppose that the method is suited for various 2-D scan trajectories – assuming continuous scanning.

We want to point out that comparison with common methods is not possible or would be unfair because they are not able to segment scans from 2-D scan trajectories by design. The limited system resolution, the variable angle of the incident laser beam relative to the interface and noise lead to a diffuse interface signal which makes the exact identification of the interface imprecise – even for an expert. Due to this lack of a quantitative gold standard, quantitative comparison below the level of system resolution is inappropriate. However, we believe that expert segmentation is gold standard to show successful segmentation of the surfaces in a qualitative manner. We did this by showing that the segmentation difference is below the axial resolution the OCT system. Regarding our future work, we believe that quantitative verification of the segmentation is only possible in the course of a comprehensive validation that involves the whole pipeline for OCT-based corneal topography and comparison with established topographers on normal and pathologic eyes.

We want to emphasise that the key of the method lies in the novel model-driven 3-D regularisation that guides the graph-based segmentation. This 3-D regularisation enables robust segmentation of scans from 2-D scan trajectories. By using hard restriction margins for ROI, slope and curvature, we aim to minimise regularisation bias. Others [6,8] use continuous penalty which potentially introduces bias by pulling the solution towards a prior, *e.g.* by adding curvature and shape terms to an energy minimisation. In contrast to established methods, the presented regularisation can be easily adapted, *e.g.* unreliable lateral-horizontal eye alignment can be addressed by adapting the initial regularisation model – in this case by increasing the tolerances of the tilt coefficient $t_{1,1}$ [1].

References

1. Braaf, B., van de Watering, T.C., Spruijt, K., van der Heijde, R.G., Sicam, V.A.D.: Calculating angle lambda (λ) using zernike tilt measurements in specular reflection corneal topography. J. Optom. **2**(4), 207–214 (2009)
2. Fu, H., Xu, Y., Lin, S., Zhang, X., Wong, D.W.K., Liu, J., Frangi, A.F., Baskaran, M., Aung, T.: Segmentation and quantification for angle-closure glaucoma assessment in anterior segment OCT. IEEE Trans. Med. Imaging (2017)
3. LaRocca, F., Chiu, S.J., McNabb, R.P., Kuo, A.N., Izatt, J.A., Farsiu, S.: Robust automatic segmentation of corneal layer boundaries in SDOCT images using graph theory and dynamic programming. Biomed. Opt. Express **2**(6), 1524–1538 (2011)
4. McNabb, R.P., LaRocca, F., Farsiu, S., Kuo, A.N., Izatt, J.A.: Distributed scanning volumetric SDOCT for motion corrected corneal biometry. Biomed. Opt. Express **3**(9), 2050–2065 (2012)
5. Wagner, J., Goldblum, D., Cattin, P.C.: Golden angle based scanning for robust corneal topography with OCT. Biomed. Opt. Express **8**(2), 475–483 (2017)
6. Williams, D., Zheng, Y., Bao, F., Elsheikh, A.: Fast segmentation of anterior segment optical coherence tomography images using graph cut. Eye Vis. **2**(1), 1 (2015)

7. Williams, D., Zheng, Y., Davey, P.G., Bao, F., Shen, M., Elsheikh, A.: Reconstruction of 3D surface maps from anterior segment optical coherence tomography images using graph theory and genetic algorithms. Biomed. Signal Process. Control **25**, 91–98 (2016)
8. Yazdanpanah, A., Hamarneh, G., Smith, B.R., Sarunic, M.V.: Segmentation of intraretinal layers from optical coherence tomography images using an active contour approach. IEEE Trans. Med. Imaging **30**(2), 484–496 (2011)

Automatic Retinal Layer Segmentation Based on Live Wire for Central Serous Retinopathy

Dehui Xiang[✉], Geng Chen, Fei Shi, Weifang Zhu, and Xinjian Chen[✉]

School of Electronics and Information Engineering, Soochow University,
Jiangsu 215006, China
{xiangdehui,xjchen}@suda.edu.cn

Abstract. Central serous retinopathy is a serious retinal disease. Retinal layer segmentation for this disease can help ophthalmologists to provide accurate diagnosis and proper treatment for patients. In order to detect surfaces in optical coherence tomography images with pathological changes, an automatic method is reported by combining random forests and a live wire algorithm. First, twenty four features are designed for the random forest classifiers to find initial surfaces. Then, a live wire algorithm is proposed to accurately detect surfaces between retinal layers even though OCT images with fluids are of low contrast and layer boundaries are blurred. The proposed method was evaluated on 24 spectral domain OCT images with central serous retinopathy. The experimental results showed that the proposed method outperformed the state-of-art methods.

Keywords: Central serous retinopathy · Optical coherence tomography · Random forest and live wire

1 Introduction

Central serous retinopathy (CSR) is a serious complex disease that usually leads to blindness. CSR occurs due to the accumulation of serous fluid under interdigitation zone of the retina [1] and may also lead to retinal pigment epithelium detachment as shown in Fig. 1. There are two types of CSR [2,3]. In Type 1 CSR, only serous fluid accumulates under the interdigitation zone. In Type 2 CSR, retinal pigment epithelium detachment may appear under the serous fluid and may also occur near the center of the macula besides the accumulation of serous fluid. These fluids lead to large morphological changes of retinal layers. In addition, thickness and optical intensity of retinal layers may change abruptly due to the occurrence of CSR [4–6]. CSR is one common type of macular disorder and the macula is responsible for the central vision. It is important to provide accurate diagnosis and treatment of CSR.

Optical coherence tomography (OCT) is a noninvasive and non-contact imaging modality for morphological analysis and diagnosis of retinal abnormality,

© Springer International Publishing AG 2017
M.J. Cardoso et al. (Eds.): FIFI/OMIA 2017, LNCS 10554, pp. 118–125, 2017.
DOI: 10.1007/978-3-319-67561-9_13

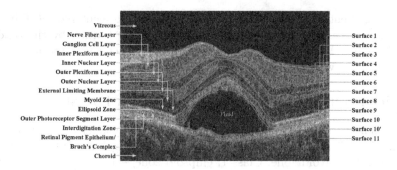

Fig. 1. OCT image with central serous retinopathy and manual annotation of retinal surfaces and layers.

such as CSR, macular hole, diabetic macular edema, glaucoma and age-related macular degeneration. The rapid development of OCT technology, especially recent developed spectral domain (SD) OCT, has led to produce higher resolution real 3-D volume images of the retina, and identify more anatomical layers of the retina [1]. The great improvements of SD-OCT devices make it possible diagnose and monitor retinal disease more accurately based on abnormality quantification and retinal layer thickness computation both in research centers and clinic routines. Figure 1 shows a macular centered OCT B-scan image with CSR. The vitreous, retina, fluid and choroid were annotated with arrows. The surfaces are numbered 1 to 11 from top to bottom. The retinal layers are nerve fiber layer (NFL), ganglion cell layer (GCL), inner plexiform layer (IPL), inner nuclear layer (INL), outer plexiform layer (OPL), outer nuclear layer (ONL), external limiting membrane (ELM), myoid zone, ellipsoid zone, outer photoreceptor segment layer (OPSL), interdigitation zone, retinal pigment epithelium (RPE)/Bruch's complex and choroid. The abnormalities include serosity (fluid), pigment epithelial detachment (PED) caused fluid.

To quantify the thickness of retinal layers in OCT with CSR, it is important to develop a reliable and automatic segmentation of retinal layers since manual segmentation is time-consuming for huge amount of OCT images in clinic applications. However, there are several challenges in retinal layer segmentation. First, the internal structures of retinas are complex and difficult to be recognized as shown in Fig. 1. Inner boundaries of retinal layers are non-smooth and there are more than twelve layers. Second, there may be several types of fluid, e.g., serosity, PED caused fluid. This leads to low contrast and blurred boundaries in OCT images between retinal layers, and also great structural changes of retinal layers. Therefore, layer segmentation may fail in using traditional surface detection methods, such as the graph search algorithm [7–10]. Therefore, new methods that can segment retinal layers are needed for quantitative analysis of CSR.

In this paper, we focus on segmentation for retinas with CSR in OCT images, which is associated with serosity and PED caused fluid. An automatic, supervised

3-D layer segmentation method is proposed for macular-centered OCT images with CSR. Shapes and intensities of retinal layers are learned by the random forest classifiers. The initial surfaces constrain the refinement of retinal surfaces by using the live wire algorithm.

2   Initial Surface Detection via Random Forest

The retinal layers in OCT images with CSR are manually labeled as eight classes. Class 1: NFL, Class 2: GCL, Class 3: IPL, Class 4: INL, Class 5: OPL, Class 6: ONL + ELM + myoid zone, Class 7: ellipsoid zone + OPSL + interdigitation zone + RPE/Bruch's complex + fluid, and Class 0: choroid. Unlike normal retinal layers, fovea is often extruded upward by serosity in OCT images with CSR. It is impossible to find the center of the fovea by computing the thinnest position as in [11]. We use three spatial features: x, y and z coordinates after surface 1 is detected. These three features denote the geometric information of each voxel related to the interface of vitreous and NFL. The intensity of the original image is considered as one feature. The original image is denoised with the curvature anisotropic diffusion filtering to reduce speckle noise and preserve boundary between adjacent layers. In the clinical images, the intensity range varies from one patient to another and the contrast between neighboring layers is often low. To address these problems, the filtered and smoothed image is normalized in several intervals as,

$$I_N\left(\boldsymbol{x}\right) = \begin{cases} I_{N,\max}; & I_f\left(\boldsymbol{x}\right) \geq I_{f,s} + I_{f,r}; \\ \frac{I_{N,\max}}{I_{f,r}}\left(I_f\left(\boldsymbol{x}\right) - I_{f,s}\right); & I_{f,s} < I_f\left(\boldsymbol{x}\right) < I_{f,s} + I_{f,r}; \\ 0; & I_f\left(\boldsymbol{x}\right) < I_{f,s}. \end{cases} \quad (1)$$

where $I_f\left(\boldsymbol{x}\right)$ is the intensity of a voxel, the intensity interval is $[I_{f,s}, I_{f,s} + I_{f,r}]$, $I_{N,\max}$ is the maximal normalized intensity. Five normalized features are used and allow the classifier to easily differentiate the darker layers and the brighter layers, and particularly recognize NFL, IPL, OPL, ellipsoid zone + OPSL + interdigitation zone + RPE/Bruch's complex.

Although the sub-range normalized intensities are useful layer features, structural features can also provide helpful information according to intensities of neighborhood voxels. The bright layer possibility in the Hessian scale space is defined as

$$L\left(\boldsymbol{x},\sigma_t\right) = \begin{cases} |\lambda_3\left(\boldsymbol{x},\sigma_t\right)| \exp\left(-\frac{\alpha\lambda_1^2(\boldsymbol{x},\sigma_t)+\beta\lambda_2^2(\boldsymbol{x},\sigma_t)}{\lambda_3^2(\boldsymbol{x},\sigma_t)}\right), & \lambda_3\left(\boldsymbol{x},\sigma_t\right) < 0 \\ 0, & \lambda_3\left(\boldsymbol{x},\sigma_t\right) \geq 0 \end{cases} \quad (2)$$

The dark layer possibility is defined as

$$L\left(\boldsymbol{x},\sigma_t\right) = \begin{cases} |\lambda_3\left(\boldsymbol{x},\sigma_t\right)| \exp\left(-\frac{\alpha\lambda_1^2(\boldsymbol{x},\sigma_t)+\beta\lambda_2^2(\boldsymbol{x},\sigma_t)}{\lambda_3^2(\boldsymbol{x},\sigma_t)}\right), & \lambda_3\left(\boldsymbol{x},\sigma_t\right) > 0 \\ 0, & \lambda_3\left(\boldsymbol{x},\sigma_t\right) \leq 0 \end{cases} \quad (3)$$

where $\boldsymbol{x}$ denotes the voxel coordinates. α and β are symmetric parameters, which control the ratio between the two minor components λ_1, λ_2 and the principal component λ_3.

To take into account the varying sizes of the layers, the scale-dependent layer possibility function $L(x, \sigma_t)$ is computed for varying thickness for all voxels x of the 3D image domain. The thickness values are discretized values between the minimal scale $\sigma_{t,min}$ and the maximal scale $\sigma_{t,max}$, using a linear scale. The multiscale layer response is obtained by selecting the maximum response over the range of all scales as

$$L_m(x, \sigma_t) = \max_{\sigma_{t,\min} \leq \sigma_t \leq \sigma_{t,\max}} \sigma_t^2 \times L(x, \sigma_t) \tag{4}$$

The bright layer responses allow the classifier to learn the possibility of NFL, IPL, OPL, ellipsoid zone + OPSL + interdigitation zone + RPE/Bruch's complex while the dark layer responses allow the classifier to learn the possibility of GCL, INL, ONL + ELM + myoid zone and choroid. For each scale, the bright layer responses and the dark responses are computed and the maximal responses from the minimal scale and current scale are also computed. Totally, fourteen layer-like features are generated for the classifier. The eigenvectors of the Hessian matrix corresponding to the three eigenvalues $\lambda_1, \lambda_2, \lambda_3$ are orthogonal to each other. One eigenvector is the normal of the layer and the other two eigenvector are tangent. Therefore, layer response features are robust to the deformation and rotation of retinal layers even with the existence of diseases such as fluid. All the voxels of the 3D OCT image are classified by trained random forest classifiers.

3   Surface Refinement via Live Wire

The surface is defined as terrain-like interface $S(x, y) \in \{1, 2, \cdots, Z\}$, where each point (x, y) has one and only one $z \in \{1, 2, \cdots, Z\}$ value. Single surface detection in OCT image is then transformed into finding a minimum cost path in $x - z$ plane and $y - z$ plane successively with an initial surface. The initial anchors are equidistantly sampled from the initial surface in one direction with the sampling step lw_s. To search the shortest path between two successive anchors, a graph is constructed in the preprocessing section. Edge features and feature transform functions selected are used to compute the cost of all edges. The shortest oriented path $\langle e_1, e_2, \cdots, e_{n_o} \rangle$ is found. n_o is the number of edges on the shortest oriented path between two neighboring anchors $\mathbf{a}_o$ and $\mathbf{a}_{o+1}$. $o = 1, \cdots, \lfloor \frac{a_x}{lw_s} \rfloor$ and a_x is X in $x - z$ plane or Y in $y - z$ plane. The corresponding local energy can be defined as,

$$e_{lw}(\mathbf{a}_o, \mathbf{a}_{o+1}) = \sum_{u=1}^{n_o} c_{ij}(e_u) \tag{5}$$

where the weighting function $c_{ij}(e_u)$ for the edge e_u is constructed as

$$c_{ij}(u) = \frac{\sum\limits_{k=1}^{n_k} \sum\limits_{l=1}^{n_l} \omega_k c_k(f_l(u))}{\sum\limits_{k=1}^{n_k} \omega_k}, \tag{6}$$

where, f_l is the feature function, which define the edge feature for e_u. The edge features consist of $n_l = 7$ features. c_k is the transfer function, which maps a edge feature to the feature cost. The transfer functions consist of $n_k = 6$ functions, the linear mapping function, the inverted linear mapping function, gaussian function, the inverted gaussian function, the hyperbolic function and the inverted modified hyperbolic function. ω_k is the weight parameter. Then, the total energy of a boundary curve can be defined as,

$$E_{lw} = \sum_{o=1}^{\lfloor \frac{a_x}{lw_s} \rfloor} e_{lw}\left(\mathbf{a}_o, \mathbf{a}_{o+1}\right) \tag{7}$$

Initial anchors $\mathbf{a}_o$ are equidistantly sampled with the step lw_s from the initial surfaces. The live wire algorithm is applied to refine the initial curve. The total energy of the refined boundary curve $\mathbf{a}'$ is computed according to Eq. (7). The step lw_s is reduced and $\mathbf{a}'$ is considered as the initial curve. The process is stopped if the total energy difference ΔE between two iterations and $lw_s \leq 1$. The retinal surface is detected by the live wire algorithm as pseudo 3D terrain-like mesh. The live wire algorithm are employed in $x - z$ plane and then in $y - z$ plane. The Canny edge detection algorithm is used to obtain the initial surface 1. The live wire algorithm is used to refine surfaces 1 to 11.

4   Experiments

4.1   Data

The OCT images were obtained from the Jiangsu Province Hospital by using a Cirrus HD-OCT 4000 scanner. Macula-centered SD-OCT scans of 24 eyes from 24 subjects diagnosed with CSR were acquired as testing images. Another 6 macula-centered SD-OCT images with CSR were used as training images for the segmentation of abnormal retinal images. All the OCT volume images contain $512 \times 128 \times 1024$ voxels and the voxel size is $11.74 \times 47.24 \times 1.96 \ \mu m^3$.

4.2   Evaluation

To evaluate the layer segmentation results, a retinal specialist manually anno-tated the surfaces in the B-scan images to form the segmentation reference. Due to the time consumption of manual annotation, only 15 out of the 128 B-scans were randomly chosen and annotated for each 3D OCT volume in the testing data set. All the 128 B-scans were manually annotated for each 3D OCT volume in the training data set, and then each 3D OCT volume was labeled with the eight classes according to the annotated surfaces for random forest classifiers training.

   To evaluate performance of surface detection methods, average unsigned sur-face distance was computed for each surface by measuring absolute Euclidean distances in the z-axis between surface detection results of the algorithms and the reference surface [10]. To demonstrate the improvement of our method, our algorithm (RFLW) was compared to the state-of-art methods: the Iowa reference algorithm (IR) [7] and the multi-resolution graph search algorithm (MGS) [10].

4.3   Results

An OCT volume image only with CSR is shown in Fig. 2. The green curves are manual annotated surfaces. The red curves are the detected surfaces via the surface detection algorithms. The yellow curves are the eight initial surfaces by using the random forest method.

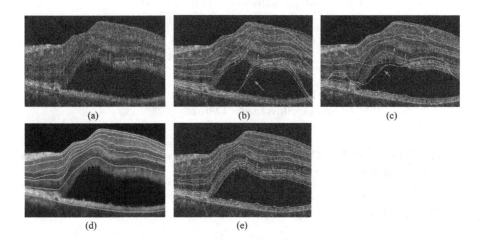

Fig. 2. Automatic surface detection (green curves are the segmentation reference, red curves are detected surfaces) of an OCT image with CSR. (a) The original image; (b) Surfaces detected via the IF algorithm; (c) Surfaces detected via the MGS algorithm; (d) The eight initial surfaces with the filtered image; (e) Surfaces detected via the RFLW algorithm. (Color figure online)

Table 1 shows the mean and standard deviation of average signed surface detection errors for each surface. The results in Table 1 show great improvement over the IR algorithm [7] and the MGS algorithm [10] even a large proportion of the layers exhibits dramatic morphological changes. For the RFLW algorithm, the average unsigned surface detection errors of surface 1 to 11 were dramatically reduced compared to the IR algorithm and the MGS algorithm as shown in the third column of Table 1. Surface detection errors were the largest at surface 5 to 7 while detection errors of the rest surfaces were smaller.

The proposed algorithm was implemented in C++ and tested on a PC with Intel i5-3450 CPU@3.10GHz and 16GB of RAM. In training stage, the average running time of the algorithm was about 6 h for the 6 CSR OCT images. In testing stage, the average running time of the random forest algorithm was 304 ± 34 s for the 24 CSR OCT images. The average running time of the IF algorithm

Table 1. Comparison of surface detection with average unsigned surface distance (Mean±SD μm^a) for CSR images

Surface	IR	MGS	RFLW
1	10.3 ± 16.7	4.4 ± 7.6	2.6 ± 0.9
2	18.7 ± 20.6	10.5 ± 21.0	5.1 ± 1.0
3	21.7 ± 18.5	16.6 ± 20.0	5.0 ± 1.2
4	22.3 ± 17.4	14.8 ± 19.3	3.0 ± 1.4
5	25.2 ± 17.0	24.5 ± 21.2	5.0 ± 1.3
6	27.1 ± 15.0	24.1 ± 15.9	6.7 ± 2.7
7	51.4 ± 40.5	18.9 ± 17.0	8.6 ± 5.0
8	48.3 ± 37.4	16.8 ± 13.8	9.3 ± 5.7
9	47.6 ± 34.7	16.8 ± 11.4	10.7 ± 5.4
10	30.0 ± 43.7	14.3 ± 9.7	8.3 ± 3.3
10'	\	13.8 ± 30.1	7.3 ± 5.9
11	27.3 ± 47.0	11.1 ± 34.1	4.7 ± 6.6

^{a}Voxel size in z direction is 1.96 μm.

was 112 ± 31 s for CSR OCT images. The average running time of the MGS algorithm was 436 ± 93 s for CSR OCT images.

5 Conclusion

In this paper, a supervised method was proposed for the automated segmentation of retinal layers on OCT scans of eyes with CSR. Surface 1 is detected by using the Canny edge detection algorithm and the live wire algorithm. Only twenty four features are generated for the training and testing of the random forests classifiers, and then eight initial surfaces are detected as constraints. By utilizing the original intensities of OCT images and the layer-like shape information, the live wire algorithm is used to find the final surface. The proposed method was evaluated on 24 spectral domain OCT images with central serous retinopathy. The experimental results showed that the proposed method outperformed the state-of-art methods. Although the proposed method was used in OCT image with CSR, it can be also transferred to other sources of OCT images. The proposed method will be tested in normal OCT images and OCT images with other retinal diseases.

Acknowledgment. This work has been supported in part by the National Basic Research Program of China (973 Program) under Grant 2014CB748600, and in part by the National Natural Science Foundation of China (NSFC) under Grant 81371629, 61401293, 61401294, 81401451, 81401472.

References

1. Staurenghi, G., Sadda, S., Chakravarthy, U., Spaide, R.F., et al.: Proposed lexicon for anatomic landmarks in normal posterior segment spectral-domain optical coherence tomography: the IN OCT consensus. Ophthalmology **121**(8), 1572–1578 (2014)
2. Field, M.G., Elner, V.M., Park, S., Hackel, R., Heckenlively, J.R., Elner, S.G., Petty, H.R.: Detection of retinal metabolic stress due to central serous retinopathy. Retina **29**(8), 1162 (2009). (Philadelphia, Pa.)
3. Hassan, B., Raja, G., Hassan, T., Akram, M.U.: Structure tensor based automated detection of macular edema and central serous retinopathy using optical coherence tomography images. JOSA A **33**(4), 455–463 (2016)
4. Matsumoto, H., Sato, T., Kishi, S.: Outer nuclear layer thickness at the fovea determines visual outcomes in resolved central serous chorioretinopathy. Am. J. Ophthalmol. **148**(1), 105–110 (2009)
5. Ahlers, C., Geitzenauer, W., Stock, G., Golbaz, I., Schmidt-Erfurth, U., Prünte, C.: Alterations of intraretinal layers in acute central serous chorioretinopathy. Acta Ophthalmol. **87**(5), 511–516 (2009)
6. Novosel, J., Wang, Z., de Jong, H., van Velthoven, M., Vermeer, K.A., van Vliet, L.J.: Locally-adaptive loosely-coupled level sets for retinal layer and fluid segmentation in subjects with central serous retinopathy. In: 2016 IEEE 13th International Symposium on Biomedical Imaging (ISBI), pp. 702–705. IEEE (2016)
7. Iowa reference algorithms: Human and murine 3d OCT retinal layer analysis and display (Iowa institute for biomedical imaging, Iowa city, IA)
8. Garvin, M.K., Abramoff, M.D., Wu, X., Russell, S.R., Burns, T.L., Sonka, M.: Automated 3-d intraretinal layer segmentation of macular spectral-domain optical coherence tomography images. IEEE Trans. Med. Imaging **28**(9), 1436–1447 (2009)
9. Song, Q., Bai, J., Garvin, M.K., Sonka, M., Buatti, J.M., Wu, X.: Optimal multiple surface segmentation with shape and context priors. IEEE Trans. Med. Imaging **32**(2), 376–386 (2013)
10. Shi, F., Chen, X., Zhao, H., Zhu, W., Xiang, D., Gao, E., Sonka, M., Chen, H.: Automated 3-d retinal layer segmentation of macular optical coherence tomography images with serous pigment epithelial detachments. IEEE Trans. Med. Imaging **34**(2), 441–452 (2015)
11. Lang, A., Carass, A., Hauser, M., Sotirchos, E.S., Calabresi, P.A., Ying, H.S., Prince, J.L.: Retinal layer segmentation of macular oct images using boundary classification. Biomed. Opt. Express **4**(7), 1133–1152 (2013)

Retinal Image Quality Classification Using Fine-Tuned CNN

Jing Sun[1], Cheng Wan[1(✉)], Jun Cheng[2], Fengli Yu[1], and Jiang Liu[3]

[1] Nanjing University of Aeronautics and Astronautics, Nanjing, China
wanch@nuaa.edu.cn
[2] Institute for Infocomm Research, A*STAR, Singapore, Singapore
[3] Ningbo Institute of Material Technology and Engineering,
Chinese Academy of Sciences, Ningbo, China

Abstract. Retinal image quality classification makes a great difference in automated diabetic retinopathy screening systems. With the increase of application of portable fundus cameras, we can get a large number of retinal images, but there are quite a number of images in poor quality because of uneven illumination, occlusion and patients movements. Using the dataset with poor quality training networks for DR screening system will lead to the decrease of accuracy. In this paper, we first explore four CNN architectures (AlexNet, GoogLeNet, VGG-16, and ResNet-50) from ImageNet image classification task to our Retinal fundus images quality classification, then we pick top two networks out and jointly fine-tune the two networks. The total loss of the network we proposed is equal to the sum of the losses of all channels. We demonstrate the super performance of our proposed algorithm on a large retinal fundus image dataset and achieve an optimal accuracy of 97.12%, outperforming the current methods in this area.

Keywords: No-reference image quality assessment (NR-IQA) · Convolutional neural networks (CNN) · Retinal image · Fine-tuning

1 Introduction

Retinal fundus images play an important role in ophthalmology diagnosis. In screening systems for diseases such as diabetic retinopathy (DR), glaucoma, age-related macular degeneration (AMD), and vascular abnormalities, a clear fundus image is a prerequisite for the right diagnosis of the disease. Research communities have put great efforts towards the automation of computer screening systems which are able to promptly detect DR in fundus images. The success of these automatic diagnostic systems heavily rely on the quality of input images. However, in reality, due to some unavoidable disturbances, for instance, differing lighting condition, the type of image acquisition equipment, the situation of different individuals, the images we acquired will be blurred and affect the final accuracy of diagnosis. Consequently, it is indispensable to conduct image quality assessment (IQA) in the computer-aided screening system for ophthalmology diagnosis. Figure 1 shows four instances of poor quality images which will restrict the

© Springer International Publishing AG 2017
M.J. Cardoso et al. (Eds.): FIFI/OMIA 2017, LNCS 10554, pp. 126–133, 2017.
DOI: 10.1007/978-3-319-67561-9_14

subsequent analysis and DR diagnosis. These images are caused by occlusion, patients movements, underexposure or overexposure.

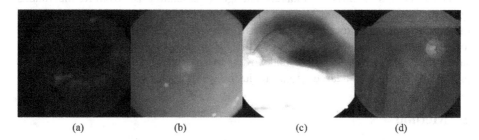

(a)   (b)   (c)   (d)

Fig. 1. Four instances of poor quality images in the retinal fundus image dataset.

Subjective evaluation and objective evaluation are two existing image quality evaluation methods [1]. In subjective method, quality is evaluated by organized groups of human observers to mark the distorted images, which is time-consuming and expensive. In general, objective image quality measures can be classified into three categories: full reference (FR) IQA, reduced-reference (RR) IQA and no-reference (NR) IQA. But, in practical applications, ideal image selected as the reference image is often not available or it costs too much, so NR-IQA is desirable. Many algorithms have been proposed in the literature for no-reference retinal fundus images quality assessment [2]. Earlier methods adopt hand-crafted features. Lee et al. [3] use a quality index Q which is calculated by the convolution of a template intensity histogram to measure the retinal image quality. Lalonde et al. [4] adopt the features which are based on the edge amplitude distribution and the pixel gray value to automatically assess the quality of retinal images. Yu et al. [5] propose a no-reference image quality assessment method to extract features and introduce the support vector machine (SVM) into image quality assessment. All these methods do not generalize well to a new dataset since they rely on some kind of hand-crafted features that are based on either geometric or structural quality parameters.

For the past decade, a deep architecture [6] has gained a great attention in various fields and convolutional neural networks is a new breakthrough due to its representational power. Different from the traditional handcraft-feature extracted methods, a deep learning model can find the hidden or latent high-level information inherent in the original features, which can be helpful to build a more robust model. [7–9] propose a new method for no-reference image quality assessment, and the structure of Le Kang's CNN has one convolutional layer with max and min pooling, two fully connected layers and an output node. However, these methods do not apply to retinal fundus images. [8, 9] leverage on learned supervised information using convolutional neural networks achieving high accuracy. Ruwan Tennakoon et al. adopt a shallow CNN architecture learning features for image quality classification, and use transfer learning achieving the same classification accuracy but they only fine-tune the AlexNet [10] architecture. Mahapatra D et al. propose a CNN architecture with five layers of convolution and max pooling operations. It needs a huge number of data to train the network otherwise it is going to lead to overfitting.

In this paper, we aim to conduct accurate classification for retinal fundus images quality. In our work, we explore four CNN architectures (AlexNet, GoogLeNet, VGG-16, and ResNet-50) from ImageNet image classification task to our Retinal fundus images quality classification, then we pick top two networks out and jointly fine-tune the two networks. The total loss of the network we proposed is equal to the sum of the losses of all channels. Our analysis shows that the proposed method can learn the necessary information relevant for IQA, and we demonstrate the superior performance of our proposed algorithm on a large retinal fundus image dataset.

2   Method

2.1   Image Preprocessing

The resolution of the original sample is 2592×1994 to 4752×3168. First, all the images are resized to 256×256 pixels. And then, in order to avoid the negative effects of different conditions such as lighting on the fundus images, the images are normalized as follows:

$$I(x,y) = \alpha I^o(x,y) + \beta Gaussian(x,y,\omega) * I^o(x,y) + \gamma \tag{1}$$

Where $*$ denotes the convolution operator, $Gaussian(x,y,\omega)$ represents the Gaussian filter with a standard deviation of ω, and the size of the Gaussian lowpass filter is $1 + floor(1 \times \omega)$. Where $floor(X)$ called the greatest integer function gives the largest integer less than or equal to X. The value of $\alpha, \beta, \omega, \gamma$ are designed empirically as $\alpha = 4, \beta = -4, \omega = 10, \gamma = 128$ respectively. In addition we clip the images to 90% size to reduce the black space on both sides of the retinal fundus images. We will evaluate the effect of image preprocessing in Sect. 3 showing that the preprocessed dataset achieves higher classification accuracy than the original dataset. The preprocessed images are shown in Fig. 2.

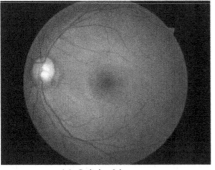   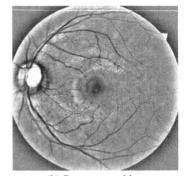

(a) Original image   (b) Preprocessed image

Fig. 2. One example from the training set.

2.2 Data Augmentation

Data augmentation is widely used in training a robust CNN network. We process the images by image rotation and horizontal reflections to increase the number of images. The training set are augmented with: random rotation 0–360°, random horizontal and vertical flips and random horizontal and vertical shifts, while the test set is only preprocessed without any augmentation. Through these operations, the training set is increased about 8 times.

2.3 Network Architecture

In practice, deep convolutional neural networks (DCNN) would not be randomly initializing trained from the beginning completely for the reason that the dataset with sufficient size to meet the needs of deep networks are quite rare. Therefore, it is common to pre-train a deep CNN based on a large dataset, and the weights of the trained DCNN are used as initial setting. In this work, the networks we used are all trained by the method of transfer learning. The four state-of-the-art CNN architectures and the Jointly Fine-tuned CNN model we proposed used for retinal fundus image quality classification are outlined below.

AlexNet: The AlexNet, proposed in [10] achieves significantly great performance in ImageNet Large Scale Visual Recognition Challenge (ILSVRC) 2012 and wins by a large margin with the next non-CNN method. The network consists of 5 convolutional layers, maxpooling layers, dropout layers, and 3 fully connected layers.

GoogLeNet: This is an architecture used by Szegedy et al. [11], which uses several "Inception" modules to create a deeper network with 22 layers while having much fewer parameters than other networks such as VGG and AlexNet.

VGG-16: The VGG-16 only uses 3×3 filters in convolutional layers and combine them as sequence of convolution to emulate the effect of lager receptive fields and decrease the number of parameters. Overall, VGG-16 is made up of 13 convolutional layers, five maxpooling layers and three fully-connected layers.

ResNet-50: ResNet, the winner of ILSVRC2015 with an incredible error rate of 3.6%, presents residual learning framework that each layer consists of a residual block and a skip connection bypassing to ease the training of networks. This architecture substantially deeper than those used previously with 50, 101 or 152 layers. In this paper, we evaluate the performance of ResNet-50. ResNet-50 has six modules called conv1, conv2 x, conv3 x, conv4 x, conv5 x and fc. Conv1 is a convolutional layer. Conv2 x, conv3 x, conv4 x and conv5 x consist of residual blocks with the number of 3, 4, 6, 3 respectively. And fc is a fully-connected layer.

Jointly Fine-tuned CNN: We pick top two networks (GoogLeNet and VGG-16) out and jointly fine-tune the two networks. This method was proposed in [12]. The total loss (Loss_All) of the network we proposed is equal to the sum of the losses of all channels. It is given by:

$$Loss\_All = Loss\_V + Loss\_G \tag{2}$$

Where Loss_V denotes the loss of VGG-16 and Loss_G denotes the loss of GoogLeNet. Since all networks update weights in parallel through backpropagation according to the total loss, they all influence each other's weight and bias values. The Jointly Fine-tuned CNN architecture we proposed is illustrated in Fig. 3. Through the two-channel CNN architecture, we get two accuracy rates: GoogLeNet accuracy rate and VGG-16 accuracy rate of Jointly Fine-tuned CNN architecture. We use JCNN_GoogLeNet Acc and JCNN_VGG-16 Acc denote them respectively.

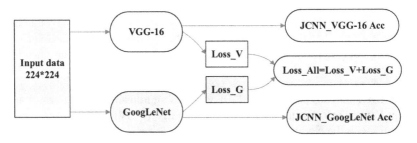

Fig. 3. The jointly fine-tuned CNN architectures.

2.4 Training

In this work, we train networks by the method of full fine-tune. It is done by removing the last fully connected layer and being replaced by a new one with 2 outputs and the learning rate of the last fully connected layer is increased ten times. In full fine-tune, the learning rate of every layer is left untouched except the last one. The purpose is to make the network has a good initial setting and iterate new data for the new fully connected layer for better learning. For AlexNet, GoogLeNet, VGG-16, and ResNet-50 architectures, the training data is directly put into the networks with pre-training weight parameters and the training process is carried on a workstation with a NVIDIA-GTX1080 GPU. The size of input data is 227×227 for AlexNet, and other networks is 224×224.

For the Jointly Fine-tuned CNN architectures, we fine-tune the GoogLeNet and VGG-16 networks at the same time, and each channel of CNN has the same data of input. The final loss is equal to the sum of the losses of all channels. It allows the backward propagation training method to broadcast the classifier gradients to all networks.

3   Experimental Result

The dataset used to verify the effectiveness of the proposed method is provided by the Kaggle coding website [13] (http://www.kaggle.com). The images in the dataset come from different models and types of cameras. Some images are shown as one would see the retina anatomically. Others are shown as one would see through a microscope condensing lens. It contains over 80000 images of diabetic retinopathy and a resolution of 2592 × 1994 to 4752 × 3168, but the proportion of the poor quality images in all images of Kaggle is small. We randomly select 2894 original samples and 2170 original samples from the dataset as training set and test set respectively. For the training set there are 1607 samples with label 1 and 1287 samples with label 0. After data augmentation, total 26046 images are used to train the CNN. The test set contains 1085 samples with label 1 and 1085 samples with label 0. All images are tagged by the professionals including doctors and experts in fields concerned based on if we can make diagnosis with the image, and the labels are determined under the majority's rule, in which label 1 represents the image with good quality and the attributes for carrying on the following DR screening and analysis, and label 0 stands for the poor quality images with the opposite attributes. The experiment results of this work are shown in Tables 1 and 2. We evaluate the performance of four state-of-the-art networks and the methods we proposed (denoted by JCNN) in this work.

Table 1.   Accuracy (Acc) and area under curve (AUC) for different methods.

Algorithm	Acc	AUC
AlexNet	96.53%	0.993
GoogLeNet	97.04%	0.994
VGG-16	96.87%	0.995
ResNet-50	96.20%	0.992
JCNN_GoogLeNet	97.00%	0.995
JCNN_VGG-16	**97.12%**	**0.995**

Table 2.   Comparison of image quality classification accuracy rate of GoogLeNet, GoogLeNet-NP, GoogLeNet-NA.

Algorithm	GoogLeNet	GoogLeNet-NP	GoogLeNet-NA
Accuracy	**97.04%**	96.12%	96.49%

We select the optimal accuracy rate (JCNN_VGG-16 Acc) as the final result of the JCNN architecture we proposed. The results show that jointly fine-tuning two-channel CNN architecture can achieve better accuracy than only fine-tuning a single convolutional neural networks, and GoogLeNet is superior to the other single channel networks. JCNN_GoogLeNet Acc achieves 97.00% which is close to GoogLeNet Acc, and JCNN_VGG-16 has achieved optimal accuracy of 97.12%, increasing 0.25% relative to VGG-16. Furthermore, all the fine-tuned networks have good performance, outperforming current methods we utilized on our dataset. This indicates that the knowledge learned from natural image can still transfer to make medical image quality classification effectively. The methods we proposed has been able to learn the necessary information for image quality classification in retinal images from convolutional neural networks.

For the Jointly Fine-tuned CNN (VGG16 + GoogLeNet), it makes the best network. This is a sensible choice because (1) the two network are among the best available networks, and (2) they are constructed based on two different architectural assumptions, making them relatively uncorrelated from the misclassification behavior standpoint.

We use GoogLeNet as the default architecture and evaluate the impact of image preprocessing and data augmentation. GoogLeNet has fewer parameters and higher accuracy than other single channel networks. Table 2 illustrates the accuracy rates of GoogLeNet, GoogLeNet-NP (model without preprocessing), GoogLeNet-NA (the model without data augmentation). We find that with the help of good preprocessing, the accuracy of the model increases about 1%. Data Augmentation is beneficial in our experiments, as evidenced by GoogLeNet(97.04%) versus GoogLeNet-NA (96.49%).

Figure 4 shows some classification results of fundus images. (a) and (b) show the correct classification results that the good-quality-images are classified as 1. (c) and (d) show the poor-quality-images are classified as 0. (e, f) and (g, h) shows the incorrect classification results that good-quality-images are classified as 0 and the poor-quality-images are classified as 1, respectively. It is worth noting that despite a few erroneous labels, our approach could learn a reliable feature representations and separates different image classes.

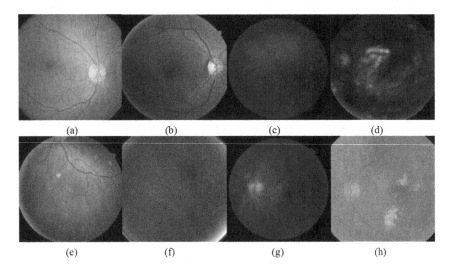

Fig. 4. Eight examples from the classification results.

4   Conclusions

In this paper, we evaluate the performance of different CNN architectures in retinal image quality classification and extensively evaluate two important factors on CNN architectures, preprocessing, data augmentation. It is evident from the results that the GoogLeNet architecture fine-tuned from ImageNet, with good image preprocessing and data augmentation performs better accuracy in the four state-of-the-art CNN architectures. Data augmentation and preprocessing is essential for medical image applications. Our experiments show the method we proposed that we pick top two networks out and jointly fine-tune the two networks is more useful for medical image analysis, with better performance than the other four CNNs. More importantly, the results of classification demonstrate that the knowledge learned from natural image can still transfer to make medical image quality classification effectively even though the disparity between them.

References

1. Ye, P.: Unsupervised feature learning framework for no-reference image quality assessment. In: IEEE Conference on Computer Vision and Pattern Recognition, vol. 157(10), pp. 1098–1105 (2012)
2. Wang, J.: A novel contourlet-based no-reference image quality assessment metric. In: International Research Association of Information and Computer Science 2014, pp. 3339–3352 (2014)
3. Lee, S.C., Wang, Y.: Automatic retinal image quality assessment and enhancement. In: Proceedings Spie, pp. 1581–1590 (1999)
4. Lalonde, M., Gagnon, L., Boucher, M.C.: Automatic visual quality assessment in optical fundus images. In: Proceedings of Vision Interface, vol. 18, pp. 437–450 (2001)
5. Yu, L., Tian, X., Li, T., Tian, J.: No-reference image quality assessment based on svm for video conferencing system. In: Lei, J., Wang, F.L., Li, M., Luo, Y. (eds.) Communications in Computer & Information Science 2016, vol. 345, pp. 555–560. Springer, Heidelberg (2012). doi:10.1007/978-3-642-35211-9_70
6. Suk, H.-I., Shen, D.: Deep learning-based feature representation for AD/MCI classification. In: Mori, K., Sakuma, I., Sato, Y., Barillot, C., Navab, N. (eds.) MICCAI 2013. LNCS, vol. 8150, pp. 583–590. Springer, Heidelberg (2013). doi:10.1007/978-3-642-40763-5_72
7. Kang, L., Ye, P.: Convolutional neutral networks for no-reference image quality assessment. In: IEEE Conference on Computer Vision and Pattern Recognition 2014, pp. 1733–1740 (2014)
8. Tennakoon, R., Mahapatra, D., Roy, P.: Image quality classification for DR screening using convolutional neural networks. In: Chen, X., Garvin, K. (eds.) OMIA 2016, pp. 113–120 (2016)
9. Mahapatra, D.: Retinal image quality classification using neurobiological models of the human visual system. In: Chen, X., Garvin, K. (eds.) OMIA 2016, pp. 97–104 (2016)
10. Krizhevsky, A., Sutskever, I.: ImageNet classification with deep convolutional neural networks. In: International Conference on Neural Information Processing Systems 2012, vol. 25, pp. 1097–1105 (2012)
11. Szegedy, W., Liu, Y.: Going deeper with convolutions. In: Computer Vision and Pattern Recognition 2015, pp. 1–9 (2015)
12. Mohammadi, M., Das, S.: SNN: Stacked Neural Networks. arXiv:1605.08612 (2016)
13. Pratt, H., Coenen, F.: Convolutional neural networks for diabetic retinopathy. Proc. Comput. Sci. **90**, 200–205 (2016)

Optic Disc Detection via Deep Learning in Fundus Images

Peiyuan Xu[1], Cheng Wan[1(✉)], Jun Cheng[2], Di Niu[1,3], and Jiang Liu[3]

[1] Nanjing University of Aeronautics and Astronautics, Nanjing 210000, China
wanch@nuaa.edu.cn
[2] Institute for Infocomm Research, A*STAR, Singapore, Singapore
[3] Ningbo Institute of Materials Technology and Engineering,
Chinese Academy of Sciences, Ningbo, China

Abstract. In order to realize the localization of optic disc (OD) effectively, a new end-to-end approach based on CNN was proposed in this paper. CNN is a revolutionary network structure which has shown its power in fields of computer vision like classification, object detection and segmentation. We intend to make use of CNN in the study of fundus images. Firstly, we use a basic CNN on which specialized layers are trained to find the pixels probably in OD region. Then we sort out candidate pixels furtherly via threshold. By calculating the center of gravity of these pixels, the location of OD is finally determined. The method has been tested on three databases including ORIGA, MESSIDOR and STARE. In totally 1240 images to be tested, the OD of 1193 are successfully located with the rate of 96.2%. Besides the accuracy, the time cost is another advantage. It takes only 0.93 s to test one image on average in STARE and 0.51 s in MESSIDOR.

Keywords: Optic disc localization · Convolution neural networks · Retinal fundus image

1 Introduction

The optic disc (OD) is one of the main physiological structures of the retina, from which optic nerve and blood vessels stretch to the surrounding areas. In fundus camera pictures, these blocks are reflected as a round bright yellow area, where few but thick blood vessels also exist. Researchers pay attention to the automatic detection of the OD for the reason that diagnosis of some ocular fundus lesions are based on its correct detection [1, 2]. The main application of this approach is to pre-process the retinal images for further studies such as the segmentation of optic disc or the detection of Macular region. Till now, to detect OD, there have occurred several analysis techniques, which can be divided into two categories: early methods mainly take the characteristics of the OD like brightness, contrast, shape etc. for example, the method in [3] locate the OD by searching for the center of rectangle region in which the amplitude of variation of gray level is highest. In [4, 5], Hough transform, which is convenient for specific shape object detection, is used to detected the OD region. These early methods can simply and timely get the results because the OD is usually brighter than other areas in fundus camera pictures and occurs as a regular ellipse. However, considering that the retinal images are not always high quality and several diseases may lead to the change of OD [19, 20], these

© Springer International Publishing AG 2017
M.J. Cardoso et al. (Eds.): FIFI/OMIA 2017, LNCS 10554, pp. 134–141, 2017.
DOI: 10.1007/978-3-319-67561-9_15

methods might fail. The other methods can be described as the methods based on vascular feature detection. The OD, where the main blood vessels converge in the retinal, can be easily detected when vascular features are known. In [6], two parabolas are used to describe the blood vessels in the left and right direction of OD. The center of OD is just located in the public vertex of two parabolas. In [7], the OD region is determined via calculating the confluence of blood vessels. Though the methods above could get relatively high detection accuracy, they should make sure that the detection of vessels is exact, which in low quality or abnormal images can be hard to realize. Besides, the OD detection algorithms based on vascular feature detection are usually complex and time-costing.

Except for two main methods mentioned above, there are several methods considering multiple features in OD region. The description of multi-source information about OD characteristics is undoubtedly helpful to improve the accuracy and robustness of OD detection. However, simple threshold or models could not make full use of these information. To overcome this drawback, supervised learning method, which requires great effort to design such a template that can integrate multiple information, are used. Supervised learning method increases the complexity of the OD detection algorithm, which is not suitable for real time applications.

Overall, the speed and accuracy of OD detection are hard to balance. The methods with appearance characteristics, which are fast, could not get a high accuracy in abnormal fundus images. In contrast, the methods based on vascular feature detection could get a relatively high accuracy in no matter normal or abnormal fundus images, with the cost of high algorithmic complexity and long locating time. Therefore, how to improve the accuracy and reduce the complexity of the algorithm as well is worth in further research. In this paper, we propose an end-to-end method for automatic localization of OD based on the Convolution Neural Network (CNN). The OD features are learned through combination of features from different layers of CNN. After this, each pixel of image will get a probability to judge whether it belongs to OD region. In order to avoid interference, only points with high probability are picked as candidate points. Then, we calculate the center of these points and finally the location of OD is determined. The rest of this paper is organized as follows. In Sect. 2 we show the details of our proposed method. Section 3 shows the experimental results and discussions. In Sect. 4, the conclusions are mentioned here.

2   Proposed Method

2.1   Preprocessing

All images in training set are firstly subtracted the mean value of each color channel. Then, these images are resized into a fixed size of 400×600, which makes the training faster and reduce the computing complexity. Considering the condition of GPU, this size can be set as other values. There's no need to pre-process the images in testing set for the reason that pre-process will not lead to obvious changes in testing results. However, restricted to hardware condition, images of ORIGA and MESSIDOR are resized into the same size as training set. The images of STARE are kept as the same.

2.2   Feature Representation by CNN

We leverage a successful deep learning architectures called VGG network, which originally used for the classification of natural images. VGG network is similar to AlexNet, which is a classic CNN. They both consist of 5 blocks. Between each block, there is pooling layer. Each block of VGG network contains several convolution layers with 3×3 size filters, differs from AlexNet which only has one convolution layer with 7×7 size filter. This can be seen as imposing a regularization on the 7×7 filters, forcing them to have a decomposition through the 3×3 filters [8]. because of the reduce of filter size, VGG has much more channels than AlexNet, which is considered to lead to higher accuracy.

Considering that the CNN are used as feature detector, we remove the fully connected layers of VGG network. The architecture remained are mainly consisted by convolutional layers with Rectified Linear Unit (ReLU) activations and max pooling layers. These layers have been pre-trained on millions of images. Features detected by deep blocks are rougher than shallow blocks duo to the decrease in size. We decide to combine features from 3 deeper blocks rather than any one of them to get better results. These features are then forwarded into deconvolution layers and crop layers to be the same size as original images. The flow chart of our method is shown in Fig. 1.

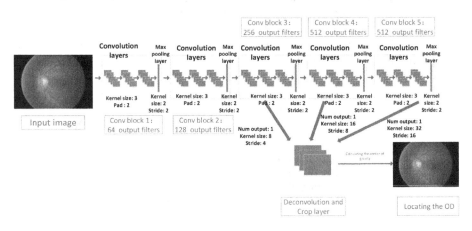

Fig. 1. The proposed model architecture

The train starts by loading the weights of VGG network. Then, input images are put into the designed network. We extract the features of last three pooling layers, which are then forwarded into corresponding deconvolution layers. the last layers, combined by these deconvolution layers, output the probabilities of each pixel of the whole image. The class of each pixel can be determined by setting a threshold. To avoid interference, we set a high threshold $T = 0.9$, which means the network judges this pixel as OD with the probability of 0.9. Finally, by calculating center of gravity of the pixels above, we realize the localization of OD. In this condition, even there are several pixels are missclassified, the center will still in OD region. The center of gravity can be calculated as following:

$$X_c = \frac{\sum P(x_i)}{\sum P_i} \qquad Y_c = \frac{\sum P(y_i)}{\sum P_i} \tag{1}$$

where P_i represents the value, x_i, y_i are the location of pixel.

To train the network, the cross entropy loss is adopted to update the weights through descent back-propagation. Cross entropy loss is used to measure the similarity between two probability distributions. It can be defined as following:

$$J(\theta) = -\frac{1}{m} \sum_{i=1}^{m} y^{(i)} \log(h_\theta(x^{(i)})) + (1 - y^{(i)}) \log(1 - h_\theta(x^{(i)})) \tag{2}$$

where, input images are $X^{(i)} = (1, x_1^{(i)}, x_2^{(i)}, \cdots, x_p^{(i)})^T$ and $y^{(i)}$ are predicted labels, θ denotes the parameters of CNN. Here, $\theta = (\theta_0, \theta_1, \theta_2, \cdots, \theta_p)^T$. The hypothesis function is defined as $h_\theta(x^{(i)}) = \frac{1}{1 + e^{-\theta^T x^{(i)}}}$.

At training time, we fine-tune the entire network with 880 images (305 from ORIGA and 575 from MESSIDOR, which will be introduced later) for 150000 iterations. The input images are operated via CNN with batches of size 1. We use a small learning rate ($lr = 10^{-9}$, which will decrease as training time increases). Stochastic gradient descent is used to minimize error function with momentum $= 0.9$.

At testing time, the OD detector is realized on 2.8 GHz Intel Xeon E5-1603 v4 CPU with GTX 1080 using python. The last layer of network outputs the probability of each pixel of testing image. Then we set a threshold $T = 0.9$, which removes most of noise and ensure that pixels remained are mostly in OD region. Finally, we get the location of OD via calculating the center of these pixels. Considering that some researchers like [9, 10] proposed that in different fundus images, the diameter of OD is about 1/5 to 1/8 of the ROI region. So, based on the center point determined, we draw a Rectangular box with length of about 1/4 of ROI region (here we set length = 100 in ORIGA and MESSIDOR. In STARE, we set as 150).

3 Experiments and Results

3.1 Databases

The approach has been tested on the following three datasets. ORIGA [11], MESSIDOR [12] and STARE [13]. MESSIDOR and STARE are available publically, among which MESSIDOR totally includes 1200 images with three sizes: 1440×960, 2200×1488, 2304×1536. Differs from MESSIDOR which contains relatively high quality images with few lesion, STARE includes many images with lesion and low quality. A large number of OD detection methods have been tested and compared on this image dataset. ORIGA is a database with 650 images. All images in ORIGA with the size of 3072×2048 are captured via a high resolution retinal fundus camera and well selected, which ensure the quality.

3.2 Results and Discussions

Table 1 shows the accuracy of our method in different datasets. Of all the 1240 fundus images, 1193 images can find the right OD location and the success rate is 96.2%. In addition, only the rectangle box contains the whole OD region, which comes from label image, can be seen as success. In Table 2 we compare different methods in MESSIDOR. Experimental results show that our method could achieve the accuracy of 99.43% with 0.51 s per image, which is better than other methods. In Table 3, it can be seen that the method based on vascular characteristics like [17] could achieve a high accuracy with the cost of long processing time. The methods making use of appearance information like [5] are not competitive in accuracy comparing with other methods for that the information they use are not stable during different images. Considering both accuracy and processing speed, our method or method in [18] are more practical. The results of other methods mentioned above are original ones in their papers.

Table 1. The accuracy of our method in different datasets

Datasets	Images	Abnormality	Accuracy
ORIGA	314	–	100%
MESSIDOR	526	54.5%	99.43%
STARE	400	91%	89%
Total	1240	–	96.2%

Table 2. The accuracy of different methods in MESSIDOR database

Methods	Accuracy	Running time
Yu [14]	99%	6.6 s
Alghamdi [15]	99.20%	–
Zubair et al. [16]	98.65%	3.5 s
Our method	99.43%	0.51 s

Table 3. The accuracy of different methods in STARE database

Methods	Accuracy	Running time
Foracchia [17]	97.5%	120 s
ZHANG [18]	91.4%	13.2 s
Haar [5]	67.9%	–
Alghamdi [15]	86.71%	–
Our method	89%	0.93 s

Our method could get a high accuracy except STARE. This is because STARE is a dataset containing many images with serious lesions. In STARE, many optic discs of fundus images are damaged and some optic discs of fundus images can only be partially observed. Besides, images with the bright yellow lesions which is similar to the OD in appearance are also contained. Of all images failed to detected by our method, images with low contrast are the most common situation.

Restricted to the length of the article, only some of the representative fundus images were selected, which can be seen in Fig. 2. In these samples, all kinds of conditions, in which OD are hard to be detected correctly, are included. (a), (b), (e) and (f) are images with regions produced by lesions. (d), (j), (l) are images caused by bleeding in small or large scales. (i) and (l) are images in which OD were covered by lesions. (k) is the classic image that OD region locates in the edge of ROI in fundus image. (c), (g) and (h) are those with low contrast. This shows the power of our method in detecting OD region from abnormality images.

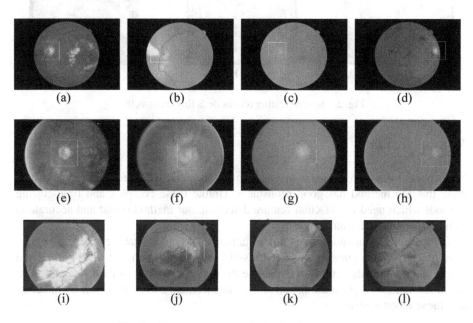

Fig. 2. Several testing results hard to be detected.

In Fig. 3, we show some images detected incorrectly. From the samples, (a)–(c) are because of low contrast, which accounts for the most of error detected images. in (d)–(e), OD region, covered by lesion, is hard to identify. Though detecting is failed, the region given by our method is surrounding the OD. We can conjecture that our method has learned some information of vessels. In (f), our method judges the lesion region as OD which are quite similar in appearance, from which we could infer that the main features CNN learns are mainly about the appearance of OD. Further research is needed to make the network learns more about vessels.

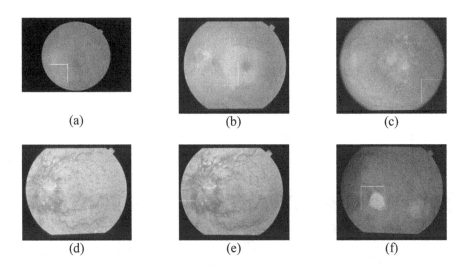

(a)   (b)   (c)

(d)   (e)   (f)

Fig. 3. Several testing results detecting incorrectly.

4   Conclusion

In this paper, we proposed a new approach for OD detection. Current experiment results show that the method has good robustness. Unlike those complex and time-costing methods which need for vascular feature detection, our method is fast and accurate in both normal and abnormal images.

In the future, we are going to evaluate our method on more database in order to obtain more objective and comprehensive test results. What's more, model will be improved by exploiting other algorithms to overcome the drawback of our method. We also want to add the method of pre-training and image enhancement before the whole architecture to achieve a better result.

References

1. Zhang, Z., Lee, B.H., Liu, J., Wong, D.W.K., et al.: Optic disc region of interest localization in fundus image for Glaucoma detection in ARGALI. In: Industrial Electronics & Applications, pp. 1686–1689 (2010)
2. Cheng, J., Liu, J., Xu, Y., Yin, F., Wong, D.W.K., Tan, N.M., Tao, D., Cheng, C.Y., Aung, T., Wong, T.Y.: Superpixel classification based optic disc and optic cup segmentation for glaucoma screening. IEEE Trans. on Med. Imaging **32**(6), 1019–1032 (2013)
3. Boyce, J.F., Cook, H.L., et al.: Automated location of the optic disk, fovea, and retinal blood vessels from digital color fundus images. Br. J. Ophthalmol. **83**(8), 902–910 (1999)
4. Barrett, S.F., Naess, E., Molvik, T.: Employing the hough transform to locate the optic disk. Biomed. Sci. Instrum. **37**(1), 81–86 (2001)
5. Haar, F.T.: Automatic localization of the optic disc in digital color images of the human retina. Utrecht University, Utrecht (2005)

6. Osareh, A.: Automated identification of diabetic retinal exudates and the optic disc. University of Bristol, Bristol (2004)
7. Lalonde, M., Beaulieu, M., Gagnon, L.: Fast and robust optic disk detection using pyramidal decomposition and Hausdorff based template matching. IEEE Trans. Med. Imaging **20**(11), 1193–1200 (2001)
8. Simonyan, K., Zisserman, A.: Very deep convolutional networks for large-scale image recognition. In: Computer Science (2014)
9. Li, H., Chutatape, O.: Automatic location of optic disk in retinal images. In: International Conference on Image Processing, vol. 2, pp. 837–840 (2001)
10. Klein, R., Klein, B., Moss, S., Davis, M., et al.: The Wisconsin epidemiologic study of diabetic retinopathy II. Arch. Ophthalmol. **102**(4), 520–526 (1984)
11. Zhang, Z., Yin, F., Liu, J., Wong, D.W.K., Tan, N.M., Lee, B.H., Cheng, J., Wong, T.Y.: Origa-light: an online retinal fundus image database for glaucoma analysis and research. In: International Conference of the IEEE Engineering in Medicine and Biology Society, pp. 3065–3068 (2010)
12. Decencière, E., et al.: Feedback on a publicly distributed database: the Messidor database. Image Anal. Stereology **33**(3), 231–234 (2014)
13. Hoover, A.: Locating blood vessels in retinal images by piecewise threshold probing of a matched filter response. IEEE Trans. Med. Imaging **19**(3), 203–210 (2000)
14. Yu, H., Barriga, E.S., Agurto, C., et al.: Fast localization and segmentation of optic disk in retinal images using directional matched filtering and level sets. IEEE Trans. Inf. Technol. Biomed. **16**(4), 644–657 (2012)
15. Alghamdi, H., Tang, H., Waheeb, S., Peto, T.: Automatic optic disc abnormality detection in fundus images: a deep learning approach. In: OMIA 2016, Held in Conjunction with MICCAI 2016, Athens, Greece, Iowa Research Online, pp. 17–24 (2016)
16. Zubair, M., Yamin, A., Khan, S.A.: Automated detection of optic disc for the analysis of retina using color fundus image. In: IEEE International Conference on Imaging Systems and Techniques, Beijing (2013). doi:10.1109/IST.2013.6729698
17. Foracchia, M., Grisan, E., Ruggeri, A.: Detection of optic disc in retinal images by means of a geometrical model of vessel structure. IEEE Trans. Med. Imaging **23**(10), 1189–1195 (2004)
18. Zhang, D.B., Yi, Y., Zhao, Y.Y.: Projection based optic disc detection method for retinal fundus images. Chin. J. Biomed. Eng. **32**(4), 477–483 (2013)
19. Anastasi, M., Lodato, G., Cillino, S.: VECPs and optic disc damage in diabetes. Doc. Ophthalmol. Adv. Ophthalmol. **66**(4), 331–336 (1987)
20. Artes, P.H., Chauhan, B.C.: Longitudinal changes in the visual field and optic disc in glaucoma. Prog. Retinal Eye Re. **24**(3), 333 (2005)

3D Choroid Neovascularization Growth Prediction with Combined Hyperelastic Biomechanical Model and Reaction-Diffusion Model

Chang Zuo[1], Fei Shi[1], Weifang Zhu[1], Haoyu Chen[2], and Xinjian Chen[1(✉)]

[1] School of Electronic and Information Engineering, Soochow University,
Suzhou, Jiangsu Province, China
xjchen@suda.edu.cn
[2] Shantou International Eye Center, Shantou, Guangdong Province, China

Abstract. Choroid neovascularization (CNV) usually causes varying degrees of irreversible retinal degradation, central scotoma, metamorphopsia or permanent visual lose. If early prediction can be achieved, timely clinical treatment can be applied to prevent further deterioration. In this paper, a CNV growth prediction framework based on physiological structure revealed in noninvasive optical coherence tomography (OCT) images is proposed. The method consists of three steps: pre-processing, CNV growth modeling and prediction. For growth modeling, a new combination model is proposed. The hyperelastic biomechanical model and reaction-diffusion model with treatment factor are combined through mass effect. For parameter optimization, the genetic algorithm is applied. The proposed method was tested on a data set with 6 subjects, each with 12 longitudinal 3-D images. The experimental results showed that the average TPVF, FPVF and Dice coefficient of $80.0 \pm 7.62\%$, $23.4 \pm 8.36\%$ and $78.9 \pm 7.54\%$ could be achieved, respectively.

Keywords: CNV growth prediction · Reaction-diffusion model · Hyperelastic bio-mechanical model

1 Introduction

Choroid neovascularization (CNV) is the proliferation of blood vessels from the choroid capillary, which extends through the stomium of the Bruch membrane. It is the cause of wet age-related macular degeneration (AMD), and can be commonly seen in central serous retinopathy (CSC) or pathologic myopic. The symptoms can be decreased visual acuity, central scotoma, metamorphopsia or permanent visual lose. Although contributing factors of CNV are not well understood, elimination of intraretinal and subretinal fluid usually helps for visual acuity gains. Vascular endothelial growth factor (VEGF) [1] is considered

---

This work has not been submitted to any conference or journal.

© Springer International Publishing AG 2017
M.J. Cardoso et al. (Eds.): FIFI/OMIA 2017, LNCS 10554, pp. 142–149, 2017.
DOI: 10.1007/978-3-319-67561-9_16

to be crucial with the development of CNV. The usual practice of treating CNV is repeated anti-VEGF injections.

The goal of CNV growth prediction is to accurately model the process, which can be achieved by modeling the change of physiological structure modeling based on optical coherence tomography (OCT) volumes. If early noninvasive prediction can be achieved, quantitative analysis can be performed to help determine the number of injections needed and the best injection time. Such personalized anti-VEGF treatment can both improve the curative effect and reduce the risk of intravitreal injections.

The traditional methods for prediction of CNV progress were overly focused on measurement and comparison but modeling, such as comparison of choroidal thickness [2], and estimation on echographic parameters with confocal indocyanine green angiography (ICGA) imaging [3]. Their evaluation indicators are relatively simple and show less predictive information. As for model-based CNV growth prediction, researches involved were limited. In [4, 5], a reaction-diffusion equation based finite-element-method (FEM) was proposed. By solving the partial differential equations (PDE), growth model can be simulated. However, the performance may be limited by use of the linear mechanical model, which is proper for small deformation (<5%) but not for large one. On the other hand, tumor growth modeling was more widely researched. The method in [6] was established on the isotropic material hypothesis but the framework in diffusion couldn't solve the nonlinear deformation of CNV growth. In [7], a mixed model was used, but it was not actually an integrated model, but a combination of the results of two separate models. What's more, the different image modality makes it difficult to apply these methods for CNV growth prediction based on OCT images.

Aiming at above growth modeling issues, we propose a method based on 3D longitudinal optical coherence tomography (OCT) image. By combining reaction-diffusion equation and hyperelastic biomechanical model, vascular proliferation and the resulting interaction between CNV and its surroundings can be effectively modeled. In this paper, personalized treatment factor is added in reaction-diffusion equation, which makes drug-induced treatment also contribute to the growth modeling. Besides, mass effect [8] is used for combining reaction-diffusion equation with biomechanical model of hyperelastic materials [9]. Therefore, the combined model we propose can provide both different structural information and functional information of hyper-viscoelastic materials simultaneously in CNV growth prediction.

2   Methods

The flow-chart of the proposed method is showed in Fig. 1. The prediction takes place for the last time point, and is based on model learning from the previous time points. It is mainly composed of three steps: pre-processing, CNV growth modeling and prediction. In growth modeling (Fig. 1(a)), mass effect is applied for combining the hyperelastic biomechanical (H-B) model with the reaction-diffusion (R-D) equation with treatment factor. The genetic algorithm (GA) is used for optimizing the parameters [10]. In prediction stage (Fig. 1(b)), the model parameter of the last time point is obtained by curve fitting the optimized parameters from the previous time points, and then the

predicted CNV region is calculated based on the combined model. The prediction accuracy is evaluated by comparing the prediction with the ground truth label of CNV region.

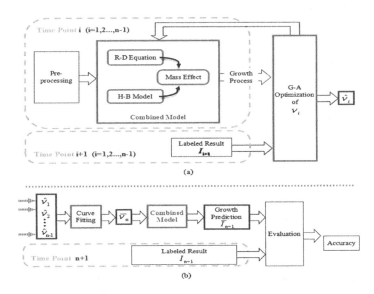

Fig. 1. Flowchart. (a) pre-processing and modeling, (b) prediction. R-D equation is combined
with H-B model by using mass effect. GA optimization is based on prediction from time point i
and the ground truth label of time point i + 1. v_i stands for the parameters to be estimated. $\hat{v}_i$ is the
optimal parameter.

2.1   Pre-processing

Pre-processing is applied to deal with the displacement of the longitudinal data and to
locate the position of regions of interest. It includes registration, segmentation and
meshing. Registration is first conducted on 3D OCT images using a rigid transformation
[5]. To model the characteristics of different physiological structures, each 3D image is
manually segmented into four parts: CNV region, outer retinal layer, inner retinal layer
and choroid layer. Then ISO2Mesh method [11] is used to mesh CNV volumes and
retinal layers.

2.2   CNV Growth Modeling

In modeling part, both structural and nonlinear functional information is required.
Reaction-diffusion model describes the substances distributed in space and their
temporal development. It is utilized to describe CNV invasion or shrinking, which can
be solved using FEM. For proliferation, most biological tissues can be modeled as hyper-
viscoelastic materials. Thus the hyperelastic biomechanical model with mass effect is
used to simulate mutual forces between CNV region and the surrounding tissues.

Invasion and proliferation with reaction-diffusion equation. In this paper, the FEM-based [12] reaction-diffusion equation with logistic growth [13] is used for CNV growth modeling, which can be formulated as:

$$\frac{\partial c}{\partial t} = \nabla \cdot (\mathbf{D}\nabla c) + \rho c(1 - c) - f_{\text{thera}} \tag{1}$$

The first and second term stand for CNV invasion and the logistic proliferation [14], where c is the CNV concentration. the anisotropic diffusion tensor $\mathbf{D}$ contains three components: D_x, D_y, D_z. ρ is the proliferate rate. When anti-VEGF treatment is applied, the third term is added in the equation as the therapy term.

$$f_{\text{thera}} = (\frac{\alpha}{1 + e^{\lambda \cdot t}} + FSV) \cdot c \tag{2}$$

where $\frac{\alpha}{2} + FSV$ stands for the initial concentration value, FSV is a constant representing the final stability value, t is the time point of treatment and λ is the ratio for efficacy. At the beginning of treatment (with small t), the concentration curve can be approximately linear [15]. Substituting (2) into (1), we have (3):

$$\frac{\partial c}{\partial t} = \nabla \cdot (\mathbf{D}\nabla c) + \rho c(1 - c) - (\frac{\alpha}{1 + e^{\lambda \cdot t}} + FSV) \cdot c \tag{3}$$

The initial value c is set empirically as 4.0×10^3 [4], which is also the threshold for the final prediction of CNV volume.

Hyperelastic Biomechanical model. The hyperelastic mechanical model can be used for simulating stress-strain in large and nonlinear deformations [16]. We use Saint-Venant-Kirchhoff constitutive law to model the slightly incompressible and isotropic material of CNV:

$$\varepsilon = \frac{1}{2}(F^T F - I) \tag{4}$$

$$\psi(\varepsilon) = \frac{1}{2}\kappa(J - 1)^2 + \frac{1}{2}\mu Tr(I_1 - 3) \tag{5}$$

In strain energy density function (4), ε is the Green-Lagrange strain tensor, and F is the deformation gradient with $J = det(F)$. By $F = (J^{1/3}I)\bar{F} = J^{1/3}\bar{F}$, F decomposed multiplicatively to a isochoric deformation component $\bar{F}$, and $J^{1/3}I$ is the volumetric deformation tensor [9]. In (5), the first and the second term account for the volumetric and isochoric elastic response. I_1 is the first invariant of the right Cauchy-Green deformation tensor. Tr represents the trace, κ and μ are the bulk modulus and shear modulus respectively. The second Piola-Kirchhoff (PKII) stress tensor ($\partial\psi/\partial\varepsilon$) can provide the nonlinear stress-strain relation [16]. In our model, the four regions (CNV, inner retina, outer retina, and choroid as segmented) have different mechanical parameters, e.g. diffusion coefficient, elastic tensor, etc.

Mass effect. As deformation rate of CNV growth is small enough to remain in internal equilibrium, the static equilibrium equation is used to simulate mass and volume changes during the process, which relates the normalized anisotropic concentration (c) in reaction-diffusion equation and the σ in hyperelastic mechanical model [9]:

$$div(\sigma) + f = 0; \; f = -\xi \nabla c \tag{6}$$

where $\sigma = J^{-1} FSF^T$ represents the Cauchy stress tensor, f stands for the gradient force generated by c, and ξ represents a constant that depends on the biological property.

2.3   Genetic Algorithm for Parameter Optimization

In this study, we use GA for parameter optimization of $v_i = \{D_x, D_y, D_z, \rho, a, c\}$ so that the following objective function [13] is minimized.

$$R(v_i) = \sum_i w_1 \cdot (1 - TPVF) + w_2 \cdot FPVF \tag{7}$$

In (7), w_1 and w_2 represent weights of the true-positive volume fraction (TPVF) and false-positive volume fraction (FPVF), and $w_1 + w_2 = 1$. $TPVF = \dfrac{ov_{i+1,c}}{I_{i+1,c}}$ and $FPVF = \dfrac{\bar{I}_{i+1,c} - ov_{i+1,c}}{I_{i+1,c}}$, where $ov_{i+1,c} = \bar{I}_{i+1,c} \cap I_{i+1}$ is the overlapping between ground truth label in time point $n = i + 1$ (I_{i+1}) and the prediction $(\bar{I}_{i+1,c})$ based on $I_{i,c}$. In this paper $w_1 = w_2 = 0.5$ are used.

In GA, the population size, iteration times/generations and tolerance was set as 20, 200 and 1e-100 respectively. For other parameters, empirical values are adopted [9, 17] with $\kappa_{CNV} = 7$ kPa, $\kappa_{choroid} = 6$ kPa, $\kappa_{outer\_layer} = 6$ kPa, $\kappa_{inner\_layer} = 0.7$ kPa and $\mu_{CNV} = \mu_{choroid} = 5 \times 10^3$ N/m^2, $\mu_{others} = 1 \times 10^3$ N/m^2.

2.4   Prediction

For each time point from 1 to $n - 1$, the optimal parameters $\hat{v}_i$ ($i = 1 \sim n - 1$) is obtained by GA based on comparison of the prediction $\bar{I}_{i+1,c}$ and the ground truth label I_{i+1}.

Then B-spline interpolation is used for curve fitting $\{\hat{v}_1, \hat{v}_2 \dots \hat{v}_{n-1}\}$ to achieve parameter $\bar{v}_n$ of the last time point. Based on $\bar{v}_n$, the prediction image of the last time point $\bar{I}_{n+1}$ is calculated using the combined H-B and R-D model. Finally, the prediction accuracy is evaluated by comparing $\bar{I}_{n+1}$ with the ground truth label I_{n+1}.

3   Experimental Results

In our study, subjects were randomly put into two groups: treatment group (T-group) and reference group (R-group) in Fig. 2, respectively. They had different treatment plans of repeated injection of anti-VEGF drugs — Conbercept (KH902) — 0.5 mg/eye/time (Fig. 2). OCT images of patients were collected by ZEISS OCT scanner with $512 \times 1024 \times 128$ voxels of $11.72 \times 5.86 \times 15.6$ um^3 voxel size.

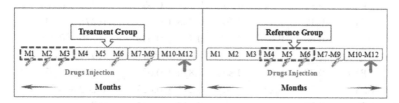

Fig. 2. Two different therapy groups during the same interval: M1 to M12 mean Month1 to Month12. Monthly treatment is illustrated in purple. In months that not marked, placebo was injected. The orange arrow means the last month, which is the time of assessment.

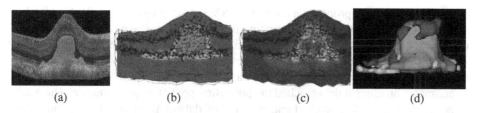

(a) (b) (c) (d)

Fig. 3. Results. (a) Segmentation results: green, blue, yellow, red and cyan in B-scan represent CNV area, intra-retinal fluid, choroid layer, outer and inner retinal layer. (b) The sectional view of concentration slice after growth modeling. (c) The Mises stress distribution slices. (d) Comparison of prediction result (blue) and ground truth label (yellow) of CNV region, where green represents the overlapping. (Color figure online)

The results of CNV growth prediction are shown in Table 1 and Fig. 3. Representation of concentration is illustrated in Fig. 3(b). The warmer color in the center represents the denser area. Stress distribution shown in Fig. 3(c) reflected the pressure on the surroundings and the border of the CNV region. Navy blue indicates almost no forces are transmitted to the outside. Dark red means great stress in that region. The 3D overlapping between prediction result and ground truth in Fig. 3(d) indicates high accuracy.

Table 1 shows the promising performance of the proposed method in terms of TPVF, FPVF and Dice coefficient. The results are compared with those achieved by single reaction-diffusion (R-D) model [5]. For both groups, by the proposed combined model, the average accuracy has been improved. The performance was worst for the 2nd patient. In this case, in each period, the volume morphology had striking differences with the previous once, which brought accuracy decrease. The experimental results showed that the average TPVF, FPVF and Dice coefficient of $80.0 \pm 7.62\%$, $23.4 \pm 8.36\%$ and $78.9 \pm 7.54\%$ could be achieved, respectively.

Table 1. Results of CNV prediction in TPVF, FPVF and Dice coefficient (DC).

	Patient-Label			Mean ± Std	
T-group	*1*	*2*	*3*	*Combined model*	*R-D model*
TPVF	0.86	0.641	0.83	0.777 ± 0.097	0.732 ± 0.031
FPVF	0.12	0.39	0.264	0.258 ± 0.11	0.275 ± 0.046
DC	0.861	0.628	0.808	0.765 ± 0.099	0.730 ± 0.036
R-group	*1*	*2*	*3*	*Combined model*	*R-D model*
TPVF	0.797	0.871	0.802	0.824 ± 0.034	0.776 ± 0.026
FPVF	0.182	0.249	0.205	0.211 ± 0.027	0.242 ± 0.021
DC	0.806	0.836	0.8	0.814 ± 0.016	0.768 ± 0.024

4   Conclusion and Discussion

In this paper, we have proposed a novel 3D CNV growth prediction method, which by using mass effect in slow deformation combines a bio-mechanical model of hyperelastic material with reaction diffusion equation with personalized treatment factor. Genetic algorithm is applied for parameter optimization. Prediction results can help ophthalmologists to assess the progress of CNV, and to make personalized treatment plans. Experiments on clinical data reached the promising prediction performance. There are some limitations in this work. First, the size of dataset is small. We are currently collecting more data and we'll test the method in a bigger dataset in future work. From current results, we are unable to conclude how differently the proposed algorithm performs for the two groups. Clinically, the sensitivity to treatment varies from person to person. Therefore, we infer that the accuracy of the prediction is more subject-related, and is also affected by image quality. In the future, to make the method more robust, we'll improve both the pre-processing and the flexibility of the model. Secondly, in this preliminary study, manual segmentation was used in pre-processing. Future work will also include developing automatic segmentation methods to reduce manual intervention while keeping the accuracy of prediction.

References

1. Spilsbury, K., Garrett, K.L., Shen, W.Y., Constable, I.J., Rakoczy, P.E.: Overexpression of Vascular Endothelial Growth Factor (VEGF) in the retinal pigment epithelium leads to the development of choroidal neovascularization. Am. J. Pathol. **157**(1), 135–144 (2000)
2. Ahn, S.J., Woo, S.J., Kim, K.E., Park, K.H.: Association between choroidal morphology and anti-vascular endothelial growth factor treatment outcome in myopic choroidal neovascularization. Invest. Ophthalmol. Vis. Sci. **54**(3), 2115–2122 (2013)
3. Mueller, A.J., Freeman, W.R., Schaller, U.C., Kampik, A., Folberg, R.: Complex microcirculation patterns detected by confocal indocyanine green angiography predict time to growth of small choroidal melanocytic tumors. Ophthalmology **109**(12), 2207–2214 (2002)

4. Zhu, S., Chen, X., Shi, F., Xiang, D., Zhu, W., Chen, H.: 3D choroid neovascularization growth prediction based on reaction-diffusion model. In: Gimi, B., Krol, A. (eds.) Proceedings of SPIE 9788, Medical Imaging 2016: Biomedical Applications in Molecular, Structural, and Functional Imaging, San Diego, California, United States, vol. 9788 (2016)
5. Zhu, S., Shi, F., Xiang, D., Zhu, W., Chen, X., Chen, H.: Choroid neovascularization growth prediction with treatment based on reaction-diffusion model in 3D OCT images. IEEE J. Biomed. Health Inf. **PP**(99), 2168–2194 (2017)
6. Clatz, O., Sermesant, M., Bondiau, P.-Y., Delingette, H., Warfield, S.K., Malandain, G., Ayache, N.: Realistic simulation of the 3D growth of brain tumors in MR images coupling diffusion with biomechanical deformation. IEEE Trans. Med. Imaging **24**(10), 1334–1346 (2005)
7. Chen, X., Summers, R.M., Yao, J.: Kidney tumor growth prediction by coupling reaction-diffusion and biomechanical model. IEEE Trans. Biomed. Eng. **60**(1), 169–173 (2013)
8. Mohamed, A., Davatzikos, C.: Finite element modeling of brain tumor mass-effect from 3D medical images. In: Duncan, J.S., Gerig, G. (eds.) MICCAI 2005. LNCS, vol. 3749, pp. 400–408. Springer, Heidelberg (2005). doi:10.1007/11566465_50
9. Wong, K.C.L., Summers, R.M., Kebebew, E., Yao, J.: Tumor growth prediction with hyperelastic biomechanical model, physiological data fusion, and nonlinear optimization. In: Golland, P., Hata, N., Barillot, C., Hornegger, J., Howe, R. (eds.) MICCAI 2014. LNCS, vol. 8674, pp. 25–32. Springer, Cham (2014). doi:10.1007/978-3-319-10470-6_4
10. Deb, K., Pratap, A., Agarwal, S., Meyarivan, T.: A fast and elitist multiobjective genetic algorithm: NSGA-II. IEEE Trans. Evol. Comput. **6**(2), 182–197 (2002)
11. Fang, Q.: ISO2Mesh: a 3D surface and volumetric mesh generator for MATLAB/octave. http://iso2mesh.sourceforge.net/cgi-bin/index.cgi. Accessed 16 Jan 2017
12. Bathe, K.J.: Finite Element Procedures. Prentice Hall, Upper Saddle River (1996)
13. Hoge, C., Davatzikos, C., Biros, G.: An image-driven parameter estimation problem for a reaction-diffusion glioma growth model with mass effects. J. Math. Biol. **56**(6), 793–825 (2008)
14. Friedman, J., Hastie, T., Tibshirani, R.: Additive logistic regression: a statistical view of boosting. Ann. Stat. **28**(2), 337–407 (1998)
15. Martin, D.F., Klein, M., Haller, J.: Preclinical and phase 1A clinical evaluation of an anti-VEGF pegylated aptamer (EYE001) for the treatment of exudative age-related macular degeneration. Retina J. Retin. Vitr. Dis. **22**, 143–152 (2002)
16. Holzapfel, G.A.: Nonlinear Solid Mechanics: A Continuum Approach for Engineering. Wiley, New York (2000)
17. Rangarajan, N., Kamalakkannan, S.B., Hasija, V., Shams, T., Jenny, C., et al.: Finite element model of ocular injury in abusive head trauma. J. Am. Assoc. Pediatr. Ophthalmol. Strabismus **13**(4), 364–369 (2009)

Retinal Biomarker Discovery for Dementia in an Elderly Diabetic Population

Ahmed E. Fetit[1(✉)], Siyamalan Manivannan[1], Sarah McGrory[2], Lucia Ballerini[3,4], Alexander Doney[1], Thomas J. MacGillivray[3], Ian J. Deary[2], Joanna M. Wardlaw[4], Fergus Doubal[4], Gareth J. McKay[5], Stephen J. McKenna[1], and Emanuele Trucco[1]

[1] VAMPIRE Project, CVIP, Computing (SSE), University of Dundee, Dundee, UK
afetit@dundee.ac.uk
[2] Centre for Cognitive Ageing and Cognitive Epidemiology, University of Edinburgh, Edinburgh, UK
[3] VAMPIRE Project, Centre for Clinical Brain Sciences, University of Edinburgh, Edinburgh, UK
[4] Centre for Clinical Brain Sciences, University of Edinburgh, Edinburgh, UK
[5] Centre for Public Health, Queen's University Belfast, Belfast, UK

Abstract. Dementia is a devastating disease, and has severe implications on affected individuals, their family and wider society. A growing body of literature is studying the association of retinal microvasculature measurement with dementia. We present a pilot study testing the strength of groups of conventional (semantic) and texture-based (non-semantic) measurements extracted from retinal fundus camera images to classify patients with and without dementia. We performed a 500-trial bootstrap analysis with regularized logistic regression on a cohort of 1,742 elderly diabetic individuals (median age 72.2). Age was the strongest predictor for this elderly cohort. Semantic retinal measurements featured in up to 81% of the bootstrap trials, with arterial caliber and optic disk size chosen most often, suggesting that they do *complement* age when selected together in a classifier. Textural features were able to train classifiers that match the performance of age, suggesting they are potentially a rich source of information for dementia outcome classification.

Keywords: Retina · Dementia · Microvasculature · Classification · Biomarkers

1 Introduction

Dementia is an umbrella term used to describe a set of brain disorders that trigger a loss of cognitive brain function. There are approximately 850,000 people with dementia in the UK, with numbers set to exceed one million by 2025 [1]. Alzheimer's Disease International reports an estimated 50 million people worldwide living with dementia in 2017, with the numbers affected expected to almost double every 20 years, reaching 75 million by 2030. The total worldwide estimated cost of dementia was put at US$818 billion in 2015, representing 1.09% of the global GDP.

© Springer International Publishing AG 2017
M.J. Cardoso et al. (Eds.): FIFI/OMIA 2017, LNCS 10554, pp. 150–158, 2017.
DOI: 10.1007/978-3-319-67561-9_17

Identifying individuals at an increased risk of developing dementia later in life earlier and detecting pre-clinical stages of cognitive decline may provide opportunities to preserve brain function and delay disease progression. The potential of retinal imaging to support early detection and risk stratification is under investigation, with studies relating the retina microvasculature with changes in the cerebral microvasculature (see [3, 11] for recent reviews). Anatomically and developmentally, the retina is an extension of the brain, hence the retinal microvasculature could work as an easily observed proxy reflecting the condition of the cerebral vasculature [2, 4, 5, 10, 11].

McGrory et al. [3] reviewed the application of fundus camera imaging to assess the associations between retinal microvascular changes and dementia, including various subtypes (i.e. Alzheimer's disease (AD), vascular and frontotemporal dementia). *Vis-á-vis* the heterogeneity among studies in terms of experimental design and the retinal parameters assessed, the most consistent finding identified was that a decreased fractal dimension (a global measure of branching complexity of the retinal vascular tree) tends to associate with AD, as reported by Williams et al. [4] who analyzed data from 507 participants, and Frost et al. [5] who used data from the Australian Imaging, Biomarkers and Lifestyle study of ageing.

We consider two categories of features computable from fundus camera imaging: **(i) clinically semantic features**, or measurements with direct clinical interpretation, e.g. optic disc radius, arterial/venular caliber, tortuosity; and **(ii) clinically non-semantic features**, or measurements that do not have a direct clinical interpretation, but may capture valuable patterns in terms of biomarkers. For these we use texture, a characterization of the spatial variation of pixel intensities, e.g. entropy and contrast computed from co-occurrence matrices [18].

We contribute to the ongoing debate on the value of retinal vascular features for assessing dementia and predicting its risk [3] with the results of a bootstrap analysis with regularized logistic regression and cross-validation in a cohort of elderly diabetic patients. This analysis determines which semantic feature *sets* are selected most often in building sparse logistic regression models, indicating their value for associations. The dementia outcome is defined as whether or not a patient record indicates dementia within a certain time frame relative to the retinal scan.

2   Materials and Methods

2.1   Dataset

Fundus camera images (3504 × 2336 pixels) were obtained from the Genetics of Diabetes Audit and Research Tayside (GoDARTS) bio-resource, Scotland [12]. Images of 2,103 diabetic individuals were available, of which 1,742 patients matched our quality control criteria reported elsewhere [13]. Association with dementia was determined through linkage with prescription, hospital admission and other medical record repositories, using the date of the first recorded event of dementia in the patient records. Of the 1,742 participants included, 237 were identified as having developed dementia by the date the records were inspected. These patients' earliest recorded dementia event ranged from 2,144 days (5.87 years) before the retinal image capture to 2,929 days (8.02 years) after. The mean and median times to dementia event were 952 and 1033 days post-capture (2.6 and 2.8 years), respectively; standard deviation was 1,055 days (2.9 years). Sex and age at retinal photograph were included in our pilot analysis. The mean and median age at scan were 75.7 and 76.1 years for dementia-associated patients, and 69.3 and 71.4 years for the remaining subjects. Of the dementia-associated patients, 105 were female and 132 were male; of the remaining subjects 646 were female and 859 were male. The study was carried out in full accordance with the current data governance and ethical approval regulations in the UK.

2.2   Feature Extraction

Clinically semantic features. A single operator (LB), trained with an established protocol, used the semi-automatic VAMPIRE 3.0 (Vascular Assessment and Measurement Platform for Images of the Retina) [14, 15] to measure optic disc (OD) radius, central retinal arteriolar equivalent (CRAE) and central retinal venular equivalent (CRVE), retinal arterio-venule-ratio (AVR), tortuosity of arteries (tortA) and veins (tortV), as well as maximum tortuosity (tortAmax and tortVmax) in right-eye images, after verifying sufficient correlation ($r > ~0.6$) of AVR, CRAE, CRVE with the left eye as done by others, e.g. [20].

Clinically non-semantic features. Using MATLAB R2016b (MathWorks, Massachusetts, USA), Grey-Level Co-Occurrence Matrix (GLCM) [18] and Grey-Level Run-Length Matrix (GLRLM) [19] features were computed. Right-eye images were used as above (high-contrast green channel). Each image was divided into four standard quadrants and 95 textural features were extracted from each quadrant. Additionally, global features summarizing the overall image texture were extracted, making it possible to build multi-scale feature pyramids.

In terms of GLCM, 1-pixel distance was chosen for displacement along the $0°$, $45°$, $90°$ and $135°$ directions. The number of grey-levels was quantized to 256 (standardizing the sizes of the GLCMs). The features were those provided by the library [6] and included autocorrelation, correlation, energy, and entropy. For the GLRLM, the number of grey-levels was also quantized to 256. Features extracted were those provided by library [9] and included short run emphasis, long run emphasis and grey-level nonuniformity. The full texture pyramid was a concatenation of the global features (95) with the four quadrants' features (380), yielding a total of 475 features per image.

2.3   Biomarker Discovery by Regularized Logistic Regression

Our goal was to deliver a pipeline for (i) assessment of the utility of retinal features for classifying dementia outcome, and (ii) automatic identification of subsets of the available semantic retinal features which give rise to models that are parsimonious and that predict dementia outcome effectively, if any.

Logistic regression was used for ease of model interpretation; model coefficients can be directly linked to feature importance. Regularization was used to perform shrinkage and drive feature coefficients towards zero. This approach is well suited for biomarker identification; it performs feature selection simultaneously with model estimation. For a particular choice of regularization parameters, λ and $\alpha \in [0, 1]$, model estimation given N training pairs $(\mathbf{x}_i, y_i)$, consists of minimizing the penalized negative log-likelihood,

$$\min_{(\beta_0, \boldsymbol{\beta}) \in \mathbb{R}^{p+1}} - \left[\frac{1}{N} \sum_{i=1}^{N} y_i \left(\beta_0 + \mathbf{x}_i^T \boldsymbol{\beta} \right) - \log \left(1 + e^{(\beta_0 + \mathbf{x}_i^T \boldsymbol{\beta})} \right) \right] + \lambda \left[\frac{(1 - \alpha) \|\boldsymbol{\beta}\|_2^2}{2} + \alpha \|\boldsymbol{\beta}\|_1 \right] \quad (1)$$

where β_0 and $\boldsymbol{\beta} = [\beta_1, \beta_2, \ldots, \beta_N]$ are the logistic model coefficients. The parameter λ controls the strength of regularization. The parameter α is the elastic-net regularization mixing parameter; $\alpha = 1$ corresponds to the lasso (also known as L_1 regularization) whereas $\alpha = 0$ corresponds to ridge regression (L_2 regularization) [8]. For highly correlated features, the lasso tends to pick one of the features and discard the others, whereas the ridge shrinks the feature coefficients towards each other. Elastic net mixes the two; for example, $\alpha = 0.5$ tends to select or exclude groups of highly correlated features together [8].

The R package *glmnet* [8] was used to perform the regularized logistic regression experiments. *glmnet* implements an efficient algorithm for computing entire regularization paths, showing the effect of varying λ on the classification error and the number of features retained in the model. Cross-validation was used to select λ; two values of interest are reported by *glmnet*: $\lambda_{\min}$, the value of λ at which the lowest validation set error is achieved, and λ_{1SE}, the λ for the most regularized model whose validation error is within one standard error of $\lambda_{\min}$. This is of interest because the difference in error obtained by $\lambda_{\min}$ and λ_{1SE} is unlikely to be significant but the number of features returned by the classifier identified by the latter is likely to be lower.

We report experiments with lasso and elastic net regularizers. Each drives some model coefficients to zero and thus performs feature selection. As different data samples give rise to different feature sets being selected, we perform a bootstrap analysis, measuring how likely features and feature subsets are to be selected as the data are perturbed [16]. Bootstrap was used similarly, for example, by Park and Hastie [17] to investigate gene interactions albeit using a different feature selection method.

Analysis of semantic features. Each bootstrap analysis comprised 500 bootstrap trials. The feature vector used comprised VAMPIRE measurements, sex and age at scan. The number of patients associating with dementia was less than 14%, resulting in a significant imbalance of the *dementia* and *no dementia* classes. Therefore, sampling with replacement was carried out to extract 100 dementia and 100 non-dementia samples from the cohort in each trial. Regularized logistic regression was implemented on the 200 samples. The regularization path was computed. Model selection used 10-fold cross-validation (CV) to choose λ. For a λ of interest (e.g. $\lambda_{\min}$), the corresponding feature coefficients ($\boldsymbol{\beta}$) and classification error obtained were reported.

We then computed the proportion of times within the 500 bootstraps that each feature had a non-zero weight, thereby providing a measure of how likely the features were to be selected. To detect interesting or frequently occurring patterns amongst groups of features across the bootstraps, we computed the number of times each possible feature-selection permutation took place (e.g., in, say, 200 of the 500 bootstraps, tortuosity and width of arteries were chosen by the model as important, while the rest of retinal features were assigned zero weights). The average classification error was calculated across the

500 bootstraps, together with the corresponding 95% CIs. This process was carried out under four different regularization settings: (a) Lasso and λ_{min}; (b) Elastic-net and λ_{min}; (c) Lasso and λ_{1SE}; (d) Elastic-net and λ_{1SE}.

Analysis of non-semantic features. A bootstrap analysis with textural features was run using the aforementioned methodology. Here, we aimed to explore whether any texture information would associate with dementia. To this end, we experimented with two settings: (a) Using the full textural pyramids; and (b) Using the local quadrant features only. We did not explore different regularization settings but ran the framework using lasso and reported results obtained with λ_{min}.

3   Results

Clinically semantic features. Figure 1 shows an example of a bootstrap trial. As can be seen in Table 1, the most powerful feature in predicting dementia association was the patient age at scan, which was assigned a non-zero weight in almost all bootstrap runs. This was expected given the elderly cohort, and that the risk of developing dementia increases with age. Retinal features were to a great extent complementary to age, given that at least one retinal feature was chosen 81–82% of the time, using λ_{min}. This percentage was lower when λ_{1SE} was used, as expected. OD radius and CRAE were highly ranked after age. In terms of classification performance (Table 2), the mean classification error (MCE) ranged between 35% and 38%, suggesting a reasonable set of discriminatory patterns available in the models used. CIs were reasonably narrow, providing a good level of certainty in the classification results obtained.

We computed the frequency of unique feature patterns across the bootstraps, shown in Fig. 2 (lasso and λ_{min}). The peak of the plot (94/500 times, 18.8%) is age only. The graph tail covers the large number of permutations possible. In 35 trials (7%), CRAE alone was selected in addition to age at scan. All retinal measurements were selected together 26 times (5.2%). All tortuosity measures tended to be selected or discarded together in the highly ranked counts. The above observations were in line with what emerged in all four regularization settings used (complete permutation reports not included for compactness).

Using a classifier trained with semantic measurements only (without age) returned a high MCE of 46% (CI: 38.5%–55%, lasso and λ_{min}). We then tested the MCE of age-only classifiers to predict the outcome with unregularized logistic regression Using the *CARET* [22] package in R (*GLM*-based implementation [7]). The MCE was 36.8% across the trials (95% CIs: 31.5%–43%). Using CRAE and age together (the second most prevalent feature subset in the feature selection experiment) gave an MCE of 35.3% (CIs: 29.5%–41%).

Clinically non-semantic features

(a) Using the textural feature pyramid without age, logistic regression models were able to classify dementia association with a MCE of 37% (CI: 30%–43%). The following quadrant features appeared in the majority of trials (at least 300): *low grey-level run emphasis (top and bottom right quadrants), grey-level non-uniformity (bottom left) and inverse difference moment normalized (45° direction, bottom right, top right and top left; 135° direction, bottom left)*. Global features also appeared in at least 300 trials: *inverse difference moment normalized (0° and 45° directions) and grey-level non-uniformity*.

(b) Using a feature vector that only comprised quadrant features achieved a comparable MCE of 38% (CI 32%–44%). The same features that appeared in (a) were also selected here in at least 300 trials, with the exception of grey-level non-uniformity. Additionally *short run emphasis (bottom left)* featured as important.

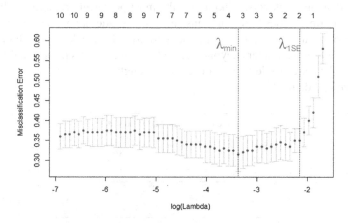

Fig. 1. Example of an individual bootstrap trial (Lasso). Varying λ affects the MCE (with 10-fold CV). Numbers above figure are the numbers of features retained in the regularized model. Interval bars are standard deviations.

4   Discussion and Conclusions

Findings. The role of fundus camera imaging as a means of identifying changes associated to dementia remains disputable [3]. This pilot used a bootstrap analysis based on regularized logistic regression to investigate the association of retinal vascular features computed with the VAMPIRE 3.0 software in fundus camera images (semantic features) as well as of textural features (nonsemantic) with a dementia outcome in an elderly population of diabetics. In the specific cohort, age was the strongest predictor; retinal features were selected in up to ~81% of the trials (both Lasso-λ_{min} and Elastic-net-λ_{min}), suggesting that they do *complement* age when selected together in a classifier. Arterial caliber and OD size were the retinal measurements selected most often, indicating highest discriminative power within the semantic set, when semantic retinal features only (not age) were considered. Textural features were able to match the performance of age and are potentially a rich source of information for dementia outcome classification. Specific features appeared in over 300 of the 500 trials of each experiment, hence further analysis of these textural features will drive our future efforts.

Study limitations and future work

Analysis. Non-linear models might be able to reveal further associations compared to linear logistic regression. Classification results were obtained with 10-fold cross-validation; a held-out test set could be adopted, although the focus of this work was investigating discriminative sets of retinal features, not maximizing classification performance. Using one eye only assumes left-right symmetric measurements, an assumption *sub judice* in the recent literature [21]. Given promising initial results using textural features, it will be interesting to also try feature representations obtained from deep learning using large retinal datasets.

Cohort. The average age at scan of dementia-class subjects was 6.4 years higher than that of non-dementia subjects, making age the most powerful predictor in this cohort. The significant time lapses between scans and dementia-defining events make it necessary to confirm results with a tighter inclusion criterion for the dementia class. We shall also include further parameters beyond age and sex, used in this pilot. Finally, strongly longitudinal data are needed to evaluate the strengths of retinal measurements for predicting risk of dementia.

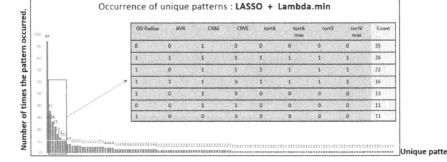

Fig. 2. Unique feature subset patterns that were selected, together with the counts of the highly ranked patterns. A '1' indicates that the feature was selected.

Table 1. Relative feature importance as the number of times a feature was selected (non-zero weight) in the 500 bootstraps. % *ret* is the percentage of times that at least one retinal feature was selected. (a) Lasso and λ_{min}, (b) Elastic-net and λ_{min}, (c) Lasso and λ_{1SE}, (d) Elastic-net and λ_{1SE}. The three most frequently selected features in each analysis are displayed in bold.

Variation	OD radius	AVR	CRAE	CRVE	tortA	tortA max	tortV	tortV max	Age at scan	Sex	% ret
(a)	**243**	156	**392**	151	192	172	180	193	**500**	188	81%
(b)	**263**	195	**310**	168	189	217	215	211	**500**	211	82%
(c)	**61**	34	**113**	36	37	33	40	30	**499**	44	36%
(d)	66	50	**138**	61	42	46	**67**	47	**500**	58	43%

Table 2. Classification error output from the bootstrap analysis. The feature vector comprised VAMPIRE semantic measurements, sex and age at scan.

Variation	Average classification error across bootstraps	95% CI of classification error
Lasso and λ_{min}	0.35	0.29–0.40
Elastic-net and λ_{min}	0.35	0.30–0.41
Lasso and λ_{1SE}	0.37	0.32–0.43
Elastic-net and λ_{1SE}	0.38	0.32–0.44

Acknowledgement. This work was supported by EPSRC grant EP/M005976/1 "Multi-modal retinal biomarkers for vascular dementia".

References

1. https://www.alzheimers.org.uk/info/20025/policy_and_influencing/251/dementia_uk
2. Patton, N., et al.: Retinal vascular image analysis as a potential screening tool for cerebrovascular disease: a rationale based on homology between cerebral and retinal microvasculatures. J. Anat. **206**(4), 319–348 (2005)
3. McGrory, S., et al.: The application of retinal fundus camera imaging in dementia: a systematic review. Alzheimer's Dement. **6**, 91–107 (2016)
4. Williams, M.A., et al.: Retinal microvascular network attenuation in Alzheimer's disease. Alzheimer's Dement. **1**(2), 229–235 (2015)
5. Frost, S., et al.: Retinal vascular biomarkers for early detection and monitoring of Alzheimer's disease. Trans. Psychiatry **3**(2), e233 (2013)
6. https://uk.mathworks.com/matlabcentral/fileexchange/22187-glcm-texture-features. Accessed May 2017
7. https://stat.ethz.ch/R-manual/R-devel/library/stats/html/glm.html. Accessed June 2017
8. Friedman, J., et al.: Regularization paths for generalized linear models via coordinate descent. J. Stat. Softw. **33**(1), 1–22 (2010)
9. Cheung, C.Y., et al.: Microvascular network alterations in the retina of patients with Alzheimer's disease. Alzheimer's Dement. **10**(2), 135–142 (2014). https://uk.mathworks.com/matlabcentral/fileexchange/52640-gray-level-run-length-image-statistics
10. Thomson, K.L., et al.: A systematic review and meta-analysis of retinal nerve fiber layer change in dementia, using optical coherence tomography. Alzheimer's Dement. Diagn. Assess. Dis. Monit. **1**(2), 136–143 (2015)
11. Heringa, S.M., et al.: Associations between retinal microvascular changes and dementia, cognitive functioning, and brain imaging abnormalities: a systematic review. J. Cerebr. Blood F. Met. **33**(7), 983–995 (2013)
12. http://medicine.dundee.ac.uk/godarts
13. MacGillivray, T.J., et al.: Suitability of UK Biobank retinal images for automatic analysis of morphometric properties of the vasculature: a VAMPIRE study. PlosONE **10**, e0127914 (2015)
14. MacGillivray, T.J., et al.: VAMPIRE: Vessel Assessment and Measurement Platform for Images of the Retina. Human Eye Imaging and Modeling. CRC Press, New York (2012)
15. Trucco, E., et al.: Novel VAMPIRE algorithms for quantitative analysis of the retinal vasculature. In: Proceedings from the 4th IEEE Biosignals and Biorobotics Conference (ISSNIP/BRC), pp. 1–4 (2013)

16. Efron, B., Tibshirani, R.: An Introduction to the Bootstrap. Chapman & Hall/CRC, Boca Raton (1993)
17. Park, M.Y., Hasite, T.: Penalized logistic regression for detecting gene interactions. Biostatistics **9**(1), 30–50 (2008)
18. Haralick, R.M., et al.: Textural features for image classification. IEEE Trans. Syst. Man Cybern. **SMC-3**(6), 610–621 (1973)
19. Galloway, M.M.: Texture analysis using gray level run lengths. Comput. Graph. Image Process. **4**(2), 172–179 (1975)
20. Jie, D., et al.: Retinal vascular caliber and the development of hypertension: a meta-analysis of individual participant data. J. Hypertens. **32**(2), 207–215 (2014)
21. Cameron, J.R., et al.: Lateral thinking: inter-ocular symmetry and asymmetry in neurovascular patterning, in health and disease. Progress in Retinal Eye Research, April 2017, epub ahead of print. doi:10.1016/j.preteyeres.2017.04.003
22. https://cran.r-project.org/web/packages/caret/caret.pdf. Accessed June 2017

Non-rigid Registration of Retinal OCT Images Using Conditional Correlation Ratio

Xueying Du[1,2(✉)], Lun Gong[1,2(✉)], Fei Shi[3], Xinjian Chen[3], Xiaodong Yang[1], and Jian Zheng[1]

[1] Suzhou Institute of Biomedical Engineering and Technology, Chinese Academy of Sciences, Beijing, China
duxy_1993@163.com, 2421280977@qq.com,
{xiaodongyang,zhengj}@sibet.ac.cn
[2] University of Chinese Academy of Sciences, Beijing, China
[3] School of Electronics and Information Engineering, Soochow University, Suzhou, China
{shifei,xjchen}@suda.edu.cn

Abstract. In this work, we propose a novel similarity measure for non-rigid retinal optical coherence tomography image registration called conditional correlation ratio (CCR). CCR calculates the correlation ratio (CR) between the moving and fixed image intensities, given a certain spatial distribution. The proposed CCR-based registration is robust to noise and less sensitive to the number of samples used to estimation the density function. Compared to mutual information (MI) and CR, both the quantitative indicators using Hausdorff distance (HD) and M-Hausdorff distance (MHD) and the qualitative indicator using checkerboard images show that CCR is more suitable to align the retinal OCT images.

Keywords: Optical coherence tomography · Non-rigid registration · Spatial information · Conditional correlation ratio

1 Introduction

Optical coherence tomography(OCT) is a medical imaging technique which based on low-coherence interferometry [1]. OCT has been used to detect and track a number of eye diseases such as glaucoma, diabetic retinopathy and age-related macular degeneration, because of high resolution, convenience and the advantage of noncontact imaging of the human retina [2]. In clinical application, to successfully achieve the purpose of detection of eye diseases, it is very important to be able to directly compare motion parameters of lesions at different time-points and vendors. Also the OCT images from normal population can produce non-rigid deformation because of the fluctuation of intraocular pressure [3]. Thus, there is great potential to work on a robust registration technique of retinal OCT images.

X. Du and L. Gong—contributed equally to this work. Both committed to the study and are co-first authors

M.J. Cardoso et al. (Eds.): FIFI/OMIA 2017, LNCS 10554, pp. 159–167, 2017.
DOI: 10.1007/978-3-319-67561-9_18

There are two main categories to register the retinal OCT images. One is based on the feature point matching. Niemeijer et al. [4] presented a rigid registration method which used the 3D SIFT feature extractor to find salient feature points. Wu et al. [5] used Myronenko's Coherent Point Drift and automated vessel shadow segmentation to achieve non-rigid registration. However, these methods are not always effective for the low signal to noise ratio of retinal OCT image. Another way is to consider the intensity information as the registration criterion. Chen et al. [6] proposed a registration algorithm based on intensity classes by combining the two-dimensional rigid registration in B-mode scans and the one-dimensional non-rigid registration in A-mode scans. Qiangding Wei et al. [7] proposed a non-rigid B-spline-based registration method using mutual information (MI) after aligning retinal OCT volumes by the coherent point drift.

However, the traditional MI only uses the intensity classes to establish the statistical relationship but ignores the spatial information of voxels. Therefore, the optimal alignment may not correspond to the minimum dispersion of the joint histogram. A common way to incorporate the spatial information is to estimate the joint probability density function given a certain spatial distribution of voxel as a priori. Studholme et al. [8] extended the spatial information as an additional channel by using a box function to fit the spatial distribution in the user-defined local region when calculating MI. Dirk Loeckx [9] proposed the conditional mutual information (CMI), which defined the spatial distribution using the degree B-spline kernels. Although this strategy is hard to select appropriate size of bins to calculate local information. If we choose a large bin, the local spatial information will be lost. But if the bin is too small, the result of MI will be inaccurate. Considering the advantages of less sensitive to the sample size and noise of CR, RaPTOR (Robust PaTch-based correlation Ratio) [10] was presented by computing the CR from small patches selected freely. However, the spatial kernel in RaPTOR gave the voxels in the patch a same weight, only distinguish whether the voxels belong to same patch and ignore the spatial information of voxels in the patch. Another flaw is that RaPTOR used simplified CR to reduce the computational complexity, causing a reduction of computational accuracy.

Therefore, this paper proposes a non-rigid registration method based on the similarity measure of conditional correlation ratio (CCR). Our approach first computes CR locally to achieve resistance to the large spatial intensity inhomogeneity in the image. A spatial kernel was chosen to consider the spatial information of voxels in the patch by giving the voxels a different weight. Then, L-BFGS is used as optimizer. Finally, the quantitative experiments using Hausdorff distance (HD) and M-Hausdorff distance (MHD) and qualitative indicator using checkerboard chart are chosen to verify the performance of our algorithm.

2   Methodology

2.1   The Similarity Measure Metrics of Conditional Correlation Ratio (CCR)

Let $V = \{\mathbf{x} = (x, y, z) \mid 0 \le x < S_x, 0 \le y < S_y, 0 \le z < S_z\} \subseteq R^3$ denote the image domain, and let the moving image and fixed image be $M(\mathbf{x})$ and $F(\mathbf{x})$ respectively.

The unknown transformation that aligns $M(\mathbf{x})$ and $F(\mathbf{x})$ is represented by T. The registration problem can be formulated as minimizing a cost function C

$$C = D(F(\mathbf{x}), M(T(\mathbf{x})) + w \cdot C_{smooth}(T(\mathbf{x})) \tag{1}$$

where D represents the similarity metric. C_{smooth} is the constraint of the grid that ensures its smoothness, as introduced in [11]. w is the weight of the constraint used to balance the metric and the penalty term. C_{smooth} is given by

$$C_{smooth}(T(\mathbf{x})) = \frac{1}{N} \sum_{\mathbf{x} \in V} [(\frac{\partial^2 T}{\partial x^2})^2 + (\frac{\partial^2 T}{\partial y^2})^2 + (\frac{\partial^2 T}{\partial z^2})^2 + 2 \cdot (\frac{\partial^2 T}{\partial x \partial y})^2 + 2 \cdot (\frac{\partial^2 T}{\partial x \partial z})^2 + 2 \cdot (\frac{\partial^2 T}{\partial z \partial y})^2] \tag{2}$$

where $\mathbf{x}$ represents the samples used to calculate the cost function and N is the total number of samples.

We choose a free-form deformation parameterized by the location of cubic B-spline nodes to model the transformation field. Given the node spacing (n_x, n_y, n_z) and the location of all the nodes $\phi = [\phi_x, \phi_y, \phi_z]$, the transformation of a pixel at the coordinate (x, y, z) is given by

$$T(\phi, \mathbf{x}) = \sum_{a=0}^{3} \sum_{b=0}^{3} \sum_{c=0}^{3} B_a(\alpha) B_b(\beta) B_c(\gamma) \phi_{i+a, j+b, k+c} \tag{3}$$

where $i = \lfloor x/n_x \rfloor - 1$, $j = \lfloor y/n_y \rfloor - 1$, $k = \lfloor z/n_z \rfloor - 1$ and $\alpha = x/n_x - \lfloor x/n_x \rfloor$, $\beta = y/n_y - \lfloor y/n_y \rfloor$, $\gamma = z/n_z - \lfloor z/n_z \rfloor$, $\lfloor \cdot \rfloor$ is the truncation operation and $B(\cdot)$ represents B-spline basis functions.

Correlation ratio. For two random variables X and Y, correlation ratio (CR) measures the functional dependence between X and Y [12]. Let $E(Y|X)$ be the conditional expectation of Y in terms of X, and $Var[\cdot]$ denotes the variance. Then, CR is defined as follows

$$\eta(Y|X) = \frac{Var[E(Y|X)]}{Var[Y]} = 1 - \frac{Var[Y - E(Y|X)]}{Var[Y]} \tag{4}$$

CR takes on values between 0 and 1. The larger the value is, the closer the functional relationship is. In fact, because of noting $\eta(Y|X) \neq \eta(X|Y)$, CR is asymmetric. In our method, the intensity values of moving image are set to X, and the intensity values of fixed image are set to Y.

Conditional correlation ratio. Compared with the traditional CR, our approach called CCR extends the joint histogram with spatial information and calculates CR from small patches by binning of the intensities in the fixed image. This method uses a local estimation of the joint histogram by subdividing the fixed image and performing a set of local registrations within average block r. For convenient calculation, we choose mesh knots of free-form deformation as r. Thus, the new similarity measure named CCR between the fixed image and moving image over all patches is given by

$$CCR = 1 - \eta(F \mid M; r) = \sum_r \left\{ \frac{p(r)}{\sigma_r^2} \left[\sum_f f^2 P_r(f) - \sum_m (\bar{f}_m)^2 P_r(m) \right] \right\} \quad (5)$$

with

$$\sigma_r^2 = \sum_f f^2 p_r(f) - (\bar{f}_r)^2, \bar{f}_r = \sum_f f p_r(f), \bar{f}_m = \frac{1}{p_r(f)} \sum_f f p_r(m,f)$$

To extend the joint histogram with spatial information, we incorporate a spatial kernel ω_r into the calculation of probability density function (PDF) based on the parzen-window. $h(\cdot)$ is the kernel function which described in detail in [12].

$$P_r(m,f) = \sum_{x \in V} \omega_r(\mathbf{x} - r) h(m - M(\mathbf{x})) h(f - F(\mathbf{x})) \quad (6)$$

$$P_r(m) = \sum_f P_r(m,f), \quad P_r(f) = \sum_m P_r(m,f), p(r) = \sum_{x \in V} \omega_r(\mathbf{x} - r)$$

where $r, M(\mathbf{x})$ and $F(\mathbf{x})$ can be considered as spatial bins. Here, we use the degree B-spline kernels as ω_r. The specific formula is shown as follows

$$\omega_r(\mathbf{x} - r) = B_{k_x}(x_x - r_x) B_{k_y}(x_y - r_y) B_{k_z}(x_z - r_z) \quad (7)$$

where we use $k_{x,y,z}$ th degree B-spline kernels for the spatial kernel in each dimension, and patch spacing chooses (n_x, n_y, n_z) which is same as that used in free from deformation. Finally, the above equations can be substituted in (5) to obtain the cost function.

2.2 Derivatives and Optimization

To minimize the cost function C, we use the gradient-based optimization algorithm named L-BFGS. The gradient of C with respect to the control points ϕ can be derived as follows

$$\frac{\partial C}{\partial \phi} = \frac{\partial CCR}{\partial \phi} + w \cdot \frac{\partial C_{smooth}}{\partial \phi} \quad (8)$$

The derivative of constraint C_{smooth} was obtained in [11]. Next, the derivative of CCR is given in detail. Given the moving image M and the fixed image F, the derivative of the similarity metric with respect to the control points ϕ is given as follows

$$\frac{\partial CCR}{\partial \phi} = \sum_r \sum_f \frac{p(r)}{\sigma_r^2} [(\bar{f}_m)^2 \frac{\partial p_r(m)}{\partial \phi} - \sum_m 2 \cdot \bar{f}_m \cdot f \cdot \frac{\partial p_r(m,f)}{\partial \phi}] \qquad (9)$$

with

$$\frac{\partial p_r(m)}{\partial \phi} = \sum_x \omega_x(x-r) \frac{\partial h}{\partial \tau}\Big|_{\tau=m-M(x)} \cdot (-1) \cdot \frac{\partial M}{\partial T} \cdot \frac{\partial T}{\partial \phi}$$

$$\frac{\partial p_r(m,f)}{\partial \phi} = \sum_x \omega_x(x-r) \frac{\partial h}{\partial \tau}\Big|_{\tau=m-M(x)} \cdot h(f - F(x)) \cdot (-1) \cdot \frac{\partial M}{\partial T} \cdot \frac{\partial T}{\partial \phi}$$

where $\partial M/\partial T$ is the gradient of the moving image and the $\partial T/\partial \phi$ is the gradient of the deformation field with respect to ϕ. Both the definitions in detail are obtained in [11].

3 Experimental Results

In this section, the proposed method was tested on 8 pairs OCT images of normal eyes. Each image pair acquired from a different time points of one person with a size of $256 \times 256 \times 128$. To demonstrate the excellent performance of our algorithm, we compared the proposed method against CR and MI which were wildly used in registration. For all experiments, the number of bins used to calculate PDF is set to 64 and the weight of penalty term is 0.1. A three-level multi-resolution framework was used to improve search efficiency. The mesh spacing for the B-spline transformation and the estimation of PDF is 6 voxels. To verify the robustness to noise, all the experimental data were not filtered.

The checkerboard images were used to qualitatively analyze the registration performance. HD and MHD [13] were exploited to quantitatively measure how well the retinal layers between the fixed and moving images were aligned. The lower these values are, the better correspondence between the retinal layers has been achieved. The retinal layers of each OCT image were automatically segmented according to [14]. Figure 1 showed that an OCT image divided into 10 retinal layers with 11 surfaces.

Table 1 exhibited the quantitative metrics of HD and MHD calculated by the 11 surfaces. For each case, the mean of MHD obtained by CCR has a significantly decrease compared to CR and MI. For case 5, it was clear that the mean of MHD obtained by CR was larger than non-registration, while CCR still demonstrated good performance. It further validated the robustness of CCR to different data. From the metric of HD, it was easy to find that the means obtained by CR and MI were worse compared to non-registration, while that obtained by CCR was still the least for all cases. It verified that CCR covered the shortage of MI which was sensitive to noise and the shortage of CR which was restrictive to the functional mapping between the intensities.

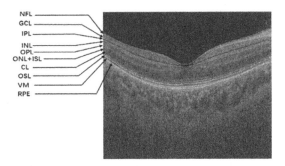

Fig. 1. OCT image of a normal eye and 10 retinal layers

Table 1. The mean ± SD(11 surfaces) of HD and MHD among four algorithms from five cases (Unit: Pixel)

		Non-registration	MI	CR	CCR
case 1	HD	9.24 ± 0.55	14.5 ± 2.58	9.91 ± 0.88	5.49 ± 1.89
	MHD	2.1 ± 0.27	1.13 ± 0.21	0.95 ± 0.29	0.73 ± 0.11
case 2	HD	7.88 ± 0.98	9.82 ± 2.49	15.6 ± 3.58	5.49 ± 2.64
	MHD	2.06 ± 0.1	0.88 ± 0.32	0.91 ± 0.22	0.57 ± 0.16
case 3	HD	5.85 ± 0.75	10.7 ± 2.59	8.08 ± 2.04	4.12 ± 1.15
	MHD	1.27 ± 0.02	0.91 ± 0.19	0.72 ± 0.13	0.52 ± 0.07
case 4	HD	4.45 ± 0.5	7.92 ± 1.02	5.97 ± 0.4	3.12 ± 1.56
	MHD	0.83 ± 0.02	0.68 ± 0.12	0.55 ± 0.1	0.52 ± 0.09
case 5	HD	7.24 ± 0.68	3.82 ± 0.74	15.1 ± 1.94	3.43 ± 1.56
	MHD	1.57 ± 0.04	0.53 ± 0.09	1.90 ± 0.15	0.52 ± 0.11
case 6	HD	10.14 ± 0.33	13.27 ± 1.15	14 ± 0.6	6.22 ± 1.09
	MHD	3.44 ± 0.02	1.06 ± 0.22	0.87 ± 0.09	0.58 ± 0.08
case 7	HD	8.45 ± 1.58	9.03 ± 2.35	7 ± 2.79	4.61 ± 1.17
	MHD	1.96 ± 0.06	0.69 ± 0.12	0.58 ± 0.10	0.61 ± 0.08
case 8	HD	7.64 ± 0.31	13.47 ± 0.41	16.98 ± 1.33	5.22 ± 0.28
	MHD	1.96 ± 0.02	1.88 ± 0.16	1.67 ± 0.13	0.65 ± 0.06

To demonstrate the alignment effect more directly, we alternately displayed the fixed and transform image by the checkerboard image with case 1 and case 3 as examples (as shown in Fig. 2). Figure 2(a) and (b) were fixed and moving images, respectively, and (c) was the checkerboard image of them without registration. (d) ~ (f) severally displayed the checkerboard images which alternately fused the fixed image and transform image obtained by MI, CR and CCR. It was clear that CCR not only has a good alignment in the outmost surfaces (NFL and RPE), it could also capture the more accurate displacement for the inner surfaces.

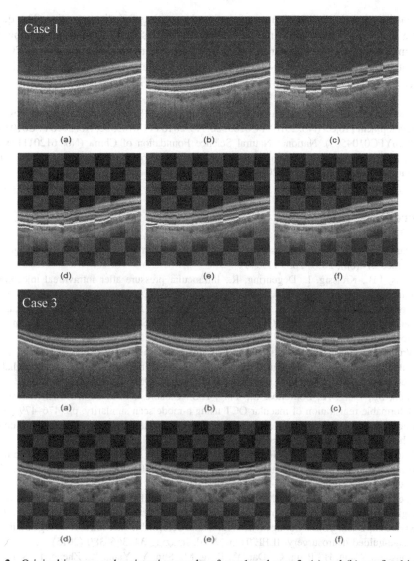

Fig. 2. Original images and registration results of case1 and case 3, (a) and (b) are fixed image and moving image, (c) ~ (f) are respectively registration results of non-registration, MI, CR, CCR using checkboard image between fixed image and transformation image

4   Conclusion

In this paper, we present a novel similarity measure called conditional correlation ratio (CCR) for retinal OCT image registration. CCR uses a local estimation of the joint histogram by subdividing the image and performing a set of local registrations. Therefore, it not only inherits the virtues of CR such as the robustness to noise and less sensitive to number of samples compared to MI, but also covers the disadvantage of

CR that it is restrictive to assume a functional mapping for all intensities. The quantitative metrics of clinic experiments show that CCR is more robust and suitable for OCT image registration compared to CR and MI. The main limitation is that CCR is calculated over a series of sub-blocks and the computation time is expensive. In the future, we will synchronize the code in parallel using GPU.

Acknowledgement. This work was supported in part by the National Program on Key Research and Development Project (No. 2016YFC0103500, No. 2016YFC0103502, No. 2016YFC0104500, No. 2016YFC0104505), National Natural Science Foundation of China (No. 61201117), the Natural Science Foundation of Jiangsu Province (No. BK20151232), and the Youth Innovation Promotion Association CAS (No. 2014281).

References

1. Tearney, G.J.: In vivo endoscopic optical biopsy with optical coherence tomography. Science **276**(80), 2037–2039 (1997)
2. Jonas, J.B., Kreissig, I., Degenring, R.: Intraocular pressure after intravitreal injection of triamcinolone acetonide. Br. J. Ophthalmol. **87**, 24–27 (2003)
3. Niemeijer, M., Garvin, M.K., Lee, K., van Ginneken, B., Abràmoff, M.D., Sonka, M.: Registration of 3D spectral OCT volumes using 3D SIFT feature point matching. In: Proceedings of the SPIE 7259, 72591I (2009)
4. Wu, J., Gerendas, B.S., Waldstein, S.M., Langs, G., Simader, C., Schmidt-Erfurth, U.M.: Stable registration of pathological 3D SD-OCT scans using retinal vessels. In: Ophthalmic Medical Image Analysis First International Workshop, OMIA 2014, pp. 1–8 (2014)
5. Chen, M., Lang, A., Sotirchos, E., Ying, H.S., Calabresi, P.A., Prince, J.L., Carass, A.: Deformable registration of macular OCT using a-mode scan similarity, pp. 476–479 (2013)
6. Chen, Q.W., F.S.; W.Z.; D.X.; H.C.; X.: Nonrigid registration of 3D longitudinal optical coherence tomography volumes with choroidal neovascularization (2017)
7. Studholme, C., Drapaca, C., Iordanova, B., Cardenas, V.: Deformation-based mapping of volume change from serial brain MRI in the presence of local tissue contrast change. IEEE Trans. Med. Imaging **25**, 626–639 (2006)
8. Loeckx, D., Slagmolen, P., Maes, F., Vandermeulen, D., Suetens, P.: Nonrigid image registration using conditional mutual information. IEEE Trans. Med. Imaging **29**, 1–2 (2010)
9. Rivaz, H., Chen, S.J.S., Collins, D.L.: Automatic deformable MR-ultrasound registration for image-guided neurosurgery. IEEE Trans. Med. Imaging **34**, 366–380 (2015)
10. Gong, L., Wang, H., Peng, C., Dai, Y., Ding, M., Sun, Y., Yang, X., Zheng, J.: Non-rigid MR-TRUS image registration for image-guided prostate biopsy using correlation ratio-based mutual information. Biomed. Eng. Online **16**, 8 (2017)
11. Roche, A., Malandain, G., Pennec, X., Ayache, N.: The correlation ratio as a new similarity measure for multimodal image registration. In: Wells, William M., Colchester, A., Delp, S. (eds.) MICCAI 1998. LNCS, vol. 1496, pp. 1115–1124. Springer, Heidelberg (1998). doi:10.1007/BFb0056301
12. Xu, R., Member, S., Chen, Y., Tang, S., Morikawa, S.: Parzen-window based normalized mutual information for medical image registration. IEICE – Trans. Inf. Syst. **E91-D**(1), 132–144 (2015)

13. Suh, J.W., Kwon, O.-K., Scheinost, D., Sinusas, A.J., Cline, G.W., Papademetris, X.: CT-PET weighted image fusion for separately scanned whole body rat. Med. Phys. **39**, 533–542 (2012)
14. Shi, F., Chen, X., Zhao, H., Zhu, W., Xiang, D., Gao, E., Sonka, M., Chen, H.: Automated 3-D retinal layer segmentation of macular optical coherence tomography images with serous pigment epithelial detachments. IEEE Trans. Med. Imaging **34**, 441–452 (2015)

Joint Optic Disc and Cup Segmentation Using Fully Convolutional and Adversarial Networks

Sharath M. Shankaranarayana[1(⊠)], Keerthi Ram[2], Kaushik Mitra[1], and Mohanasankar Sivaprakasam[1,2]

[1] Dept of Electrical Engineering, IIT-Madras, Chennai, India
ee15s050@ee.iitm.ac.in
[2] Healthcare Technology Innovation Centre, IIT-Madras, Chennai, India

Abstract. Glaucoma is a highly threatening and widespread ocular disease which may lead to permanent loss in vision. One of the important parameters used for Glaucoma screening in the cup-to-disc ratio (CDR), which requires accurate segmentation of optic cup and disc. We explore fully convolutional networks (FCNs) for the task of joint segmentation of optic cup and disc. We propose a novel improved architecture building upon FCNs by using the concept of residual learning. Additionally, we also explore if adversarial training helps in improving the segmentation results. The method does not require any complicated preprocessing techniques for feature enhancement. We learn a mapping between the retinal images and the corresponding segmentation map using fully convolutional and adversarial networks. We perform extensive experiments of various models on a set of 159 images from RIM-ONE database and also do extensive comparison. The proposed method outperforms the state of the art methods on various evaluation metrics for both disc and cup segmentation.

Keywords: Deep learning · Fully Convolutional Networks · Glaucoma · Optic disc and cup segmentation · Adversarial networks

1 Introduction

Glaucoma is a potentially blinding disorder affecting a large number of people worldwide. One of the most important steps in the diagnosis of glaucoma is the assessment of the Optic Disc (OD) and optic cup, using 2D color fundus images. Cupping is a phenomena in which there is an enlargement of the cup due to loss in optic nerve fibers. The enlargement of the cup with respect to OD, measured as vertical cup-to-disc ratio (CDR) is one of the most important indicators of the disease. This necessitates accurate segmentation of the optic cup and disc. This task is typically performed by a highly skilled human grader and the task is highly time consuming and expensive along with a high degree of variability between the graders. This requires the need to automate the task of segmentation.

© Springer International Publishing AG 2017
M.J. Cardoso et al. (Eds.): FIFI/OMIA 2017, LNCS 10554, pp. 168–176, 2017.
DOI: 10.1007/978-3-319-67561-9_19

There have been numerous works on the task of optic disc and cup segmentation [6]. Existing techniques for the determination of optic disc boundary are either based on morphological techniques [8] or based on deformable energy based models [9,10]. Some of the drawbacks of existing approaches is their dependency on initialization and their inability to detect weak edges in neuroretinal rim.

Optic cup segmentation on the other hand is considered to be a challenging task even for the human graders. Some of the existing works are based on energy based models similar to optic disc segmentation techniques [11,14], using graph cuts [12]. Such techniques may not be effective in case of images with very low contrast.

On the other hand, deep learning based convolutional neural network (CNN) methods have been successful at many tasks such as image classification, object recognition, semantic segmentation etc. Recently, CNNs have been used for deep feature learning for only glaucoma classification [13], wherein they predict whether the given retinal image has glaucoma or not. For optic disc and cup segmentation, recently [15] use CNNs and learn filters in a greedy fashion instead of backpropagation. In their proposed method, given a retinal image with the region of interest (i.e. containing optic disc and cup), they preprocess the image and pass it through their network and get pixelwise predictions of whether the given pixel belongs to optic cup or disk or background thus obtaining a probability classification map on which they use graph cut and convex hull transformation to get the final segmentation map. Their proposed network contains fully connected layers and is also not end to end, while consisting of a pipeline of various techniques to obtain the final segmentation map. We propose an end to end, fully convolutional, encoder-decoder type network for this task. Although, such networks have been used in the medical image segmentation tasks (for example U-net) [5], they have not been used for the task of joint optic disc and cup segmentation. Building upon U-net, we propose a novel architecture called ResU-net inspired from RESNET [7], incorporating residual learning along with feature concatenation in an encoder decoder based

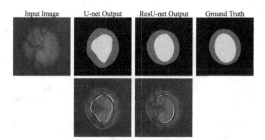

Fig. 1. First row shows the segmentation output of U-net and the proposed ResU-net architecture, along with input image and ground truth. The second row shows delineations for better comparison, green (disc) and black (cup) lines correspond to ground truth and red (disc) and yellow (cup) lines correspond to network output. (Color figure online)

architecture for segmentation task. This offers an advantage over U-net [5] since we can have deeper architectures leading to improved segmentation results (as shown in Fig. 1) and also over fully convolutional networks (FCN) like [16] in terms of lesser training time. Apart from that, we also incorporate adversarial training [1,2] for the segmentation task.

2   Methods

In the proposed framework, our goal is to learn a mapping from the fundus image containing the region of interest to the corresponding segmentation map with the segmentation map consisting of three classes- optic disc, cup and the background. Let x be the input image and y be the corresponding ground truth segmentation map, then our goal is to learn mapping $G : x \rightarrow y$, where the function G is learned using a base network. The base network is a FCN which is trained to minimize multi-class cross entropy loss $L_{mce}(G)$ given by

$$L_{mce}(G) = \mathbb{E}_{x,y \sim p_{data}(x,y)}[-\sum_{i}^{N} y_i \log (G_i(x))] \qquad (1)$$

where i represents the pixel index with total of N pixels.

2.1   Proposed Base Network Architecture (ResU-net)

The proposed architecture of the main network is shown in Fig. 2. The network, similar to U-net, [5] consists of a contracting path or an encoder (left side of the network having downsampling operations) and an expanding path or a decoder

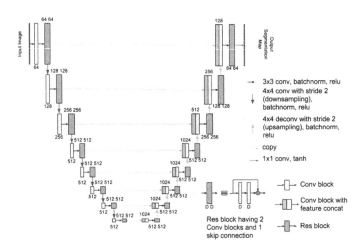

Fig. 2. Proposed Base Network Architecture (ResU-net): The network consists of residual blocks along with convolutional blocks

(right side of the network having up sampling operations). The network differs from U-net in many ways. The network uses residual blocks which is made up of 2 convolutional blocks and a skip connection, with 3 × 3 convolution operation with a stride of 1 followed by batch normalization and relu. In the encoding path or contracting path, while downsampling, we do a 4 × 4 convolution with a stride of 2 followed by batch normalization relu operation and double the number of filters in each layer after downsampling. Our architecture is also much deeper than the U-net but we double the number filters only till it reaches 512. This is done to keep the number of parameters less while still going deep. For the decoding or expanding path, we retain feature concatenation operation similar to the original U-net and again use both convolutional and residual blocks. For the first 3 decoding layers, we also use dropout with 50% rate. For upsampling we do a 4 × 4 deconvolution operation with stride 2. All convolution and residual operations are followed by batch norm and relu operations. Also the encoder part employs a leaky relu with slope 0.2 while the decoder part uses normal relu. After the last decoding layer a 1 × 1 convolution is performed to map to the number of output channels followed by *tanh* activation. Thus we see that the network incorporates best of both skip connections- feature concatenation and residual addition.

2.2 Adversarial Network

The adversarial network model for our task is motivated from [3] and is shown in Fig. 3 . In generative adversarial networks (GANs), the learning takes place by pitting two networks - Generator (G) and Discriminator (D) against each other. The task of the generator is to generate plausible representations of segmentation map from the input fundus images, and the goal of the discriminator is

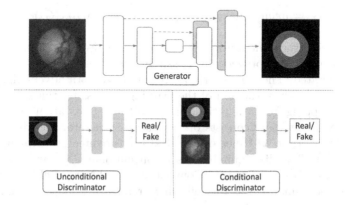

Fig. 3. The Adversarial Network Framework: here the generator has the base network architecture- either U-Net of ResU-Net and discriminator is a conventional CNN used for classifying whether the segmentation map is real or fake, and discriminator can also be conditioned on input fundus image

discriminate between the generated and ground truth segmentation maps. Generator and discriminator is jointly trained and the learning process attempts to maximize misclassification error of the discriminator. Therefore generator tries to generate more plausible representations of segmentation map that can deceive discriminator and the discriminator becomes better at its task of discriminating which in-turn improves the ability of the generator to generate better samples. Mathematically, the generator is trained to learn a mapping from observed image x to $y : G : x \rightarrow y$ in a way such that the generator, G, learns to produce outputs to fool an adversarially trained discriminator, D, The discriminator is trained to distinguish between the generated images and real images and thus classify the given input image as real of fake. The objective function is given by:

$$L_{GAN}(G,D) = \mathbb{E}_{x,y \sim p_{data}(x,y)}[log(D(y))] + \mathbb{E}_{x \sim p_{data}(x)}[log(1 - D(G(x)))], \quad (2)$$

where $\mathbb{E}_{x,y \sim p_{data}(x,y)}$ represents the expectation of the log-likelihood of the pair (x,y) being sampled from the underlying probability distribution of real pairs $p_{data}(x,y)$, while $p_{data}(x)$ corresponds to the distribution of optic cup and disc. We can also have conditional GANs where the discriminator is conditioned on the input image x, for which the objective function becomes:

$$L_{cGAN}(G,D) = \mathbb{E}_{x,y \sim p_{data}(x,y)}[log(D(x,y))] + \mathbb{E}_{x \sim p_{data}(x)}[log(1 - D(x,G(x)))] \quad (3)$$

Since it has also been found useful to combine adversarial loss with the traditional $L2/L1$ [3,4] loss, we impose this loss on the generator so that its task is not only to fool the discriminator but also produce outputs close to the ground truth in the $L1$ sense:

$$L_{L1}(G) = \mathbb{E}_{x,y \sim p_{data}(x,y)}[\|(y - G(x)\|_1] \quad (4)$$

therefore the final objective becomes

$$G^* = arg\min_{G}\max_{D}(L_{GAN/cGAN}(G,D) + \lambda(L_{L1}(G)) \quad (5)$$

where λ balances the contribution of two losses. In Eq. (5), the discriminator tries to maximize the expression by classifying whether the segmentation map is real or generated. The generator tries to minimize both adversarial loss and $L1$ loss in Eq. (5). Thus, the aim of the learning process for the generator is to find a good mapping from the retinal image to the segmentation map.

The GAN architecture consists of two parts - generator and discriminator. The generator is same as U-net or the ResU-net architecture explained in the previous section. The discriminator has a conventional CNN architecture used for classification. Let Ln denote a Convolution-BatchNorm-ReLU layer with n filters. The discriminator uses the following architecture- L64-L128-L256-L512-L512-L512.

After the last layer, a convolution is applied to map to a 1 dimensional output, followed by a Sigmoid function. BatchNorm is not applied to the first L64 layer. Discriminator employs leaky ReLUs, with slope 0.2, and all convolutions being 4×4 with a stride of 2.

3   Experiments and Results

The proposed method is evaluated on the RIM-ONE dataset. The dataset contains 159 retinal fundus images with 85 normal cases and 74 confirmed glaucoma cases. We select a region of interest around the optic disc in fundus image and corresponding region in segmentation map and resize it to size 256×256. We do a $5 - fold$ cross validation for determining classification accuracy as done in [15]. We experiment for the following cases-

1. Standard U-net architecture (U-net)
2. Standard U-net architecture as generator in GAN (U-GAN)
3. Standard U-net architecture as generator in conditional GAN (U-cGAN)
4. Proposed modified U-net architecture (ResU-net)
5. Proposed modified U-net architecture as generator in GAN (ResU-GAN)
6. Proposed modified U-net architecture as generator in conditional GAN (ResU-cGAN)

All models were trained from scratch with initialization from a Gaussian distribution with mean 0 and standard deviation 0.02 and run for 200 epochs.

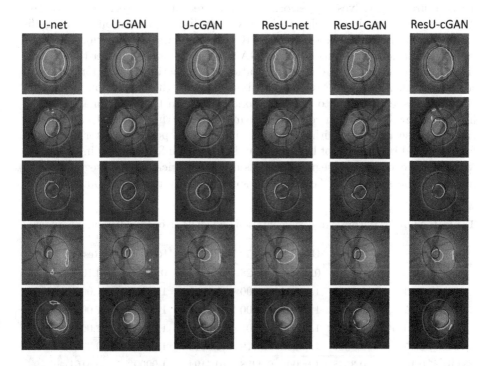

Fig. 4. The Segmentation results along with the ground truth. The green and black lines indicate the ground truth segmentation boundaries for optic disc and cup respectively and red and yellow lines indicate the segmentation boundaries for optic disc and cup respectively obtained using various methods (Color figure online)

The initial learning rate was kept to be 10^{-4} and halved every 50 epochs. We used data augmentation techniques like flip, rotate as done in any standard CNN setting. The training took an average of 4 h on a single Pascal Titan X GPU and the inference took less than half a second per image on GPU. The results for some of the test images are shown in Fig. 4

The metrics used for quantitative evaluation are- F-score, the intersection over union (IOU) the non-overlap ratio (NOR) and absolute difference δ between the Cup to disc ratios of output segmentation map and the ground truth. F-score is the harmonic mean of precision and recall. The IOU and NOR measure the extent of overlap in the segmentation regions of the output and the ground truth and is given by: $IOU = \frac{S_O \cap S_G}{S_O \cup S_G}$ $NOR = 1 - \frac{S_O \cap S_G}{S_O \cup S_G}$ where S_O and S_G are segmentation map of the output and the corresponding ground truth segmentation map respectively. The absolute cup-to-disc ratio (CDR) error is given by $\delta = |CDR_G - CDR_O|$ where CDR_G and CDR_O are the cup-to-disc ratios of ground truth and output respectively.

The results for various experiments are shown in Table 1 and Fig. 4. When comparing just the base networks, the proposed ResU-net performs significantly better than U-net. From Table 2 it can be seen that compared to other reported state of the art techniques, all our models perform significantly better. The base architectures themselves outperform the most recent CCN techniques [15,16]. Also adversarial training helps to improve the disc segmentation by a significant amount in terms F-measure and IOU, but shows lesser performance for cup segmentation. Also unconditional GANs seem to perform better than conditional GANs for the optic disc segmentation but sometimes worse for optic cup segmentation. A possible reason could be that since the cup region is small in size and as such difficult to segment, conditioning on the input image may be helpful in this case. When comparing using CDR as the metric, it can be seen that the base networks without adversarial training perform better. A reason for this could be the lack of large data and inherent difficulty in training GANs. More errors occur in cup segmentation, since it is a tricky area to segment. And moreover, the strength of GANs lie in solving highly ambiguous and ill-posed

Table 1. NOR for the optic disc segmentation and CDR error for different experiments

Method	U-net	U-GAN	U-cGAN	ResU-net	ResU-GAN	ResU-cGAN
mean NOR	0.1174	0.0509	0.1328	0.0991	**0.0388**	0.1024
NOR ≤ 0.30	1.0000	1.0000	1.0000	1.0000	1.0000	1.0000
NOR ≤ 0.25	0.9677	1.0000	1.0000	1.0000	1.0000	1.0000
NOR ≤ 0.20	0.9677	1.0000	1.0000	1.0000	1.0000	1.0000
NOR ≤ 0.15	0.8387	1.0000	0.7419	0.9355	1.0000	0.9355
NOR ≤ 0.10	0.3548	1.0000	0.2258	0.4194	1.0000	0.5161
NOR ≤ 0.05	0.0000	0.5806	0.0000	0.0968	0.8387	0.0645
mean CDR error δ	0.03820	0.0509	0.0555	**0.03370**	0.04380	0.0375

graphics problems rather than problems like segmentation where non adversarial training would probably suffice.

Table 2. Comparison with other techniques

Method	Optic disc		Optic cup	
	F-Measure	IOU	F-Measure	IOU
[8]	0.901	0.842	-	-
[11]	0.931	0.880	0.801	0.764
[14]	0.892	0.829	0.744	0.732
[15]	0.942	0.890	0.824	**0.802**
[16]	0.960	0.890	-	-
U-net	0.973	0.886	0.927	0.749
U-GAN	0.984	0.949	0.779	0.675
U-cGAN	0.971	0.867	0.878	0.718
ResU-net	0.977	0.901	**0.945**	0.786
ResU-GAN	**0.987**	**0.961**	0.906	0.739
ResU-cGAN	0.977	0.897	0.940	0.768

4   Conclusion

In this work, a new architecture for image segmentation was proposed and with extensive experimental evaluations it was shown that the method outperforms several state of the art techniques for the task of joint optic disc and cup segmentation. Adversarial training was also explored to evaluate its usefulness for the task of medical image segmentation. The proposed architecture and models can be readily applied to other medical image segmentation tasks. A good future work would be to improve segmentation results of adversarial networks by improving the design of the discriminator and also evaluate the method for other retinal image analysis tasks like vessel segmentation and hemorrhage detection.

References

1. Goodfellow, I., Pouget-Abadie, J., Mirza, M., Xu, B., Warde-Farley, D., Ozair, S., Courville, A., Bengio, Y.: Generative adversarial nets. In: NIPS (2014)
2. Radford, A., Metz, L., Chintala, S.: Unsupervised representation learning with deep convolutional generative adversarial networks. arXiv preprint arXiv:1511.06434 (2015)
3. Isola, P., Zhu, J.-Y., Zhou, T., Efros, A.A.: Image-to-image translation with conditional adversarial networks. arXiv.org, November 2016. arXiv:1611.07004

4. Pathak, D., Krahenbuhl, P., Donahue, J., Darrell, T., Efros, A.A.: Context encoders: feature learning by inpainting. In: CVPR (2016)
5. Ronneberger, O., Fischer, P., Brox, T.: U-Net: convolutional networks for biomedical image segmentation. In: Navab, N., Hornegger, J., Wells, W.M., Frangi, A.F. (eds.) MICCAI 2015. LNCS, vol. 9351, pp. 234–241. Springer, Cham (2015). doi:10.1007/978-3-319-24574-4_28
6. Almazroa, A., Burman, R., Raahemifar, K., Lakshminarayanan, V.: Optic disc and optic cup segmentation methodologies for glaucoma image detection: a survey. J. Ophthalmol. **2015**, 28 (2015). doi:10.1155/2015/180972. Article ID 180972
7. He, K., Zhang, X., Ren, S., Sun, J.: Deep residual learning for image recognition. arXiv preprint arXiv:1512.03385 (2015)
8. Aquino, A., Gegundez-Arias, M., Marin, D.: Detecting the optic disc boundary in digital fundus images using morphological edge detection and feature extraction techniques. IEEE Trans. Med. Imaging **20**(11), 1860–1869 (2010)
9. Lowell, J., Hunter, A., Steel, D., Basu, A., Ryder, R., Fletcher, E., et al.: Optic nerve head segmentation. IEEE Trans. Med. Imaging **23**(2), 256264 (2004)
10. Xu, J., Chutatape, O., Sung, E., Zheng, C., Chew, P.: Optic disk feature extraction via modified deformable model technique for glaucoma analysis. Pattern Recognit. **40**(7), 20632076 (2007)
11. Joshi, G.D., Sivaswamy, J., Krishnadas, S.R.: Optic disk and cup segmentation from monocular color retinal images for glaucoma assessment. IEEE Trans. Med. Imaging **30**(6), 1192–1205 (2011)
12. Zheng, Y., Stambolian, D., O'Brien, J., Gee, J.C.: Optic disc and cup segmentation from color fundus photograph using graph cut with priors. In: Mori, K., Sakuma, I., Sato, Y., Barillot, C., Navab, N. (eds.) MICCAI 2013. LNCS, vol. 8150, pp. 75–82. Springer, Heidelberg (2013). doi:10.1007/978-3-642-40763-5_10
13. Chen, X., Xu, Y., Yan, S., Wong, D.W.K., Wong, T.Y., Liu, J.: Automatic feature learning for glaucoma detection based on deep learning. In: Navab, N., Hornegger, J., Wells, W.M., Frangi, A.F. (eds.) MICCAI 2015. LNCS, vol. 9351, pp. 669–677. Springer, Cham (2015). doi:10.1007/978-3-319-24574-4_80
14. Cheng, J., Liu, J., et al.: Superpixel classification based optic disc and optic cup segmentation for glaucoma screening. IEEE Trans. Med. Imaging **32**(6), 1019–1032 (2013)
15. Zilly, J., Buhmann, J.M., Mahapatra, D.: Glaucoma detection using entropy sampling and ensemble learning for automatic optic cup and disc segmentation. Comput. Med. Imaging Graph. **55**, 2841 (2017)
16. Maninis, K.-K., Pont-Tuset, J., Arbeláez, P., Van Gool, L.: Deep retinal image understanding. In: Ourselin, S., Joskowicz, L., Sabuncu, M.R., Unal, G., Wells, W. (eds.) MICCAI 2016. LNCS, vol. 9901, pp. 140–148. Springer, Cham (2016). doi:10.1007/978-3-319-46723-8_17

Automated Segmentation of the Choroid in EDI-OCT Images with Retinal Pathology Using Convolution Neural Networks

Min Chen[1]($\boxtimes$), Jiancong Wang[1], Ipek Oguz[1], Brian L. VanderBeek[2], and James C. Gee[1]

[1] Department of Radiology, University of Pennsylvania,
Philadelphia, PA 19104, USA
`minchen1@upenn.edu`
[2] Department of Ophthalmology, University of Pennsylvania,
Philadelphia, PA 19104, USA

Abstract. The choroid plays a critical role in maintaining the portions of the eye responsible for vision. Specific alterations in the choroid have been associated with several disease states, including age-related macular degeneration (AMD), central serous chorioretinopathy, retinitis pigmentosa and diabetes. In addition, choroid thickness measures have been shown as a predictive biomarker for treatment response and visual function. Where several approaches currently exist for segmenting the choroid in optical coherence tomography (OCT) images of healthy retina, very few are capable of addressing images with retinal pathology. The difficulty is due to existing methods relying on first detecting the retinal boundaries before performing the choroidal segmentation. Performance suffers when these boundaries are disrupted or suffer large morphological changes due to disease, and cannot be found accurately. In this work, we show that a learning based approach using convolutional neural networks can allow for the detection and segmentation of the choroid without the prerequisite delineation of the retinal layers. This avoids the need to model and delineate unpredictable pathological changes in the retina due to disease. Experimental validation was performed using 62 manually delineated choroid segmentations of retinal enhanced depth OCT images from patients with AMD. Our results show segmentation accuracy that surpasses those reported by state of the art approaches on healthy retinal images, and overall high values in images with pathology, which are difficult to address by existing methods without pathology specific heuristics.

Keywords: Segmentation · Deep learning · Convolution neural network · Retina · EDI-OCT

1 Introduction

The choroid is the vascular layer located between the retina and sclera in the eye. It plays the vital role of providing nutrients and maintaining the portions of the

© Springer International Publishing AG 2017
M.J. Cardoso et al. (Eds.): FIFI/OMIA 2017, LNCS 10554, pp. 177–184, 2017.
DOI: 10.1007/978-3-319-67561-9_20

eye responsible for vision. Specific alterations in the choroid have been associated with several disease states, including age-related macular degeneration (AMD) [1], retinitis pigmentosa [2], Stargardts disease, diabetes [3], sarcoidosis, and Vogt-Koyanagi-Harada syndrome. In addition, choroid thickness measures have been shown as a predictive biomarker for treatment response [4] and visual function [5].

Since the introduction of enhanced depth imaging optical coherence tomography (EDI-OCT) [6], there has been an explosion of interest in studying the choroid in vivo. This has included not only the disease processes previously associated with choroidal abnormalities, but also exploring the role of the choroid in ocular conditions as diverse as myopia and angle closure glaucoma. This quick (<1 s per scan), non-contact, safe, and inexpensive imaging modality has become readily accepted by both clinicians and patients.

To date, most assessments of EDI-OCT images have involved manual evaluation of the borders of the choroid and subjective judgments of choroidal vessel caliber (large, small, dilated, attenuated) and stromal density, which has proven difficult and time consuming. Fully or semi-automated systems are needed to make it possible to use in direct patient care and in clinical studies involving large numbers of patients examined serially over time. While several techniques [7–16] have been designed for the segmentation and measurement of the choroid in OCT, existing methods are primarily focused on images with normal (or normal-appearing) retinal structures with limited pathology.

Current approaches begin by first segmenting the retinal layers using methods such as graph-cuts [8,10], dynamic programming [7,9], gradient-based edge detection [11,15], and active contours [16]. After locating the retinal layers, the choroid is found using an intensity based approach within a sub-region of the image, typically defined by the Bruchs Membrane (BM) located in the first step. Proposed approaches for segmenting the choroid in this sub-region include thresholding and region growing [8], multi-scale filtering with probabilistic estimation [9], constructing statistical [7], morphological models [10], and texture or gradient analysis [15,16].

In the presence of pathology, existing approaches become less accurate and robust due to changes to the retinal morphology caused by disease. Very few methods have been presented that addresses automated choroid segmentation in the presence of pathology. Notably, [7,9] proposed addressing the problem by making the retinal boundary segmentation more robust. Their approach first uses image derivative information and edge orientation to prevent unrealistic boundary jumps and shifts. A convex hull is then fit to the estimated boundaries to detect possible detachment of the retina. The method is shown to be robust to many cases of retinal pathology, such as drusen and retinal detachment. However, the algorithm still relies on the initial delineation of the retinal pigment epithelium, which the authors locate using the most hyper-intense boundary in the image. The method will be unreliable in cases where this assumption is violated due to artifacts or pathology. Also relevant, [17] presents an outer retinal-subretinal layer segmentation approach that addresses pathology by augmenting their graph search algorithm with a specialized fluid detection algorithm that is able to determine abnormal fluid-filled structures in the layer.

In this work, we present an approach where the detection and segmentation of the choroid and choroidal vessels are performed without the prerequisite delineation of the retinal layers. Instead we train a convolution neural network to directly identify the interior and exterior boundaries of the choroid in the image. This approach utilizes the fact that (1) the choroid is often not noticeably affected by retinal pathology, and (2) the morphology and texture of the choroid are distinct from the retina and retinal pathology. This allows us to directly identify the choroid regardless of the state of the retina in the image. Our approach aims to avoid needing to model and delineate the often unpredictable pathological changes in the retina due to disease.

2   Method

Our method consists of two primary steps. First, a convolution neural network (CNN) is trained to find the pixel-wise probability maps for the interior (Bruch's membrane) and exterior (choroid-sclera interface) boundaries of the choroid. Once these probability maps are found we use seam carving [18] to estimate the two boundaries in the image and produce the final segmentation of the choroid.

2.1   Generating Edge Probability Maps Using CNN

For our CNN architecture, we use the SegNet design presented in [19]. The network consists of an encoder network, a corresponding decoder network and a pixel-wise classification layer. The SegNet architecture was designed specifically for pixel-wise classification of images where boundary delineation is vital. One of its key features is the ability to reduce the loss of spatial resolution due to max-pooling and sub-sampling by storing the max-pooling indices in the encoder and using it in the respective decoder to upsample the input feature map. This also has the advantage of avoiding the need to learn to upsample, reducing the overall number of parameters.

For our task, we use 6 layers of encoder and 6 layers of decoder, with (8, 16, 16, 32, 32, 64) features in each encoder layer and the reverse order in the decoder layers. A 5-by-5 convolution kernel is used throughout the network. An element-wise rectified linear non-linearity (ReLU) $max(0, x)$ is applied to every layer except the final layer, which uses a softmax function to produce a probability output. Stochastic gradient descent is used for training the network, with a momentum of 0.9 and a fixed learning rate of 0.0001. We used a constant scale factor of 2 in the X and Y directions. We found that the network in general converges within 40 epochs.

Training and Testing. Two different SegNets are trained for our method, one to locate the Bruch's membrane and the second to locate the choroid-sclera interface. Each network is trained on full EDI-OCT images with manually delineations of the respective boundaries, where each pixel in the training image is marked as either *boundary* or *background*. To increase the number of training examples, small random affine perturbations are used to displace each training images. This provides additional examples that can account for anatomical variability in the eye that may not be fully represented in our data. Given an unseen image, both SegNet are applied to the image to produce two probability maps representing the likely location of the two boundaries in the images.

2.2 Seam Carving

To convert the edge probability maps into a binary segmentation of the choroid, we use a technique known as *seam carving* [18]. Given an image I with dimension $n \times m$, the goal of seam carving is to find a path of connected pixel that fully traverses across the image. For our task, we are interested in finding the horizontal seam,

$$s = \{s_j^y\}_{j=1}^m = \{(j, y(j))\}_{j=1}^m, \ s.t. \ \forall \ j, |y(j) - y(j-1)| \leq 1, \tag{1}$$

where y is the mapping $y : [1, \ldots, m] \Rightarrow [1, \ldots, n]$. This formulation ensures that the seam only has a single pixel in each column and each pixel in the seam is 8-connected to the pixels in the adjacent columns. To find this seam, we define the cost function

$$E(s) = E(I_S) = \sum_{j=1}^m e(I(s_j)), \tag{2}$$

where e is an energy function. For our purpose, $e(I(s_j))$ is the value of the probability map at location s_j. Given this energy function, the optimal seam can be found by using dynamic programming as described in [18].

The optimal seams found for our two probability maps are used as the interior and exterior boundaries of the choroid, and the pixels between the boundaries are completely filled to provide the full choroidal segmentation. This approach is advantageous over simply thresholding the probability maps, because it allows us to enforce a specific topology, connectivity, and smoothness to the segmentation.

3 Evaluation and Results

3.1 Data

62 EDI-OCT retinal images from 32 patients diagnosed with age related macular degeneration (AMD) were used for the evaluation of our method. Two images were acquired from each patient, the first image was of a retina with *dry* (atrophic) AMD from one eye, and the second image was of a retina with *wet* (exudative) AMD from the other eye. Each EDI-OCT image was a 2D cross-sectional slice centered on the fovea, with approximate dimensions of 1150 by 700 pixels. For each image, a manual segmentation of the choroid was performed by a trained rater using ITK Snap [20]. These manual segmentations serve as the ground truth used in our evaluation.

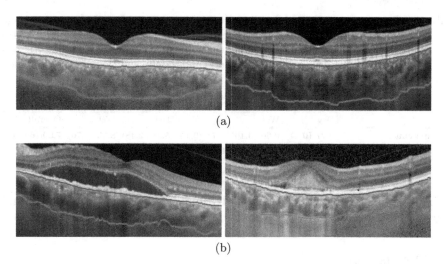

(a)

(b)

Fig. 1. Examples of the interior (Bruch's membrane, shown in red) and exterior (choroid-sclera interface, shown in green) boundaries of the choroid found by the proposed method on retinal image of eyes diagnosed with (a) dry and (b) wet AMD. (Color figure online)

3.2 Results

We evaluated our algorithm on each image using 5-fold cross-validation, where 80% of the images (50 image) were randomly selected and used for training, and the remaining 20% were used to testing. This process was repeated until all images were segmented. The same parameters as described in Sect. 2.1 were used for each SegNet network used in the evaluation. Figure 1 shows several examples of the automated choroidal boundaries detected by our method. We compared our automated results against the manual ground truth by calculating the average distance error of the Bruch's membrane (evaluted as the average absolute difference between the manual and automated boundary location in each A-scan), and the overall Dice overlap coefficient [21],

$$\mathrm{Dice}\,(A, B) = \frac{2|A \cap B|}{|A| + |B|}, \tag{3}$$

between the automated and manual segmentations.

For a baseline comparison, we also performed the same evaluation using a graph cuts based segmentation approach, which have been shown [22,23] to produce highly accurate segmentations of retinal layers in OCT images of healthy subjects. However, for our comparison, we adapted the approach to find the interior and exterior boundaries of the choroid in our 2D EDI-OCT images. No pathology-specific correction step was used to improving the BM surface in the wet AMD cases [17], but rather a single graph cut optimization with two surfaces was performed. Table 1 shows the average (and standard deviation) of

Table 1. The average (standard deviation) of the Dice overlap coefficient and average Bruch's membrane (BM) boundary distance error (in pixels) of the choroid segmentation, evaluated between each algorithm and the manual ground truth. Each metric was first evaluated over the dry and wet AMD cases separately, and then on the combined overall dataset.

	Dice overlap			BM error in pixels		
	Dry	Wet	Overall	Dry	Wet	Overall
Graph cuts	0.77 (0.11)	0.66 (0.16)	0.71 (0.15)	5.58 (2.48)	8.55 (7.76)	7.09 (6.00)
SegNet + Seam carving	0.85 (0.07)	0.81 (0.10)	0.83 (0.09)	4.19 (2.02)	7.25 (6.92)	5.72 (5.36)

each algorithm's performance over the dry and wet AMD cases separately and over the full dataset.

4   Discussion

From our results we see that, overall, our approach produced segmentations of the choroid that aligned well with the manual delineations. On average our algorithm produced a Dice overlap coefficient of 0.82 ($\pm$0.10) relative to manual segmentation. This is comparable to existing literature [8], which reports an average Dice overlap of 0.78 ($\pm$0.08) for automated segmentation of the choroid in healthy retinal. While the comparison is indirect, the result is promising considering that our dataset consisted of 2D images with retina pathology, many of which contained large intensity and morphological changes. Conversely, our images are EDI-OCT, which may have allowed the choroidal structures to be more easily segmented than standard OCT.

From Table 1 we see that on average our approach produced segmentations with higher Dice overlap and lower BM boundary errors than the graph cuts based approach. However, it would be fair to note that the graph cuts algorithm was adapted from a design developed for 3D OCT volumes of healthy subjects. Thus, the lack of 3D context in our data may explain the lower performance. Additionally, as noted above, the graph cut approach can be augmented with a specific correction technique to handle drusen, cysts and RPE detachment [17], which we have not included. This further contributes to its lower performance in the wet AMD cases. In contrast, our approach is robust to pathology and can be readily deployed even in a single 2D B-scan.

Qualitatively, our proposed algorithm is very robust to retinal pathology (as shown in Fig. 1(b)). This satisfies one of the primary goals of our approach, which was to design an algorithm that can detect the choroid independent of the state of the retina. One disadvantage of using a learning based approach to address this problem is that the success of the algorithm is predicated on the diversity of the training images. The training set must cover the wide range of appearances that the choroid can take in the image. For example, given our limited training set consisting mostly of normal appearing choroids, we can expect the algorithm to fail in the presence of choroidal pathology or imaging artifacts in the choroid.

Likewise images acquired using different systems may also pose a problem if the imaging characteristics are sufficiently different.

5   Conclusion

We have introduced an automated approach for segmenting the choroid in EDI-OCT images with retinal pathology. Our results showed high performance relative to manual segmentations, and does not require prerequisite retinal layer segmentations which are necessary for most existing algorithm. There are several direction that this work can be extended. One potential area of exploration is the use of CNN to directly segment the choroid vasculature instead of locating the choroidal edges. This can potentially allow for more accurate and robust segmentation by avoiding the need to detect the thin structure represented by the edges. In addition, 3D information from adjacent (non-EDI) OCT B-scans can potentially be incorporated into the segmentation to allow for more contextual information in the segmentation.

References

1. Chung, S.E., Kang, S.W., Lee, J.H., Kim, Y.T.: Choroidal thickness in polypoidal choroidal vasculopathy and exudative age-related macular degeneration. Ophthalmology **118**(5), 840–845 (2011)
2. Dhoot, D.S., Huo, S., Yuan, A., Xu, D., Srivistava, S., Ehlers, J.P., Traboulsi, E., Kaiser, P.K.: Evaluation of choroidal thickness in retinitis pigmentosa using enhanced depth imaging optical coherence tomography. Br. J. Ophthalmol. **97**(1), 66–69 (2013)
3. Esmaeelpour, M., Brunner, S., Ansari-Shahrezaei, S., Nemetz, S., Považay, B., Kajic, V., Drexler, W., Binder, S.: Choroidal thinning in diabetes type 1 detected by 3-Dimensional 1060 nm optical coherence tomography. Investig. Ophthalmol. Visual Sci. **53**(11), 6803–6809 (2012)
4. Kang, H.M., Kwon, H.J., Yi, J.H., Lee, C.S., Lee, S.C.: Subfoveal choroidal thickness as a potential predictor of visual outcome and treatment response after intravitreal ranibizumab injections for typical exudative age-related macular degeneration. Am. J. Ophthalmol. **157**(5), 1013–1021 (2014)
5. Moutray, T., Alarbi, M., Mahon, G., Stevenson, M., Chakravarthy, U.: Relationships between clinical measures of visual function, fluorescein angiographic and optical coherence tomography features in patients with subfoveal choroidal neovascularisation. Br. J. Ophthalmol. **92**(3), 361–364 (2008)
6. Spaide, R.F., Koizumi, H., Pozonni, M.C.: Enhanced depth imaging spectral-domain optical coherence tomography. Am. J. Ophthalmol. **146**(4), 496–500 (2008)
7. Kajić, V., Esmaeelpour, M., Považay, B., Marshall, D., Rosin, P.L., Drexler, W.: Automated choroidal segmentation of 1060 nm OCT in healthy and pathologic eyes using a statistical model. Biomed. Opt. Express **3**(1), 86–103 (2012)
8. Zhang, L., Lee, K., Niemeijer, M., Mullins, R.F., Sonka, M., Abramoff, M.D.: Automated segmentation of the choroid from clinical SD-OCT. Investig. Ophthalmol. Visual Sci. **53**(12), 7510–7519 (2012)

9. Kajić, V., Esmaeelpour, M., Glittenberg, C., Kraus, M.F., Honegger, J., Othara, R., Binder, S., Fujimoto, J.G., Drexler, W.: Automated three-dimensional choroidal vessel segmentation of 3D 1060 nm OCT retinal data. Biomed. Opt. Express 4(1), 134–150 (2013)
10. Hu, Z., Wu, X., Ouyang, Y., Ouyang, Y., Sadda, S.R.: Semiautomated segmentation of the choroid in spectral-domain optical coherence tomography volume scans. Investig. Ophthalmol. Visual Sci. 54(3), 1722–1729 (2013)
11. Tian, J., Marziliano, P., Baskaran, M., Tun, T.A., Aung, T.: Automatic segmentation of the choroid in enhanced depth imaging optical coherence tomography images. Biomed. Opt. Express 4(3), 397–411 (2013)
12. Zhang, L., Buitendijk, G.H., Lee, K., Sonka, M., Springelkamp, H., Hofman, A., Vingerling, J.R., Mullins, R.F., Klaver, C.C., Abràmoff, M.D.: Validity of automated choroidal segmentation in SS-OCT and SD-OCT. Investig. Ophthalmol. Visual Sci. 56(5), 3202–3211 (2015)
13. Vupparaboina, K.K., Nizampatnam, S., Chhablani, J., Richhariya, A., Jana, S.: Automated estimation of choroidal thickness distribution and volume based on OCT images of posterior visual section. Comput. Med. Imaging Graph. 46, 315–327 (2015)
14. Philip, A.-M., Gerendas, B.S., Zhang, L., Faatz, H., Podkowinski, D., Bogunovic, H., Abramoff, M.D., Hagmann, M., Leitner, R., Simader, C., et al.: Choroidal thickness maps from spectral domain and swept source optical coherence tomography: algorithmic versus ground truth annotation. Br. J. Ophthalmol. 1–5 (2016)
15. Chen, Q., Fan, W., Niu, S., Shi, J., Shen, H., Yuan, S.: Automated choroid segmentation based on gradual intensity distance in hd-oct images. Opt. Express 23(7), 8974–8994 (2015)
16. González-López, A., Remeseiro, B., Ortega, M., Penedo, M.G., Charlón, P.: A texture-based method for choroid segmentation in retinal EDI-OCT images. In: Moreno-Díaz, R., Pichler, F., Quesada-Arencibia, A. (eds.) EUROCAST 2015. LNCS, vol. 9520, pp. 487–493. Springer, Cham (2015). doi:10.1007/978-3-319-27340-2_61
17. Zhang, L., Sonka, M., Folk, J.C., Russell, S.R., Abramoff, M.D.: Quantifying disrupted outer retinal-subretinal layer in SD-OCT images in choroidal neovascularization. Investig. Ophthalmol. Visual Sci. 55, 2329–2335 (2014)
18. Avidan, S., Shamir, A.: Seam carving for content-aware image resizing. ACM Trans. Graph. (TOG) 26(3), 10 (2007). ACM
19. Badrinarayanan, V., Kendall, A., Cipolla, R.: Segnet: a deep convolutional encoder-decoder architecture for image segmentation. arXiv preprint arXiv:1511.00561 (2015)
20. Yushkevich, P.A., Piven, J., Hazlett, H.C., Smith, R.G., Ho, S., Gee, J.C., Gerig, G.: User-guided 3D active contour segmentation of anatomical structures: significantly improved efficiency and reliability. Neuroimage 31(3), 1116–1128 (2006)
21. Dice, L.R.: Measures of the amount of ecologic association between species. Ecology 26(3), 297–302 (1945)
22. Garvin, M.K., Abramoff, M.D., Wu, X., Russell, S.R., Burns, T.L., Sonka, M.: Automated 3-D intraretinal layer segmentation of macular spectral-domain optical coherence tomography images. IEEE Trans. Med. Imaging 28(9), 1436–1447 (2009)
23. Lang, A., Carass, A., Hauser, M., Sotirchos, E.S., Calabresi, P.A., Ying, H.S., Prince, J.L.: Retinal layer segmentation of macular OCT images using boundary classification. Biomed. Opt. Express 4(7), 1133–1152 (2013)

Spatiotemporal Analysis of Structural Changes of the Lamina Cribrosa

Charly Girot[1], Hiroshi Ishikawa[2], James Fishbaugh[1(✉)], Gadi Wollstein[2], Joel Schuman[2], and Guido Gerig[1]

[1] Tandon School of Engineering, New York University, Brooklyn, NY, USA
james.fishbaugh@nyu.edu
[2] Langone Medical Center, Department of Ophtalmology, NYU School of Medicine, New York, NY, USA

Abstract. Glaucoma, a progressive and degenerative disease of the optic nerve, is the second leading cause of blindness worldwide. Mechanical deformation of the lamina cribrosa (LC) under high intraocular pressure (IOP) can lead to axonal death of optic nerve fibers. To explore the effect of pressure on the LC, we utilize an experimental setup where longitudinal 3D optical coherence tomography (OCT) images are acquired at different levels of IOP administered via a well-controlled external force. Structural changes are measured via image deformations which map all observed images simultaneously into a common coordinate space. These deformations encode local patterns of structural and volume change across the image sequence, resulting in quantification of the spatiotemporal deformation pattern of the LC due to variation of pressure. We also describe a 3D segmentation algorithm to restrict our deformation analysis separately to the beams or pores of the LC. A single case study demonstrates the potential of the proposed methodology for non-invasive in-vivo analysis of LC dynamics in individual subjects.

Keywords: OCT · Lamina cribrosa · Spatiotemporal analysis · Glaucoma

1 Introduction

Glaucoma is a progressive and degenerative disease of the optic nerve and is the second leading cause of blindness worldwide [1]. Due to irreversible damage to the optic nerve, it is essential to diagnose glaucoma early and to sensitively monitor disease progression in order to prevent potential vision loss. The lamina cribrosa (LC) is a connective tissue meshwork where optic nerve fibers pass through from inside the eye to the outside. Because of this anatomical placement, it can make it a vulnerable location in the visual neural pathway. Mechanical deformation of the LC, especially under high intraocular pressure (IOP), can lead to axonal death of optic nerve fibers [2]. Therefore, assessment and monitoring of LC condition may provide clinically useful biomarkers to manage glaucoma.

© Springer International Publishing AG 2017
M.J. Cardoso et al. (Eds.): FIFI/OMIA 2017, LNCS 10554, pp. 185–193, 2017.
DOI: 10.1007/978-3-319-67561-9_21

Optical coherence tomography (OCT) provides 3D imaging of the ocular tissues at microscopic resolutions [3]. OCT has been extensively used in glaucoma studies and is known to provide clinically favorable quantitative measurements [4,5]. Recent advances in OCT technology opened the possibility for 3D imaging of the LC but significant challenges for analysis of such data remain. Individual OCT images show considerable noise which make it difficult to obtain consistent segmentation across a time series. Alignment of images to a common coordinate frame, accounting for eye movement and deformation, and assessment of deformations to analyze structural changes remain open issues.

In this paper, we address these challenges with an experimental setup and novel analysis method to measure structural changes of the LC with respect to different IOP conditions. The experimental setup includes applying increasing IOP and acquiring a longitudinal time-series of observations in the form of in-vivo OCT images [6]. To address the presence of noise in OCT, we explore the noise reduction properties of several filtering techniques. From the dynamic longitudinal sequence, we estimate a geometric average template image, which establishes a common reference frame for joint structural segmentation and includes deformation mappings to each observation. The diffeomorphic mappings encode local deformation and volume changes between *any two* observations in the sequence. Such measurements capture detailed non-linear patterns of structural changes to the LC and provide qualitative and quantitative assessment of regional deformations as a function of external pressure and its release. We present a case study of newly acquired prototype data to explore the effect of increasing IOP on a single individual. All methodology in this paper utilizes full volumetric (3D) images, though results are presented as 2D slices.

2   Methods

2.1   Digital Filtering

Digital filtering is important to overcome the speckle noise pattern inherent in acquisitions by narrow-band detection systems like OCT. Specifically, the presence of noise makes it difficult to accurately differentiate the beams and pores of the LC. Therefore, we seek to reduce speckle noise while also preserving edge-sharpness, to better delineate between beams and pores.

The 6 compared algorithms were: Lee filtering, non-local means, wavelet decomposition, virtual averaging [7], anisotropic diffusion, and the block matching and 3D (BM3D) filtering algorithm [8]. In our tests, BM3D provided the best results with respect to signal-to-noise ratio. Furthermore, B3MD filtered images also passed visual image quality tests performed by OCT clinical experts. Figure 1 shows a typical result from B3MD filtering.

2.2   Average Template Construction

Average template construction was initially developed by the brain mapping community for analyzing shape variability within a population [9]. From a set

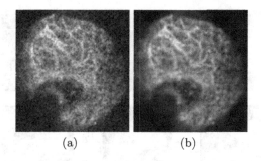

(a)   (b)

Fig. 1. Slice extracted from volumetric OCT data from (a) original noisy image and (b) BM3D filtered image.

of images, the goal is to estimate an 'average' template image. The key intuition is the template is not a simple voxelwise average of the observed images, which has the known problem of producing fuzzy averages and false structure. Rather it is a mean in the Fréchet sense, i.e. a minimizer of distance, which produces a sharp average geometrically representative of the population. Most commonly, distance is defined by the amount of deformation (via diffeomorphic transport $h : R^3 \rightarrow R^3$) required to warp one image onto another. Template estimation can be expressed by the cost function

$$E(T, \{h_i\}) = \sum_{i=1}^{N} ||T \circ h_i - I_i||_{L^2}^2 + \text{Reg}(\{h_i\}) \tag{1}$$

where T is the template image, $\{h_i\}$ is the set of diffeomorphic mappings which align the template to each image observation I_i, and Reg is a measure of regularity on the set of diffeomorphisms (more detail in [9]).

This method allows us to map all images into a common coordinate system to study local deformations only - without considering global movement (during acquisition) - and to create an average image, the template T, as shown in Fig. 2. The most important information, however, is encoded in the deformations themselves, as the diffeomorphic mappings capture individual variability as deviation from average. As shown Fig. 2, we can also compute mappings from any image to any other image by composition of diffeomorphisms, and are therefore able to measure the amount of structural change between any two observations.

The average template also serves as a necessary tool for segmentation, as it is only performed once in the template space, and then propagated to each observation by the mappings $\{h_i\}$. This segmentation procedure is essential for structural analysis, as it guarantees topological consistency across observations.

In this paper we are specifically using the method developed in [10], available in the ANTs package [11].

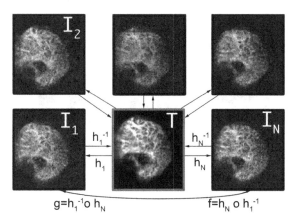

Fig. 2. Overview of average template construction. The template image T (red) is the geometric average of the set of images $\{I_i\}$ obtained via deformable mappings. T is estimated by minimizing the total amount of diffeomorphic deformation per image $\{h_i\}$ to align observations with the template. Composition of diffeomorphisms allows to compute mappings between any pair of images to analyze spatiotemporal profiles. (Color figure online)

2.3   Segmentation

Segmentation involves extracting structures composing the LC, namely the beams meshwork and the pores, which are respectively characterized as sheet-like and tube-like structures in OCT images. In [12], a generalized Frangi multiscale vesselness method was proposed to enhance M dimensional shapes in N dimensional images. It is based on the examination of the Hessian (a square matrix of local second order spatial derivatives applied to a scalar field f : $H_{i,j} = \frac{\partial f}{\partial x_i \partial x_j}$) and its eigen decomposition. The extracted three orthonormal directions (3D) encode shape structure regarding the isotropy of those directions.

If we consider $M < N$, M the shape dimension (0 for blobs, 1 for tubes, 2 for sheets), N the image dimension, and $|\lambda_1| \leq |\lambda_2| \leq ... \leq |\lambda_N|$ the eigenvalues of the $N \times N$ Hessian matrix, the following enhancement is defined:

$$R_A = \frac{|\lambda_{M+1}|}{\prod_{i=M+2}^{N} |\lambda_i|^{\frac{1}{N-M-1}}}, \quad R_B = \frac{|\lambda_M|}{\prod_{i=M+1}^{N} |\lambda_i|^{\frac{1}{N-M}}}, \quad S = \sqrt{\sum_{j=1}^{N} \lambda_j^2} \quad (2)$$

which combine to define an objectness measure as

$$O(\lambda)_\sigma = \begin{cases} (1 - e^{-\frac{R_A^2}{2\alpha^2}}) \cdot e^{-\frac{R_B^2}{2\beta^2}} \cdot (1 - e^{-\frac{S^2}{2\gamma^2}}) & \text{if } \lambda_j \leq 0 \text{ for } M \leq j \leq N \\ 0 & \text{otherwise} \end{cases} \quad (3)$$

which is evaluated over a range of spatial scales and the maximum response is selected as

$$O(\lambda) = \max \sigma \in [\sigma_{min}, \sigma_{max}] \, O(\lambda)_\sigma. \quad (4)$$

The result is a probability map for each extraction representing the probability of each voxel belonging to either beams or pores. Typical segmentation results are shown in Fig. 3. The binarization step uses a probability threshold of 0.15, but may be improved in the future with an adaptive thresholding scheme. Note that segmentation is done only once in the template space and then deformed to individual images via deformations computed in template estimation.

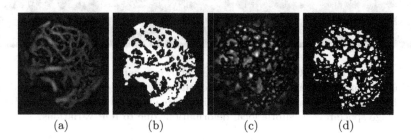

(a)   (b)   (c)   (d)

Fig. 3. (a) Structural segmentation of beam structures with $\sigma_{min} = 0.2$, $\sigma_{max} = 4.0$, $N_\sigma = 20$, (b) binary label for beams, and (c) pore structures with $\sigma_{min} = 1.0$, $\sigma_{max} = 4.0$, $N_\sigma = 20$, and (d) binary label for pores.

2.4   Spatiotemporal Analysis

The goal is to quantify the effect of increasing pressure on the structure of the lamina cribrosa. As mentioned in Sect. 2.2, the template provides a set of deformations which warp any image onto any other image in the time series. Encoded in the mappings is precisely the structural change that we wish to measure. Consider the mapping as a displacement field, i.e. vectors $f(i)$ at each voxel, which describe where intensity values in the source image move to in the target image. By taking the determinant of the Jacobian of the displacement field $J = [\frac{\partial f}{\partial x_1} ... \frac{\partial f}{\partial x_n}]$ at each voxel, we obtain information about volume change, with positive values indicating expansion, and negative values indicating contraction. This provides local information about structural change between observations.

3   Experimental Results

We explore our analysis pipeline with a case study, a longitudinal pressure experiment of one patient with 2 images acquired at each stage: baseline, IOP + 30 mmHg, IOP + 50 mmHg, and post pressure recovery. The images were filtered using the method described Sect. 2.1 with standard deviation of the noise $\sigma = 0.3$ by minimizing the MSE between the filtered image and the original image. Figure 1 shows the original and the denoised image.

Average Template Construction: The 8 images from the experiment are used to estimate an average template, as described in Sect. 2.2, shown as T in

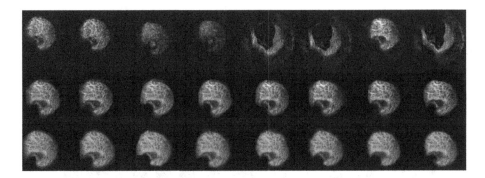

Fig. 4. Top: Original OCT image series showing same 2D slice across time depicting lack of registration. **Middle:** Observations warped to the template and thus co-registered. **Bottom:** Inverse diffeomorphic mapping from the template to each individual image space reveals subtle local deformations due to IOP variations.

Fig. 2. The advantage of this process can be seen in Fig. 4, namely the creation of a common coordinate system and the ability to isolate local deformations. The first row shows images before alignment, notice whole 2D slices are not in correspondence across observations. The second row shows the input volumes warped into the template space. These images look similar, as they have been co-registered through template estimation; computing their average is the resulting template T. The last row represent the diffeomorphisms $\{h_i\}$ applied to the template. In contrast to the second row (which shows very little change over the time series, no change in a perfect case scenario), viewing this sequence as an animation shows local structural changes across time. This is precisely what we wish to measure with respect to the longitudinal pressure experiment.

Spatiotemporal Analysis: Beams and pores were segmented in the template space with the method in Sect. 2.3. Deformations between images in the chronological order of the original timeline are reconstructed, illustrated in Fig. 5 using the composition rule (arrow from bottom left to bottom right of Fig. 2 is one example of the composition rule). Structural changes between the baseline image and IOP + 30 mmHg are shown in Fig. 6(a), with the Jacobian determinant

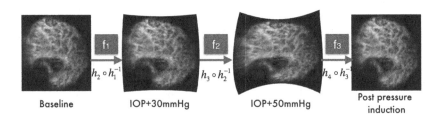

Fig. 5. Schematic of timeline reconstruction obtained by applying composition of deformations computed via template construction (deformations artificially enhanced).

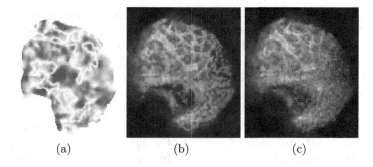

(a)   (b)   (c)

Fig. 6. Slice extracted from deformation analysis between baseline and IOP + 30 mmHg. (a) Jacobian determinant shows volume changes as local expansion (red) or contraction (blue). Volume changes masked with segmentation of beams (b) and pores (c). (Color figure online)

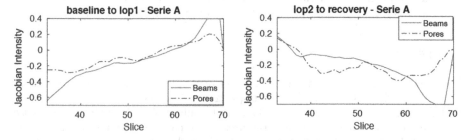

Fig. 7. Global analysis of structural changes for two scenarios shown as normalized volume evolution along the optic nerve axis for beams (red) and pores (blue). (Color figure online)

representing local contraction and expansion, as in Sect. 2.4. In Fig. 6(b) and (c), results of segmentation are used as a mask on Fig. 6(a), to produce measures of contraction and expansion isolated on beams and pores, respectively.

In addition to analyzing local deformation patterns, we also compute a global summary of deformation by integrating each slice along the optic nerve axis. Figure 7 shows the result of this analysis over the whole LC. This study aims to explore patterns of deformation of the analyzable lamina due to pressure change and can be focused on individual or small groups of pores. Positive values in these plots indicates the region is more expanded by deformation, while negative values indicate the region is more contracted.

4 Discussion

In this paper, we adapted proven image analysis methods developed by the brain mapping community to study deformation of structures in an OCT image sequence acquired under a controlled pressure experiment. Template construction provides an average image with reduced noise, and segmentation in this space followed by back-mapping to original coordinates ensures consistent 3D structural segmentation across all images of the sequence. Cascading spatial mappings and analysis of the Jacobian of deformations results in spatiotemporal analysis of patterns of dynamic changes of the LC. Future work will focus on improved interpretation of deformations by quantifying variability via repeated scans at each pressure time point, by analysis of the dynamics of beams and pores via bio-mechanical modeling, and by acquisition and testing of dynamic image series from multiple subjects diagnosed with glaucoma. The preliminary case study demonstrates proof of concept of image-based analysis of the LC and highlights its potential for improved insight into the dynamic deformation of the LC caused by external pressure. With the hypothesis that resulting measures may indicate vulnerability to axonal damage, it is our long-term goal to develop a tool for early monitoring of glaucomateous disease. To our knowledge, our framework is the first methodology to address fundamental issues related to the dynamic characteristics of the microstructure of the LC with serial OCT imaging under varying IOP followed by spatiotemporal image analysis.

References

1. Quigley, H.A., Broman, A.T.: The number of people with glaucoma worldwide in 2010 and 2020. Br. J. Ophthalmol. **90**(3), 262–267 (2006)
2. Burgoyne, C.F., Downs, J.C., Bellezza, A.J., Suh, J.K.F., Hart, R.T.: The optic nerve head as a biomechanical structure: a new paradigm for understanding the role of IOP-related stress and strain in the pathophysiology of glaucomatous optic nerve head damage. Prog. Retinal Eye Res. **24**(1), 39–73 (2005)
3. Drexler, W., Fujimoto, J.G.: State-of-the-art retinal optical coherence tomography. Prog. Retinal Eye Res. **27**(1), 45–88 (2008)
4. Gabriele, M.L., Wollstein, G., Ishikawa, H., Xu, J., Kim, J., Kagemann, L., Folio, L., Schuman, J.: Three dimensional optical coherence tomography imaging: advantages and advances. Prog. Retinal Eye Res. **29**(6), 556–579 (2010)
5. Gabriele, M.L., Wollstein, G., Ishikawa, H., Kagemann, L., Xu, J., Folio, L.S., Schuman, J.S.: Optical coherence tomography: history, current status, and laboratory work. Invest. Ophthalmol. Vis. Sci. **52**(5), 2425–2436 (2011)
6. Tran, H., Voorhees, A.P., Wang, B., Jan, N.J., Tyler-Kabara, E., Kagemann, L., Ishikawa, H., Schuman, J.S., Smith, M.A., Wollstein, G., et al.: In-vivo modulation of intraocular and intracranial pressures causes nonlinear and non-monotonic deformations of the lamina cribrosa. Invest. Ophthalmol. Vis. Sci. **57**(12), 3565–3565 (2016)
7. Chen, C., Ishikawa, H., Wollstein, G., Bilonick, R., Kagemann, L., Schuman, J.: Virtual averaging making nonframe-averaged optical coherence tomography images comparable to frame-averaged images. Trans. Vis. Sci. Techol. **5**(1) (2016)
8. Dabov, K., Foi, A., Katkovnik, V., Egiazarian, K.: BM3D image denoising with shape-adaptive principal component analysis. In: SPARS (2009)
9. Joshi, S., Davis, B., Jomier, M., Gerig, G.: Unbiased diffeomorphic atlas construction for computational anatomy. NeuroImage **23**, S151–S160 (2004)
10. Avants, B.B., Yushkevich, P.A., Pluta, J., Minkoff, D., Korczykowski, M., Detre, J.A., Gee, J.C.: The optimal template effect in hippocampus studies of diseased populations. NeuroImage **49**(3), 2457–2466 (2010)

11. Avants, B.B., Tustison, N., Song, G.: Advanced normalization tools (ants). Insight J. **2**, 1–35 (2009)
12. Antiga, L.: Generalizing vesselness with respect to dimensionality and shape. Insight J. (2007). http://hdl.handle.net/1926/576

Fast Blur Detection and Parametric Deconvolution of Retinal Fundus Images

Bryan M. Williams[1(✉)], Baidaa Al-Bander[2], Harry Pratt[1], Samuel Lawman[2],
Yitian Zhao[4,5], Yalin Zheng[1,3], and Yaochun Shen[2]

[1] Department of Eye and Vision Science, University of Liverpool, Liverpool, UK
{bryan,yzheng}@liverpool.ac.uk
[2] Department of Electrical Engineering and Electronics,
University of Liverpool, Liverpool, UK
[3] St. Paul's Eye Unit, Royal Liverpool University Hospital, Liverpool, UK
[4] Chinese Academy of Sciences, Ningbo Institute of Material Technology
and Engineering, Ningbo, China
[5] School of Optics and Electronics, Beijing Institute of Technology, Beijing, China

Abstract. Blur is a significant problem in medical imaging which can
hinder diagnosis and prevent further automated or manual processing.
The problem of restoring an image from blur degradation remains a
challenging task in image processing. Semi-blind deblurring is a useful
technique which may be developed to restore the underlying sharp image
given some assumed or known information about the cause of degradation. Existing models assume that the blur is of a particular type, such as
Gaussian, and do not allow for the approximation of images corrupted
by other blur types which are not easily incorporated into deblurring
frameworks. We present an automated approach to image deconvolution
which assumes that the cause of blur belongs to a set of common types.
We develop a hierarchical approach with convolutional neural networks
(CNNs) to distinguish between blur types, achieving an accuracy of 0.96
across a test set of 900 images, and to determine the blur strength,
achieving accuracy of 0.77 across 1500 test images. Given this, we are
able to reconstruct the underlying image to mean ISNR of 7.53.

Keywords: Deconvolution · Convolutional neural networks · Colour
fundus · Retina · Parametric

1 Introduction

Image deconvolution is a very useful tool amongst image preprocessing techniques which aims to remove blur which can hinder diagnosis with medical imaging and prevent further processing. In a current screening programme, approximately 5% of the images acquired are too blurred for assessment. It is also an
important step for other techniques in image processing such as super resolution. While there exist models for image segmentation which can cope with some
noise in an image, blur proves to be more of a problem for this as well as related

© Springer International Publishing AG 2017
M.J. Cardoso et al. (Eds.): FIFI/OMIA 2017, LNCS 10554, pp. 194–201, 2017.
DOI: 10.1007/978-3-319-67561-9_22

tasks such as registration. Parametric kernel identification can be used to deblur images making some assumptions about the blur function. There exist many models which work well without noise. However, noise is often present in images and can cause misidentification of the blur function and thus prevent accurate recovery of the image. This paper presents a model for restoring noisy, blurred images in which the blur is assumed to be of a certain type.

Assuming that the blur is spatially invariant, then denoting by h and u the blur function and true image respectively, we model the blurred image z as the convolution of the true image and kernel $z(x,y) = (h * u)(x,y) + \eta(x,y)$ where $*$ denotes the operation of convolution and η denotes noise. Deblurring (or deconvolution) [1] is the associated inverse problem which aims to recover the true image u from the received data z.

Deconvolution models may be split into 3 categories: non-blind deconvolution [2] involves recovering the true image with known blur function; blind deconvolution, [1] involves restoring the image with no knowledge of the blur function and is computationally expensive and difficult to achieve; semi-blind deblurring [3] involves recovering the hidden true image with only partial knowledge or assumptions about the blur function, such as the type of blur and offers a way of achieving an accelerated deblurring algorithm. Such models perform well and can obtain improved results over blind deblurring when the blur type may be known or estimated. Such techniques are useful in related areas such as the segmentation of blurred images and super-resolution where the blur is often of Gaussian or out of focus type. Our aim in this case is to recover the parameters and thus reconstruct the blur function.

Recently, deep neural networks (DNNs) have been emerged as a new area in machine learning analytics. Unlike conventional artificial neural networks, DNN layers are not fully connected and can learn to recognise complex nonlinear features. DNNs are also based use with graphical processing units (GPUs) which facilitate efficient training of large and complex machine learning techniques. Various deep learning architectures such as convolutional neural networks (CNNs) have been reported and developed for various applications including speech recognition [4] and bioinformatics [5] where they have been shown to produce state-of-the-art results on various tasks. Models for deconvolution employing machine learning approaches, including deep learning, have recently been reported. Schuler et al. [6] developed a method for non-blind deblurring where the deconvolution procedure is learned with a multi-layer perceptron. The method is tested on synthetic examples and real out-of-focus images. The authors later extended this to the blind case for small blur kernels [7]. Xu et al. [8] also developed a neural network approach to non-blind deconvolution by linking to optimisation-based schemes, combining deconvolution with denoising. A semi-blind motion blur [9] approach to deconvolution was presented by Sun et al. [10] who used convolutional neural networks to estimate motion blur and adapted a uniform deconvolution approach to the non-uniform problem. In this paper, we develop a framework for semi-blind deblurring with a fast technique of finding the type and strength of blur from an image using CNNs which allow us to determine the blur function quickly and accurately.

2   Method

Our algorithm is separated into training the neural network to classify our data, and separate testing which includes classifying our images given the trained networks and producing a clean image. These stages can be done separately, so that the algorithm may be trained beforehand and later tested on individual examples without needing computationally-expensive training for each image, making this potentially a very fast approach to semi-blind image deconvolution.

For the first part of the training stage of our approach, we attempt to train a convolutional neural network to distinguish blur type using the training images with no assumptions on the blur; this includes the case of no blur being present. We also train individual networks to identify blur strength, for each of a set of blur types, given only the training images and an assumption on the type of blur; for example, we may assume that the blur is out-of-focus. At the testing stage, given an example image which may be blurred or not, we use the first trained network to determine whether blur is present in the image and, if so, the type of blur which is present. If the image is determined to not be blurred, nothing more is done and the image exits the algorithm. Since most images are likely to not contain blur, this means that most images can be processed in the approximate 0.0028 s that it takes the one CNN to classify it. If the image is deemed to blurred, the blur type should already be determined at the same time. Given this information, the appropriate pre-trained second CNN is used to classify the image by blur strength. This allows us to determine the kernel function. Since the kernel function is now assumed to be known, the problem is transformed into one of non-blind deconvolution which may be solved by an existing fast method such as [2]. This algorithm is presented in Fig. 1 and the details of the CNN and deconvolution are shown below.

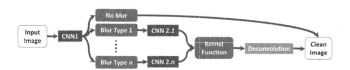

Fig. 1. Flow chart of our overall approach for testing an example image. Assuming that the CNNs are trained, the image is first classified as being corrupted by no blur or a particular type. If the image is blurred, a further CNN determines the strength of blur before the image is restored by a deconvolution process.

2.1   Classification Using Convolutional Neural Networks

Convolutional neural networks (CNNs) are among the most popular deep neural network architectures and have achieved state-of-the-art results in image pattern recognition and other applications. CNNs learn features from raw data without the need for manually designing hand-crafted features.

A CNN is comprised of a modified version of LeNet convolutional neural network implemented by LeCun [11] with successive convolution layers alternated with subsampling and activation functions to implement the feature space for the input data. Fully connected layers combined with a softmax layer normalises the probability of the examples to be classified between 0 and 1. The convolution, nonlinearity, pooling, dropout and classification in a dense layer are the main operations in a convolutional neural network and considered the basic building blocks. The convolution layers work as feature detectors by extracting features from small squares of input image using filters of a certain window size allowing the pixels to preserve the spatial relationship between them. Moreover, to introduce the nonlinearity to convolutional neural networks, which typically use linear operations in the convolution operation, the Rectified Linear Unit (ReLU) is usually used as an activation function after each convolutional layer. To reduce the dimensionality of the feature maps resulting from the convolutional layers, a spatial sub-sampling (or pooling) layer is defined by sliding a square window on the input image and taking the maximum value in each small region. In addition to that, to decrease overfitting during the training stage, a dropout layer is used as a regularisation technique. The final layer is the conventional Multi Layer Perceptron which is a fully connected layer using fully connected nodes followed by a softmax activation function. The purpose of the dense layer (fully connected layer) is to use the features extracted from proceeding layers for classifying the input image into various labels based on the training examples.

The architecture of the CNN used in this experiment was structured as follows: four convolutional layers; each two followed by a non-linear activation function, a maxpooling layer, and dropout layer with dropping probability 0.25 and finally two fully connected layers; one has 512 neurons with dropout layer with dropping probability 0.5 and the other has 5 neurons represent the number of classes to be detected as shown in Fig. 2.

The network was trained using stochastic gradient descent (SGD) with a constant learning rate of 0.001 and momentum parameter 0.9 by updating the network weights which are initialised using Glorot weight initialisation. The objective function to be minimized was cross-entropy loss function $L = -tlog(p) - (1-t)log(1-p)$.

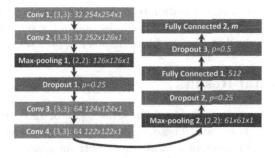

Fig. 2. Flow chart of our CNN architecture. m denotes the number of output classes.

2.2   Non-blind Image Deconvolution

Assuming that the blur kernel function is already determined, we aim to recover the sharp image by a deconvolution process. We might attempt to do this using a regularised variation approach which may be achieved by solving a minimising problem of an functional of the form

$$\min_{u(\mathbf{x})} \left\{ \|[h * u](\mathbf{x}) - z(\mathbf{x})\|_{L^2(\Omega)}^2 + |\nabla u(\mathbf{x})| \right\} \tag{1}$$

where $h(\mathbf{x})$ denotes the blur function, $u(\mathbf{x})$ denotes the clean unknown image which we aim to recover, $z(\mathbf{x})$ denotes the blurred image which we started with, $\|\cdot\|_{L^2(\Omega)}^2$ denotes the L^2-norm over the domain and ∇ denotes the gradient. The first term in the energy functional is a fitting term which has a minima when $[h * u](\mathbf{x}) = z(\mathbf{x})$ and the second part is a regularisation term, in this case total variation, which aims to deal with the effects of noise which makes this problem ill-posed. While this can achieve good results, it can be quite slow to solve using traditional solvers such as gradient descent and conjugate gradient. The quality of results from this approach can also suffer from the relative simplicity of the model. Much work has been done recently in defining constrained deconvolution models which achieve improved results over more traditional ideas as well as fast solution techniques such split-Bregman and alternate direction methods. For this work, we reconstruct our images using an approach from Williams et al. [2] which provides implicitly constrained image deconvolution and a fast solver. The problem is presented as $\min_{u,\psi;\lambda}(f(u,\psi;\lambda))$ where

$$f(u,\psi;\lambda) = \frac{1}{2}\|h * u - z\|_{L^2(\Omega)}^2 + \frac{\gamma}{2}\|T_{\mathbf{a}}(\psi) - u\|_{L^2(\Omega)}^2 + <\lambda, T_{\mathbf{a}}(\psi) - u>$$

$$+ \mu\|\psi - \zeta\|_{L^2(\Omega)}^2 + \alpha \int_\Omega \left| \nabla \left(T_{\mathbf{a}}(\psi) + \theta\|\psi - \zeta\|_{L^2(\Omega)}^2 \right) \right| \, d\Omega, \tag{2}$$

where the first term is a deconvolution fitting term, the second and third terms aim to constrain the values of the reconstructed image $u(\mathbf{x})$ to be similar to the implicitly constrained function $T(\psi)$ [2] using a lagrange multiplier λ. The fourth term is included to encourage convexity given certain parameters where ζ should be an initial approximation of the solution and $\psi(\mathbf{x})$ is a dual variable. The final component is a regularisation term. To minimise the functional, we first calculate ζ and proceed with alternate minimisation of the remaining arguments which can each be solved efficiently. More details are presented in [2].

3   Experimental Results

We test our approach using the Messidor dataset [12] of 1200 eye colour fundus images as our sharp, true data. These were acquired from patients with varying stages of retinopathy or maculopathy at three ophthalmologic departments using a colour video 3CCD camera on a Topcon TRC NW6 non-mydriatic retinograph with a 45 degree field of view. The 8-bit images were captured at 1440 × 960,

2240×1488 or 2304×1536 pixels but, for our testing, we resize to 256×256. We split our datasets (to be defined in the results section) into training (75%) and testing (25%) sets; of the training data, 20% is reserved for validation. All tests were run on an HP Z440 Workstation with Intel Xeon E5-1620, 32GB RAM and an NVidia Titan Xp GPU which was used to train the CNNs.

We first aim to determine blur type. For this experiment, we consider the cases of no blur, out-of-focus blur and motion blur. We form a dataset for training and testing the CNNs composed of the 1200 messidor images which are sharp and uncorrupted; we consider these as class 1. We blur these images using out-of-focus blur of random diameter (strength) between 1 and 10 and consider these images as class 2. Similarly, we blur the class 1 sharp images using motion blur of random strength between 1 and 10; we consider these images as class 3. Examples are shown in Fig. 3. From each class, 900 images are used for training, of which 180 are reserved for validation, and 300 images are used for testing once the network is trained. The network was trained until the cost function reached a plateau and then tested on the combined testing set. We achieved an accuracy of 0.9589. All of the clean images were classified correctly, while 99% of the out-of-focus images were classed correctly and 88.7% of the motion blurred images were classified correctly. The remaining incorrect images were all classified as clean.

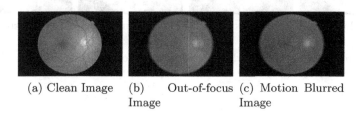

(a) Clean Image   (b)   Out-of-focus   (c) Motion Blurred
                   Image   Image

Fig. 3. Examples of training data: (a) clean image, (b) image corrupted by out-of-focus blur, (c) image corrupted by motion blur. In the cases of the blurred images, the strength of added blur corruption was random.

We now consider the feasibility of using neural networks to determine the strength of blur in an image with an obvious case which should be easily solvable. We define a set composed of the 1200 resized, clean Messidor images as class 0. We then blur these using a 20-pixel motion blur function and consider these as class 1. From each class, we randomly select 900 images for training, of which 180 are reserved for validation. The remaining 300 images from each class are combined into a test-set and are to be classified once the network is trained. The network was trained using the training and validation data to distinguish between clean images and the heavily blurred images, and achieved an accuracy of 1.00 on the 600 test images, meaning that every image was classified correctly.

Given this encouraging result, we consider the same experiment but with a more difficult case using 10-tap motion blur. Training again until the relative cost was sufficiently small, we achieve 0.988 accuracy on 600 test images. Increasing the difficulty further by decreasing this to 3-tap blur, we are still able to achieve accuracy of 0.94. These results strongly suggest that may be able to use CNNs to reliably determine the unknown strength of blur in fundus images.

We consider a multi-class approach using a set of potential strength values including no blur, 4-, 6-, 8-, and 10-tap blur since less than 4 is not considered likely to considerably distort the image and greater than 10- is unlikely to happen in practice. To form a training and testing dataset, we blur the messidor dataset by each blur function and consider the resulting corrupted images as classified by blur strength. 75% of the images of each class (4500 images in total) are used for training, of which 20% (900 images) are reserved for validation. The remaining 1500 images are used for testing. We trained the network for 100 epochs. Using all five classes, we achieve 77% accuracy. Subsequent deconvolution resulted in a mean ISNR of 7.53 across 1200 examples which is similar to the 7.80 achieved by [3]. However, it should be noted that a different and smaller dataset was used for experiments. Some results are presenting in Fig. 4.

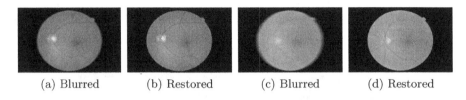

    (a) Blurred   (b) Restored   (c) Blurred   (d) Restored

Fig. 4. Two examples of blurred images (a), (c) restored by our algorithm (c), (d).

4 Conclusion

We have presented a new technique for determining the type and level of blur in images, considering in particular colour fundus images of the retina. By developing convolutional neural networks for single and multi-class problems, we have been able to determine whether an image is blurred and how strong that blur is to a high accuracy. One considerable benefit is that the method naturally includes the same number of images in each class, thereby avoiding the issue of bias requiring solutions such as weighting. Building in image deconvolution, we create an automatic semi-blind deconvolution technique which does not require manual inspection of the images to determine or estimate the type and strength of blur present. An important aspect is to test this method beyond synthetic blur which requires creation of an annotated dataset. Further work could be considered in the future to improve the accuracy for distinguishing the strength of blur so that the correct blur function may be identified, however the high accuracies found in this work are very encouraging. This approach may be extended to consider classification of other blur types which are not currently addressed.

In particular, this approach is fast, automatic, and provides a technique for determining that an image is clean, estimating the blur and strength, and recovering the clean image from the blur degradation.

Acknowledgement. This project is funded by the National Institute for Health Research's i4i Programme. This paper summarises independent research funded by the National Institute for Health Research (NIHR) under its i4i Programme (Grant Reference Number II-LA-0813-20005). B. Al-Bander acknowledges financial support from the Higher Committee for Education Development in Iraq (Grant No. 182).

References

1. Chan, T.F., Wong, C.-K.: Total variation blind deconvolution. IEEE T. Image Process. **7**(3), 370–375 (1998)
2. Williams, B.M., Chen, K., Harding, S.P.: A new constrained total variational deblurring model and its fast algorithm. Numer. Algorithms **69**(2), 415–441 (2015)
3. Almeida, M.S.C., Almeida, L.B.: Blind and semi-blind deblurring of natural images. IEEE T. Image Process. **19**(1), 36–52 (2010)
4. Abdel-Hamid, O., Mohamed, A.-R., Jiang, H., Deng, L., Penn, G., Yu, D.: Convolutional neural networks for speech recognition. IEEE/ACM TASLP **22**(10), 1533–1545 (2014)
5. Zeng, T., Li, R., Mukkamala, R., Ye, J., Ji, S.: Deep convolutional neural networks for annotating gene expression patterns in the mouse brain. BMC Bioinform. **16**(1), 147 (2015)
6. Schuler, C.J., Christopher Burger, H., Harmeling, S., Scholkopf, B.: A machine learning approach for non-blind image deconvolution. In: CVPR, 2013, pp. 1067–1074
7. Schuler, C.J., Hirsch, M., Harmeling, S., Schölkopf, B.: Learning to deblur. IEEE T. Pattern Anal. **38**(7), 1439–1451 (2016)
8. Xu, L., Ren, J.S., Liu, C., Jia, J.: Deep convolutional neural network for image deconvolution. In: NIPS, pp. 1790–1798 (2014)
9. Levin, A.: Blind motion deblurring using image statistics. In: Advances in Neural Information Processing Systems (NIPS) (2007)
10. Sun, J., Cao, W., Xu, Z., Ponce, J.: Learning a convolutional neural network for non-uniform motion blur removal. In: CVPR, pp. 769–777 (2015)
11. LeCun, Y., Jackel, L., Bottou, L., Brunot, A., Cortes, C., Denker, J., Drucker, H., Guyon, I., Muller, U., Sackinger, E., et al.: Comparison of learning algorithms for handwritten digit recognition. In: ICANN, vol. 60, pp. 53–60 (1995)
12. Decencière, E., Zhang, X., Cazuguel, G., Laÿ, B., Cochener, B., Trone, C., Gain, P., Ordonez, R., Massin, P., Erginay, A., et al.: Feedback on a publicly distributed image database: the messidor database. Image Anal. Stereol. **33**(3), 231–234 (2014)

Towards Topological Correct Segmentation of Macular OCT from Cascaded FCNs

Yufan He[1]([⊠]), Aaron Carass[1,2], Yeyi Yun[1], Can Zhao[1], Bruno M. Jedynak[3], Sharon D. Solomon[4], Shiv Saidha[5], Peter A. Calabresi[5], and Jerry L. Prince[1,2]

[1] Department of Electrical and Computer Engineering,
The Johns Hopkins University, Baltimore, MD 21218, USA
`yhe35@jhu.edu`
[2] Department of Computer Science, The Johns Hopkins University,
Baltimore, MD 21218, USA
[3] Department of Mathematics and Statistics, Portland State University,
Portland, OR 97201, USA
[4] Wilmer Eye Institute, The Johns Hopkins University School of Medicine,
Baltimore, MD 21287, USA
[5] Department of Neurology, The Johns Hopkins University School of Medicine,
Baltimore, MD 21287, USA

Abstract. Optical coherence tomography (OCT) is used to produce high resolution depth images of the retina and is now the standard of care for *in-vivo* ophthalmological assessment. In particular, OCT is used to study the changes in layer thickness across various pathologies. The automated image analysis of these OCT images has primarily been performed with graph based methods. Despite the preeminence of graph based methods, deep learning based approaches have begun to appear within the literature. Unfortunately, they cannot currently guarantee the strict biological tissue order found in human retinas. We propose a cascaded fully convolutional network (FCN) framework to segment eight retina layers and preserve the topological relationships between the layers. The first FCN serves as a segmentation network which takes retina images as input and outputs the segmentation probability maps of the layers. We next perform a topology check on the segmentation and those patches that do not satisfy the topology criterion are passed to a second FCN for topology correction. The FCNs have been trained on Heidelberg Spectralis images and validated on both Heidelberg Spectralis and Zeiss Cirrus images.

Keywords: Retina OCT · Fully convolutional network · Topology preserving

1 Introduction

Optical coherence tomography (OCT) is a widely used modality for imaging the retina as it is non-invasive, non-ionizing, and provides three-dimensional data

© Springer International Publishing AG 2017
M.J. Cardoso et al. (Eds.): FIFI/OMIA 2017, LNCS 10554, pp. 202–209, 2017.
DOI: 10.1007/978-3-319-67561-9_23

which can be rapidly acquired [6]. OCT improves upon traditional 2D fundus photography by providing depth information, which enables measurements of layer thicknesses that are known to change with certain diseases [9]. Automated methods for measuring layer thicknesses in large-scale studies are critical since manual delineation is time consuming. In recent years, many automated methods have been developed for the segmentation of retinal layers [3,7,10]. The most prominent technique in use for OCT images are graph based methods coming from the work of Garvin et al. [5]. Recent developments in deep learning have made deep convolutional networks a viable alternative to this status quo and it provides a more flexible framework for abnormal retina analysis. Fang et al. [4] used a convolutional neural network to predict the central pixel label of a given image patch, and subsequently used the graph based approach to finalize the segmentation. However, such patch based pixel-wise labeling schemes use overlapped patches which introduces redundancy and a trade-off between localization accuracy and patch size.

The more elegant architectures of fully convolutional networks (FCNs) [8] have been proposed and applied to various segmentation tasks. In FCNs, the fully connected layer of traditional convolutional neural networks is replaced with convolutional layer. The network can be trained end-to-end and pixels-to-pixels, and the outputs can have high resolution. This architecture avoids patch based pixel labeling and is thus more efficient. Roy et al. [13] designed a fully convolutional network to segment retina layers and fluid filled cavities in OCT images.

Although FCN based networks have been successful in various segmentation tasks, at its core it is providing pixel-wise labeling without using higher-level priors like topological relationships between layers or layer shape, and can thus give nonsense segmentations. In the case of OCT, or medical imaging in general, there are strict anatomical relationships that should be preserved. Approaches proposed to solve this include, Chen et al. [2] using a fully connected conditional random field (CRF) as a post-processing method for the segmentation map from a deep network; however, the CRF does not utilize the topology or shape prior information. Bentaieb et al. [1] proposed a hand-designed loss function to penalize topology disorders, but the pixel-wise labeling of FCN still cannot guarantee the topology correctness and cannot fix the topology defects. Ravishankar et al. [11] used a FCN to segment kidney and cascaded a convolutional auto-encoder to regularize the shape and works well.

We propose to segment the retina layers as well as building a framework to correct topological defects that contradict the known anatomy of healthy human retinas. We do this by cascading two FCNs. The first FCN segments the retina layers and produce the initial segmentation masks. We also proposed an algorithm to check the topology correctness of the segmentation. We then iterate the masks with topology defects over the second FCN to fix the defects and check the topology until all the segmentation masks have the correct topology or an max iteration count is reached. Since the topology fixing net fixes most of the topology defects in the first two iterations, only a small number of masks need to iterate through the second net multiple times. There are two key differences between our approach and the work of Ravishankar et al. Firstly, we iterate over the topology correction step with successive iterations correcting 98% of defects; secondly our network is structurally similar to a segmentation style network with long skip connections and is not a convolutional auto-encoder.

2   Method

2.1   Preprocessing

We first identify the Bruch's membrane and flatten the input images to it, which is a standard OCT pre-processing step. We then subdivide the B-scan into 128×128 overlapping image patches with a fixed step size (determined by the B-scan size), resulting in 10 image patches per B-scan. When we reconstruct the B-scan segmentation from those patches we average the segmentation probability map if they are overlapped. See the pre-processing portion of Fig. 1.

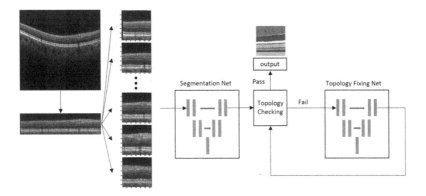

Fig. 1. Our proposed cascaded FCNs, made up of a Segmentation FCN and Topology fixing FCN that we iterate over to resolve topology errors.

2.2   Segmentation Network Architecture

Our segmentation FCN (S-Net) is based on U-net [12], and consists of a contracting encoder and an expansive decoder. The encoder takes a 128×128 image patch as input and repeatedly uses 3×3 convolutions and rectified linear unit (ReLU) activation followed by batch normalization. We conduct 2×2 max pooling at four different layers in the encoder to down sample the image patches. The decoder portion of our FCN concatenates the feature map from the corresponding encoder and up-samples it repeatedly. The final output from S-Net is a $10 \times 128 \times 128$ volume, which corresponds to probability maps for our eight layers and backgrounds above and below the retina(vitreous and choroid). Figure 2 shows a schematic of the network used, with training outlined in Sect. 2.5.

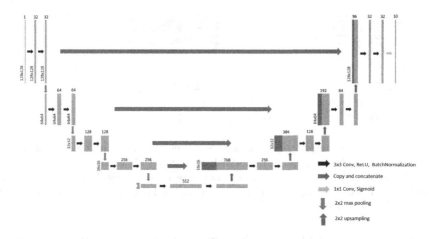

Fig. 2. A schematic of the network structure of S-Net and T-Net.

2.3 Topology Correction Network Architecture

The topology fixing net (T-Net) shares the same structure as S-Net, with the addition of an applied dropout of 0.5 after each max pooling and up-sampling layer. T-Net tries to learn the shape and correct topology of the true segmentation and use the learnt knowledge to fix the topology identified in the output of S-Net. Training for T-Net is outlined in Sect. 2.5.

2.4 Topology Checking

The segmentation masks should have a strict topology relationship, with layers being nested, and the k-th layer should only touch the $(k-1)$-th and $(k+1)$-th layers with no overlaps or gaps for $k = 1, \ldots, 8$ ($k = 0$ and 9 are the vitreous and choroid respectively). S-Net outputs a segmentation mask of size $10 \times 128 \times 128$, which we denote as $M_k(\boldsymbol{x})$ for $k = 0, \ldots, 9$, with $\boldsymbol{x}$ the A-scan index within the 128×128 image patch. We build a new mask, $M_t(\boldsymbol{x})$, as

$$M_t(\boldsymbol{x}) = \sum_{k=0}^{9} k \times M_k(\boldsymbol{x}).$$

Figure 3 shows an example $M_t(\boldsymbol{x})$ and the corresponding profile of one A-scan. We perform a backward difference within each A-scan, if the topology is correct, there are no negative values. However, if there are hierarchical disorders, gaps, or overlaps, there will be negative values. We use this analysis to identify segmentation masks with topological defects, and such masks are passed to T-Net for correction.

2.5 Training

S-Net is trained based on 128×128 Spectralis image patches, with output $10 \times 128 \times 128$ based on manual delineation of the OCT data. We train the

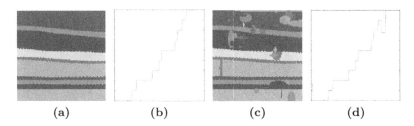

(a)	(b)	(c)	(d)

Fig. 3. Shown is an example of **(a)** $M_t(x)$, the segmentation groundtruth without any topology defects. While a single **(b)** middle A-scan of **(a)**, shows that we expect $M_t(x)$ to be a strictly increasing function when there are no topological defects. **(c)** is the image with simulated topology defects added on **(a)** and the **(d)** middle A-scan of **(c)**, showing the effects of topology errors.

FCN using back-propagation to minimize a loss function based on a modified Dice score between the ground truth and the output segmentations. T-Net, which fixes topology errors in the segmentation maps, is trained on manual delineations with simulated randomly generated topological defects. Examples of our simulated defects and the corresponding ground truth are shown in Fig. 3.

3   Experiments

3.1   Data

We have 7 Spectralis Spectral Domain OCT (SD-OCT) scans (of size $496 \times 1024 \times 49$) and each has 8 B-scans manually delineated for training. We flatten and crop each B-scan into 128×1024 size images and extract overlapped 128×128 patches by a fixed step and obtain 69 patches from each B-scan, with $7 \times 8 \times 69 = 3864$ total training patches. For validation, we have 10 manually delineated Spectralis scans (totaling 490 manually delineated B-scans) and 6 manually delineated Cirrus scans, each has 8 B-scans delineated (totaling 48 B-scans).

3.2   Comparison to Manual Segmentation

Spectralis. We compared the cascaded network (S-Net + T-Net) with the single segmentation network (S-Net) and a state-of-art random forest and graph cut based method (RF+Graph) [7]. The Dice coefficients between the segmentation results and manual delineation of eight retina layers are shown in Table 1. RF + Graph is still better than the deep network as the graph have been designed and refined for retina segmentation. However, the deep network (S-Net) has reached similar performance to the RF + Graph and the topology fixing (S-Net + T-Net) gives the deep network the correct anatomical structure. See Fig. 4 for example results.

Cirrus. The network was trained only on Spectralis images, but was also evaluated on Cirrus images, with results shown in Table 2. In this case, we used the

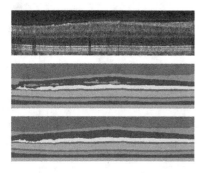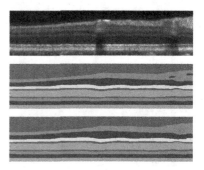

Fig. 4. The top row shows Cirrus and Spectralis B-scans, respectively. The second row shows the segmentation after S-Net, and the bottom row shows the effect of topology correction with the output from T-Net.

Table 1. Dice coefficients of eight layers evaluated against 490 manually delineated Spectralis B-scans.

Layer	RNFL	GCL+IPL	INL	OPL	ONL	IS	OS	RPE
S-Net	0.898	0.917	0.829	0.776	0.933	0.832	0.839	0.874
S-Net + T-Net	0.904	0.922	0.830	0.776	0.935	0.835	0.839	0.873
RF + Graph	0.914	0.926	0.831	0.787	0.939	0.833	0.844	0.873

Table 2. Dice coefficients of eight layers evaluated against 48 manually delineated Cirrus B-scans.

Layer	RNFL	GCL+IPL	INL	OPL	ONL	IS	OS	RPE
S-Net	0.846	0.927	0.897	0.773	0.948	0.792	0.818	0.901
S-Net + T-Net	0.860	0.939	0.899	0.776	0.951	0.800	0.820	0.844
RF + Graph	0.909	0.950	0.919	0.815	0.958	0.915	0.916	0.927

version of RF + Graph that had been trained on Cirrus data, with graph parameters specifically chosen to optimize performance on Cirrus data. It is observed that S-Net + T-Net has reached comparable performance to that of RF + Graph, which is rather striking given that the deep network had been trained only on Spectralis data. See Fig. 4 for example results.

3.3   Evaluation of Topology Correction

From Tables 1 and 2 we see only small improvements in the Dice coefficients after the T-Net because the topology disorders only affect a small number of pixels, but the topology disorders are greatly decreased. Figure 5 shows the relation between the percentage of patches with topology disorders and the iteration through the T-Net. After eight iterations most segmentation masks converge to the correct topology. Figure 6 shows some examples of T-Net.

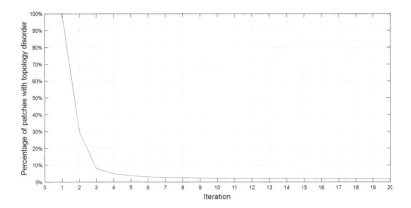

Fig. 5. Percentage of patches with topology disorder and the iterations into the topology fixing net.

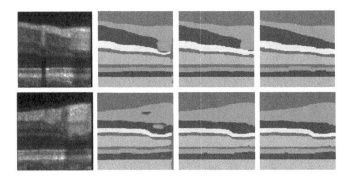

Fig. 6. From left to right: original patch, initial segmentation mask by S-Net, first iteration through T-Net, and fourth iteration through T-Net.

4 Conclusions

In the paper, we propose a cascaded FCN framework to segment both Spectralis and Cirrus retina SD-OCT images while addressing the topology relations between layers. The topology fixing net is learning the shape and topology priors of the segmentation and uses the learnt priors to fix the topology disorders. It fixes 98% of them within eight iterations. The topology errors that are not corrected are usually single wrongly labeled pixels around layer boundaries as they are not represented in the simulated training data. We expect that better topology correction can be achieved by simulating more representative topology defects and include manually selected real topology defects and original image intensities as extra information. We plan to modify the framework to incorporate the prior topological knowledge for segmenting abnormal retinas.

References

1. BenTaieb, A., Hamarneh, G.: Topology aware fully convolutional networks for histology gland segmentation. In: Ourselin, S., Joskowicz, L., Sabuncu, M.R., Unal, G., Wells, W. (eds.) MICCAI 2016. LNCS, vol. 9901, pp. 460–468. Springer, Cham (2016). doi:10.1007/978-3-319-46723-8_53
2. Chen, L.C., Papandreou, G., Kokkinos, I., Murphy, K., Yuille, A.L.: Deeplab: semantic image segmentation with deep convolutional nets, atrous convolution, and fully connected crfs. IEEE Trans. Pattern Anal. Mach. Intell. **5**(99), 1 (2017)
3. Chiu, S.J., Li, X.T., Nicholas, P., Toth, C.A., Izatt, J.A., Farsiu, S.: Automatic segmentation of seven retinal layers in SDOCT images congruent with expert manual segmentation. Opt. Express **18**(18), 19413–19428 (2010)
4. Fang, L., Cunefare, D., Wang, C., Guymer, R.H., Li, S., Farsiu, S.: Automatic segmentation of nine retinal layer boundaries in OCT images of non-exudative AMD patients using deep learning and graph search. Biomed. Opt. Express **8**(5), 2732–2744 (2017)
5. Garvin, M.K., Abràmoff, M.D., Wu, X., Russell, S.R., Burns, T.L., Sonka, M.: Automated 3-D intraretinal layer segmentation of macular spectral-domain optical coherence tomography images. IEEE Trans. Med. Imag. **28**(9), 1436–1447 (2009)
6. Hee, M.R., Izatt, J.A., Swanson, E.A., Huang, D., Schuman, J.S., Lin, C.P., Puliafito, C.A., Fujimoto, J.G.: Optical coherence tomography of the human retina. Arch. Ophthalmol. **113**(3), 325–332 (1995)
7. Lang, A., Carass, A., Hauser, M., Sotirchos, E.S., Calabresi, P.A., Ying, H.S., Prince, J.L.: Retinal layer segmentation of macular OCT images using boundary classification. Biomed. Opt. Express **4**(7), 1133–1152 (2013)
8. Long, J., Shelhamer, E., Darrell, T.: Fully convolutional networks for semantic segmentation. In: The IEEE Conference on Computer Vision and Pattern Recognition (CVPR), pp. 3431–3440, June 2015
9. Medeiros, F.A., Zangwill, L.M., Alencar, L.M., Bowd, C., Sample, P.A., Susanna Jr., R., Weinreb, R.N.: Detection of glaucoma progression with stratus OCT retinal nerve fiber layer, optic nerve head, and macular thickness measurements. Invest. Ophthalmol. Vis. Sci. **50**(12), 5741–5748 (2009)
10. Novosel, J., Thepass, G., Lemij, H.G., de Boer, J.F., Vermeer, K.A., van Vliet, L.J.: Loosely coupled level sets for simultaneous 3D retinal layer segmentation in optical coherence tomography. Med. Image Anal. **26**(1), 146–158 (2015)
11. Ravishankar, H., Venkataramani, R., Thiruvenkadam, S., Sudhakar, P., Vaidya, V.: Learning and incorporating shape models for semantic segmentation. In: 20th International Conference on Medical Image Computing and Computer Assisted Intervention (MICCAI 2017). LNCSc. Springer, Heidelberg (2017). https://www.researchgate.net/profile/Sheshadri_Thiruvenkadam/publication/314256462_Learning_and_incorporating_shape_models_for_semantic_segmentation/links/58be2ddc45851591c5e9c108/Learning-and-incorporating-shape-models-for-semantic-segmentation.pdf
12. Ronneberger, O., Fischer, P., Brox, T.: U-Net: convolutional networks for biomedical image segmentation. In: Navab, N., Hornegger, J., Wells, W.M., Frangi, A.F. (eds.) MICCAI 2015. LNCS, vol. 9351, pp. 234–241. Springer, Cham (2015). doi:10.1007/978-3-319-24574-4_28
13. Roy, A.G., Conjeti, S., Karri, S.P.K., Sheet, D., Katouzian, A., Wachinger, C., Navab, N.: ReLayNet: retinal layer and fluid segmentation of macular optical coherence tomography using fully convolutional network. CoRR abs/1704.02161 (2017)

Boosted Exudate Segmentation in Retinal Images Using Residual Nets

Samaneh Abbasi-Sureshjani[1(✉)], Behdad Dashtbozorg[1],
Bart M. ter Haar Romeny[1,2], and François Fleuret[3]

[1] Eindhoven University of Technology,
P.O. Box 513, 5600 MB Eindhoven, The Netherlands
{s.abbasi,B.Dasht.Bozorg,B.M.terhaarRomeny}@tue.nl
[2] Sino-Dutch Biomedical and Information Engineering School,
Northeastern University, P.O. Box 129, 500, Zhihui Street, Shenyang 110167, China
[3] Idiap Research Institute, Rue Marconi 19, 1920 Martigny, Switzerland
francois.fleuret@idiap.ch

Abstract. Exudates in retinal images are one of the early signs of the vision-threatening diabetic retinopathy and diabetic macular edema. Early diagnosis is very helpful in preventing the progression of the disease. In this work, we propose a fully automatic exudate segmentation method based on the state-of-the-art residual learning framework. With our proposed end-to-end architecture the training is done on small patches, but at the test time, the full sized segmentation is obtained at once. The small number of exudates in the training set and the presence of other bright regions are the limiting factors, which are tackled by our proposed importance sampling approach. This technique selects the misleading normal patches with a higher priority, and at the same time avoids the network to overfit to those samples. Thus, no additional post-processing is needed. The method was evaluated on three public datasets for both detecting and segmenting the exudates and outperformed the state-of-the-art techniques.

Keywords: Exudate segmentation · Retinal images · Residual nets · Importance sampling · Diabetic retinopathy · Diabetic macular edema

1 Introduction

Diabetes is threatening the health of many people in the world, and it normally remains undiagnosed unless its symptoms and complications appear. Among its different ophthalmic complications, diabetic retinopathy (DR) is one of the most common and the most vision-threatening complication. DR is classified to non-proliferative DR (NPDR) and proliferative diabetic retinopathy (PDR), which determines the severity level and the need for further treatments. On the other hand, diabetic macular edema (DME) defined as retinal thickening, is another important complication that might happen in eyes at any DR severity level. Diabetic eyes are typically categorized into three groups based on the

© Springer International Publishing AG 2017
M.J. Cardoso et al. (Eds.): FIFI/OMIA 2017, LNCS 10554, pp. 210–218, 2017.
DOI: 10.1007/978-3-319-67561-9_24

DME severity (healthy, moderate or severe DME). There are several signs and symptoms associated with DR and DME such as microaneurysms, hemorrhages, hard exudates and cotton-wool spots. Among these signs, exudates are the early signs of both moderate NPDR and moderate DME. They are largely made up of extracellular lipid, which has leaked from abnormal retinal capillaries, and appear as white, yellowish or waxy lesions situated mainly in the outer plexiform layer of the retina [6,13].

In this work, we propose a fully automatic method for segmenting the exudates in retinal images. Retinal images are one of the cost-effective and non-invasive sources of medical information, which are widely used for diagnosis purposes and studying the progression of the diseases. There are several works in the literature proposed for segmenting the exudates, which are mainly based on a series of preceding handcrafted feature extraction and landmark classification steps (e.g. [3,14]). The CNNs are taking over the conventional image processing approaches in various computer vision tasks, and medical applications are not excluded from this rapid change. Recently, new methods using the state-of-the-art convolutional neural networks (CNNs) have been proposed for automatic lesion and landmark detection, e.g., [1,9,11]. In the work proposed by [11], the exudate probability map created by a 10 layer CNN is combined with the output of other methods segmenting the optic disc, vessels, and bright borders to create the final masks for the exudates. While in [9], a 7-layer CNN is trained to localize the exudates and they are later used in another network for the automatic classification of DME.

In this article, we present a novel end-to-end segmentation framework using residual nets (ResNets) [5]. The depth of the neural networks is the key factor in enhancing the performance of visual recognitions tasks. A residual learning framework solves the difficulty of training very deep networks by introducing a reference to the input layer. Using this framework, it is possible to gain higher performance, while keeping the complexity the same. Since limited images with their annotations are available, we train the segmentation network with small patches and then after the kernels are learned well, we test the method on full-sized images. Bright reflections are always misleading for the network. In order to help the network to learn better from non-exudate, but exudate-looking samples, we propose a new sampling approach. This sampling technique presents the misleading negative samples to the network more often. This leads to a faster convergence compared to the uniform sampling. The paper is structured as follows: in Sect. 2, all the steps of our proposed network, sampling technique, and data preparations are explained in detail. In Sect. 3, the evaluation results are presented. At the end, the paper is concluded in Sect. 4.

2 Methodology

In this section, all the steps of our proposed technique are presented. An overview of our approach is depicted in Fig. 1. Each element in this figure will be explained in the following.

2.1 Material

There are very few public datasets with manual segmentations of exudates available. We used the e-ophtha-EX dataset [14], which contains 82 images with different image sizes ranging from 1440 × 960 px to 2544 × 1696 px. All the images are taken with the same field-of-view of 45°. Among these 82 images, 47 images contain in total 2278 annotated exudate components, and 35 images are normal images, which might contain misleading structures such as optical artifacts and vessel reflections. Since the images have different resolutions, after removing the black boundaries so that we have a square bounding box, each image, and its corresponding manual segmentation are scaled to have the resolution of 1024 × 1024 px. Then the images are enhanced by removing the local mean values using a Gaussian kernel (G_σ) with the scale of $\sigma = 1024/30$ as $I_{\text{enh}} = I - I * G_{\sigma=1024/30}$, where $*$ is the convolution operator. The top row, the left side of Fig. 1 shows a sample image before and after pre-processing together with its corresponding manual segmentation.

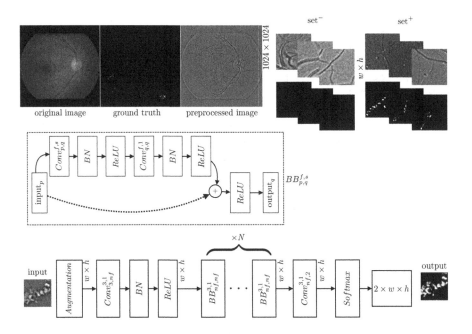

Fig. 1. An overview of our proposed architecture.

We split the data into the training/validation sets (80/20% split) at the image level. This splitting is done for both healthy and pathological images randomly. In the next step, for each of the training and validation sets, we define two different categories called set$^-$ and set$^+$. The set$^-$ includes patches that have been selected at random locations from the normal images; while the patches in set$^+$ have been selected around the centers of exudate components in the pathological images. All patches have a fixed size of $w \times h$. We selected $w = h = 128$ to have large enough patches so that different structures (blood vessels, exudates, reflections, etc.) are easily differentiable from each other. Some sample patches for both set$^-$ and set$^+$ are shown in the top row, the right side of Fig. 1. By selecting maximum 800 patches per image, there are in total 24035 patches in the training set ($|$set$^-| = 22400$ and $|$set$^+| = 1635$), and 6184 patches in the validation set ($|$set$^-| = 5600$ and $|$set$^+| = 584$).

The e-ophtha-EX set was mainly used for training the network. For evaluating the method, two other public datasets were used, the DiaRetDB1 [7] and DR2 [10] public datasets. The DiaRetDB1 includes 89 color fundus images captured using a 50° field-of-view digital fundus camera. Because the annotations have been done by different experts, we only consider the exudate annotations with the agreement higher than 75%. These annotations do not show the exact contours of the lesions and only an approximate mask of the lesion is provided. The same pre-processing as e-ophtha-EX dataset is applied on these images. The DR2 dataset includes in total 529 images and only the presence (not the location) of different types of lesions are provided. We only used 379 images including 300 normal images and 79 images with exudates. The images have the resolution of 867×575 px. We rescaled all the images to 512×512 px and pre-processed with $\sigma = 512/30$ after cropping the black boundaries.

2.2 Network Details

We use ResNets as the main blocks of our architecture. The basic ResNet block ($BB_{p,q}^{f,s}$) used in our model is shown in the middle row of Fig. 1. In this figure, $Conv_{p,q}^{f,s}$ is a 2D convolutional layer, where f, p, q, and s represent the filter size ($f \times f$), the number of input planes, the number of output planes, and the convolution step size, respectively. The batch normalization layer and the rectified linear unit are represented by BN and $ReLU$ respectively. The full model is depicted in the bottom row of Fig. 1. In this architecture, the cascade of N ResNet blocks ($BB_{nf,nf}^{3,1}$) in combination with two convolutional layers, one $ReLU$, one BN and one softmax layer is used. In this work, nf and N are set to 64 and 9 respectively, and the cross entropy criterion is used for the loss measurements. Using the filter sizes of $f = 3$ and stride $s = 1$ in all convolutional layers, the spatial resolution of the output is similar to the input, i.e. the input patch has the size of $3 \times w \times h$ and the output of the network has the size of $2 \times w \times h$. The first and second channels of the output represent for each pixel the probability of being a non-exudate or exudate pixel.

In each epoch, the input patches are augmented before feeding them to the network. The transformations include horizontal and vertical flipping with the probability of 0.5, rotation between $-10°$ to $10°$ with uniform probability and elastic transformations. The weights are initialized as in [4] and training was done from scratch. We used the stochastic gradient descent optimization technique with Nesterov momentum updates [8]. At the beginning, the learning rate was set to 0.1 and momentum to 0.9. We decreased the learning rate every time the loss stopped decreasing, and the training was done until there were no significant changes in the loss value.

2.3 Importance Sampling

One of the main difficulties in exudate detection is the high number of false positives due to the presence of reflections and other bright lesions. One way to solve this problem as proposed by [11,14] is to provide several other masks (generated in separate pipelines) for these regions and remove falsely classified non-exudate pixels from the final exudate mask. However, we propose to solve this problem directly during training the network and without introducing any additional post-processing steps. The non-exudate pixels are mainly present in set$^-$ and they result in a higher loss when comparing the output of the network to the ground truth. We propose to use the importance sampling approach so that the samples in set$^-$ having a higher loss in previous epochs, have a higher chance to be seen in the next training iteration. In this way, the misleading negative samples are presented to the network more often and the network learns to adapt its weights and parameters accordingly.

If set$^+ = \{x_1, \ldots, x_M\}$ and set$^- = \{x_1, \ldots, x_N\}$ are the sets of training samples, then we assign a weight to each sample in these two sets as $W^+ = \{w_1, \ldots, w_M\}$ and $W^- = \{w_1, \ldots, w_N\}$, so that the sum of weights for both W^+ and W^- equals 1. These weights determine the probability of being selected for the next training iteration. Since the patches with exudates need to be treated equally, we define $w_i = 1/M$ for all $w_i \in W^+$. However, for the normal patches $w_i = \frac{l_i}{\sum_{j=1}^N l_j}$ for $w_i \in W^-$, where l_j is the loss of the network achieved for the sample $x_j \in$ set$^-$ in the previous training epoch. For very few epochs at the beginning (e.g. 5) the network is trained using $2K$ samples selected only from set$^+$. This results in a good initialization of the network. Then in the rest of the iterations, K samples are selected from set$^+$ and K samples from set$^-$ according to their defined weights. After feeding the minibatch to the network and computing the derivatives of the loss with respect to the output units, one more step is needed in order to avoid the network to get too biased toward examples with high losses. We rescale the gradient of the loss on individual samples of set$^-$ with the scale of $1/\mu_j$, where $\mu_j = N \frac{w_j}{\sum_{j=1}^N w_j}$ (see [2] for more details). Finally, the weights of the network are updated accordingly.

3   Experiments

To get the segmentation for the entire image, we just pass the image through the network. The spatial resolution does not change in the network, and the patches are selected large enough to present enough contextual information; therefore, the learned kernels are sufficient for segmenting the full image. Figure 2 from left to right represents the full segmentation (probability maps) of two sample images

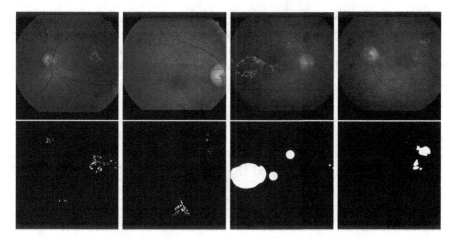

Fig. 2. Four sample segmentation results overlaid on the original images (top row) and their corresponding ground truth images (bottom row).

from the e-ophtha-EX and two images from the DiaRetDB1 dataset, overlaid on top of the original images in the first row. Their corresponding ground truth images are presented in the second row.

In order to evaluate the performance of our method, we use the same evaluation approach as proposed by [14]. In this approach, the evaluation is done either at the exudate level or at the image level. At exudate level, one exudate component (defined as a set of connected pixels) is considered to be completely segmented, if there is a certain overlap between that exudate and the ground truth. For the definition of true/false positives and true/false negatives, the reader is referred to [14]. However, the image level validation only evaluates the correct prediction of the presence of exudates in the images, which is more important from the clinical point of view. To this aim, the image level prediction probability is defined as the maximum of all individual probabilities at the pixel level.

The results are reported in Table 1. The second column represents the total number of images in each set and the number of healthy vs. images with exudates (h/ex). The third column represents the F1-score at the exudate level. The next two columns present the F1-score and the area under the ROC curve (AUC) at the image level. Finally, the last column includes the AUC only at the image level reported by the state-of-the-art techniques. The DR2 set was only used for evaluation at the image level because the exudate masks are not available for this dataset. Our proposed method achieved the F1-score of 0.832 at the exudate level on the e-ophtha-EX dataset, which is higher than the score (F1-score = 0.732) reported by [14]. Using the same evaluation approach, the authors in [11] reported the F1-score of 0.78 for the DRiDB dataset [12], which was not available to us for comparison. Based on these results, our method outperforms the state-of-the-art techniques in most of the cases. The performance on the DR2 dataset is also as high as the results reported by [10]. The F1-score values at the exudate level are very good indications showing that the number of false positives is very low, i.e., the network is differentiating the exudate pixels from misleading non-exudate ones very well. The ROC curves for different datasets are also depicted in Fig. 3.

Table 1. The evaluation results on different public datasets

Dataset	Size	Exudate	Image		Literature
	Total (h/ex)	F1-score	F1-score	AUC	AUC
e-ophtha-EX [14]	82 (47/35)	0.832	0.967	0.994	0.95 [14]
DiaRetDB1 [7]	89 (59/30)	0.819	0.880	0.965	0.95 [14]
DR2 [10]	379 (300/79)	-	0.871	0.972	0.978 [10]

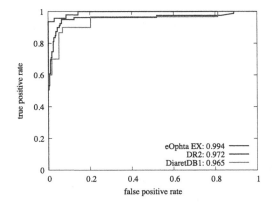

Fig. 3. The ROC curves (at the image level) obtained for different datasets.

4   Conclusion

We presented a novel method for exudate segmentation in retinal images. Our proposed network consists of 20 convolutional layers (9 ResNet blocks). The proposed importance sampling step, which prioritizes the sampling towards highly misleading non-exudate samples, helps to decrease the number of falsely detected non-exudate components to a great extent. Therefore, no additional post-processing steps are needed. Moreover, it helps to achieve a high performance, outperforming the state-of-the-art techniques, in less number of iterations. Even though the main goal of this work was to segment the exudate components, the results show that our network performs very well in deciding about the presence of exudates, which is typically enough for clinicians to take actions. This method might easily be used for detection of other types of lesions if their manual segmentations are available.

Acknowledgement. This project has received funding from the European Union's Seventh Framework Programme, Marie Curie Actions-Initial Training Network, under Grant Agreement No. 607643, "Metric Analysis For Emergent Technologies (MAnET)". It was also supported by the Hé Programme of Innovation, which is partly financed by the Netherlands Organization for Scientific Research (NWO) under Grant No. 629.001.003.

References

1. Alghamdi, H.S., Tang, H.L., Waheeb, S.A., Peto, T.: Automatic optic disc abnormality detection in fundus images: a deep learning approach. In: Proceedings of the Ophthalmic Medical Image Analysis Third International Workshop, Held in Conjunction with MICCAI, pp. 17–24 (2016)
2. Canévet, O., Jose, C., Fleuret, F.: Importance sampling tree for large-scale empirical expectation. In: International Conference on Machine Learning, pp. 1454–1462 (2016)
3. Harangi, B., Lazar, I., Hajdu, A.: Automatic exudate detection using active contour model and regionwise classification. In: Annual International Conference of the IEEE Engineering in Medicine and Biology Society, pp. 5951–5954 (2012)
4. He, K., Zhang, X., Ren, S., Sun, J.: Delving deep into rectifiers: Surpassing human-level performance on imagenet classification. In: Proceedings of the IEEE International Conference on Computer Vision, pp. 1026–1034 (2015)
5. He, K., Zhang, X., Ren, S., Sun, J.: Deep residual learning for image recognition. In: Proceedings of the IEEE Conference on Computer Vision and Pattern Recognition, pp. 770–778 (2016)
6. The International Council of Ophthalmology (ICO): ICO Guidelines for Diabetic Eye Care, January 2017
7. Kälviäinen, R., Uusitalo, H.: DIARETDB1 diabetic retinopathy database and evaluation protocol. In: Medical Image Understanding and Analysis, p. 61 (2007)
8. Nesterov, Y.: A method for unconstrained convex minimization problem with the rate of convergence O(1/k2). Sov. Math. Dokl. **27**(2), 372–376 (1983)
9. Perdomo, O., Otalora, S., Rodríguez, F., Arevalo, J., González, F.A.: A novel machine learning model based on exudate localization to detect diabetic macular edema. In: Proceedings of the Ophthalmic Medical Image Analysis Third International Workshop, Held in Conjunction with MICCAI, pp. 137–144 (2016)
10. Pires, R., Jelinek, H.F., Wainer, J., Valle, E., Rocha, A.: Advancing bag-of-visual-words representations for lesion classification in retinal images. PloS One **9**(6), e96814 (2014)
11. Prentašić, P., Lončarić, S.: Detection of exudates in fundus photographs using deep neural networks and anatomical landmark detection fusion. Comput. Methods Programs Biomed. **137**, 281–292 (2016)

12. Prentašić, P., Lončarić, S., Vatavuk, Z., Bencic, G., Subasic, M., Petkovic, T., Dujmovic, L., Malenica-Ravlic, M., Budimlija, N., Tadic, R.: Diabetic retinopathy image database (DRiDB): a new database for diabetic retinopathy screening programs research. In: 8th International Symposium on Image and Signal Processing and Analysis, pp. 711–716. IEEE (2013)
13. Raman, R., Nittala, M.G., Gella, L., Pal, S.S., Sharma, T.: Retinal sensitivity over hard exudates in diabetic retinopathy. J. Ophthalmic Vis. Res. **10**(2), 160 (2015)
14. Zhang, X., Thibault, G., Decencière, E., Marcotegui, B., Laÿ, B., Danno, R., Cazuguel, G., Quellec, G., Lamard, M., Massin, P., et al.: Exudate detection in color retinal images for mass screening of diabetic retinopathy. Med. Image Anal. **18**(7), 1026–1043 (2014)

Development of Clinically Based Corneal Nerves Tortuosity Indexes

Fabio Scarpa[(⊠)] and Alfredo Ruggeri

Department of Information Engineering, University of Padova, Padua, Italy
fabio.scarpa@unipd.it

Abstract. In-vivo specular microscopy provides information on the corneal health state. The correlation between corneal nerve tortuosity and pathology has been shown several times. However, because there is no unique formal definition of tortuosity, reproducibility is poor. Recently, two distinct forms of corneal nerve tortuosity have been identified, describing either short-range or long-range directional changes. Using 30 images and their manual grading provided by 7 experts, we automatically traced corneal nerves with a custom computerized procedure and identified the combination of geometrical measurements that best represents each tortuosity definition (Spearman Rank Correlation equal to 0.94 and 0.88, respectively). Then, we evaluated both of these tortuosity indexes in 100 images from 10 healthy and 10 diabetic subjects (5 images per subject). A Linear Discriminant Analysis showed a very good capability (accuracy 85%) to differentiate healthy subjects from pathological ones by using both tortuosity indexes together.

Keywords: Corneal nerves · Corneal images · Specular microscopy · In vivo microscopy · Tortuosity

1 Introduction

The cornea is the transparent tissue located in the front of the vertebrate eye and it is responsible for about two-thirds of the eye's refractive power [1], and as so, it has an important role in vision acuity. Much of the cornea's diagnostic potential relies on the usage of in vivo confocal microscopy (IVCM) to image the corneal nerves. The cornea is a richly innervated structure [2]. It is known as one of the most sensitive tissues in the human body. Peripheral nervous system unmyelinated fibers form a dense plexus known as the subbasal nerve plexus (SBP) that can be easily and quickly be visualized by IVCM. Numerous studies have found important correlations between nerve parameters, such as, density, branching, or tortuosity, and a wide range of ocular and/or systemic diseases. Recently, a particular increasing interest in the latter has surged. Tortuosity is now a widely studied corneal nerve property. Many studies have found links to dry eye disease [3], keratoconus [4], and even diabetes [5, 6]. However, there is still no standard tortuosity measurement or even definition.

© Springer International Publishing AG 2017
M.J. Cardoso et al. (Eds.): FIFI/OMIA 2017, LNCS 10554, pp. 219–226, 2017.
DOI: 10.1007/978-3-319-67561-9_25

The clinical perception of corneal nerve tortuosity was recently shown to have two distinct forms [7]. These are defined by short-range (low amplitude, high frequency) or long-range (high amplitude, low frequency) directional changes.

In this study, we automatically traced corneal nerves with our own computerized procedure [9] and identified a combination of mathematical tortuosity measurements that could correctly represent either the short-range tortuosity (SRT) or the long-range tortuosity (LRT) definition. Then, we investigated if one or both forms of tortuosity are capable of highlighting differences between healthy and diabetic individuals, and if these differences allow to correctly classify the health state of each individual.

2   Material

Two datasets were used in this study. They consisted in IVCM images acquired using the Heidelberg Retina Tomograph (HRT-II) with the Rostock Cornea Module (Heidelberg Engineering GmbH, Heidelberg, Germany), covering a field of 400 × 400 µm (384 × 384 pixels).

Images were originally collected at various clinical centers and anonymized by removing all patient information. As the acquisition of these images was approved by the respective local ethical review committees, occurred with informed consent, and followed the tenets of the Declaration of Helsinki, no specific further ethical approval was sought for the retrospective analysis of the resulting compilation of images.

2.1   Ground Truth Dataset for Tortuosity Indexes Definition

A set of 30 nerve confocal images, ordered by experts according to short- or long-range tortuosity definition, was used as ground truth in the present study.

The dataset and the manual analysis procedure are described in detail in [7]. Shortly, images from healthy (10) and diseased (20) subjects were included (one image per subject). Seven expert graders from different institutions visually assessed and ordered them by increasing nerve tortuosity, according to either tortuosity definition (Fig. 1). Their average ordered rankings were assumed as ground truth.

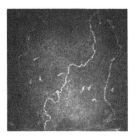 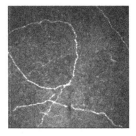

Fig. 1. Corneal nerves image with the highest tortuosity rank for the short-range (left) and the long-range tortuosity (right) measurement.

2.2   Dataset for Investigation on Healthy and Diabetic Individuals

A set of 100 nerve confocal images was used to investigate the capability of indexes above to discriminate between healthy and pathological individuals. Images from 10 healthy and 10 diabetic subjects (Type 1 or 2) with neuropathy were included in this dataset. For each subject, 5 non-overlapped images from the central part of the cornea were included.

3   Methods

In [8], the centerlines of all visible nerves in each image were fully manually traced by an experienced observer and two combination of mathematical tortuosity measurements that correctly represent SRT and LRT definitions, respectively, were identified. In this study we automatically traced corneal nerves. Automatically traced nerves differed from the manually traced ones because of possible errors in the tracing procedure, i.e. false nerves, missing nerves, splitting of a nerve in multiple segments, etc. Thus, we reproduced what done in [8] to identify the combinations of mathematical tortuosity measurements that correctly represent short- and long-range tortuosity definitions from automatically traced nerves.

3.1   Corneal Nerve Tracing

We automatically traced corneal nerves with our own computerized procedure [9]. Briefly, it consists of a thresholding step followed by a supervised classification based on support vector machines (SVM). As in [8], we applied three different smoothing functions, with increasing scale ($\sigma = 1, 2, 3$), to highlight differences between the two tortuosity classes. As a result, each nerve segment is defined by an ordered set of xy positions as $[(x_i^\sigma, y_i^\sigma); i = 1,..., n]$, with n being the total number of coordinates.

3.2   Nerve Tortuosity Metrics

Multiple metrics of tortuosity have been proposed over the years. Typically, tortuosity measurements fall into one of four categories: length-, angle-, curve-, or twist-based measurements. In order to have o global view of tortuosity, we have specifically selected measurements from each of these groups.

Length-based Tortuosity

One of the first and most widely used measurements of tortuosity is the Arc over Chord Length ratio (*AOC*) [10]. It is computed as the ratio between the length of nerve segment (*L*) over the length of its chord (*L_c*) as:

$$AOC = \frac{L}{L_c} \tag{1}$$

where

$$L = \sum_{1}^{n} \sqrt{\left(\Delta x_i^\sigma\right)^2 + \left(\Delta y_i^\sigma\right)^2} \tag{2}$$

$$L_c = \left\| \left(x_1^\sigma, y_1^\sigma\right) - \left(x_n^\sigma, y_n^\sigma\right) \right\| \tag{3}$$

Another length-based measurement is used in this study. It is computed as:

$$LR = \frac{L}{L_{SG}} \tag{4}$$

where L_{SG} is the length of the nerve segment filtered using a 2-degree Savitzky-Golay filter, computed as in Eq. (2).

Angle-based Tortuosity

The sum of angles metric (SOAM) is used. It is computed as:

$$SOAM = \sum_{2}^{n-1} \arccos \frac{V1_i \cdot V2_i}{\|V1_i\| \cdot \|V2_i\|} \tag{5}$$

where V1 and V2 are vectors computed, for each point (x_i^σ, y_i^σ), as:

$$V1_i = \left(x_i, y_i\right) - \left(x_{i-1}, y_{i-1}\right) \tag{6}$$

$$V2_i = \left(x_{i+1}, y_{i+1}\right) - \left(x_i, y_i\right) \tag{7}$$

Curve-based Tortuosity

The absolute curvature is used. It quantifies the curvature k_i over the entire nerve segment [11], as:

$$AC = \sum_{3}^{n} |k_i| \tag{8}$$

$$k_i = \frac{\Delta x_i^\sigma \Delta^2 y_i^\sigma - \Delta^2 x_i^\sigma \Delta y_i^\sigma}{\left[\left(\Delta y_i^\sigma\right)^2 + \left(\Delta y_i^\sigma\right)^2\right]^{3/2}} \tag{9}$$

Twist-based Tortuosity

The tortuosity index (*TI*) was considered. In [12], the number of twists is associated with the number of changes in the curvature (k_i) sign. According to these sign changes, each nerve segment is partitioned into m sub-segments ($s = s_1 \oplus s_2 \ldots \oplus s_m$). *TI* is then computed as

$$TI = \frac{m-1}{m} \sum_1^m \left(\frac{L_c^{S_j}}{L^{S_j}} - 1 \right) \tag{10}$$

where L^{S_j} and $L_c^{S_j}$ are arch and chord length, respectively, of sub-segment s_j ($j = 1,\ldots,n$). In addition, High-pass Twist Tortuosity (*HTT*) was considered:

$$HTT = \sum_1^m A_j \tag{11}$$

where m is the total number of local maximums and A_j is the amplitude of the local maximum j ($j = 1,\ldots,m$) of the curve obtained by the difference between the nerve curve and its 2-degree Savitzky-Golay filtered version.

3.3 Normalization

In this study we applied different normalization factors. As so, each tortuosity metrics is weighted by: 1 (no normalization); L; L_c; L_{SG}; and ΣL (the sum of all segment lengths – image based normalization).

3.4 Aggregation

Different methods were used to combine all the individual nerve tortuosity into a single image-level value: (1) average value for all nerves; (2) maximum value for all nerves; (3) 75th percentile; (4) average value of the (at most) 3 longest nerves; (5) average value of all nerves whose length is within 15% of the longest nerve.

3.5 Combination of Tortuosity Metrics

Each of the multiple variations of the proposed tortuosity metrics (features) was computed using the automatic nerve tracing in all the 30 images described in Sect. 2.1. Spearman Rank Correlation (SRC) was then applied in order to rank all the features according to the two ground-truth ordered rankings (for LRT or SRT). According to [8], the 20 features with the highest SRC coefficient were then selected for each tortuosity definition. A linear regression model was used to combine the selected features into one tortuosity index for SRT and one for LRT.

4   Results

4.1   Evaluation of Short- and Long-Range Tortuosity Indexes

SRT and LRT indexes were computed for each of the 30 images described in Sect. 2.1 and used to order them according to increasing tortuosity. Spearman Rank Correlation (SRC) was computed as a measure of fitness between automated and manual tortuosity grading. We were able to achieve SRC coefficients of 0.945 and 0.886 for SRT and LRT, respectively.

It is of interest to note that higher SRC coefficients (0.985 and 0.959 for SRT and LRT, respectively) were obtained in [8], where manual nerve tracing was used. This may be an indication that automated tracing, used in this paper, may produce errors that affect SRT and LRT assessment.

4.2   Evaluation on Healthy and Diabetic Individuals

SRT and LRT were then computed using the automatic nerve tracing on each image of the healthy and diabetic subjects described in Sect. 2.2. This dataset was used to define neither the features nor their linear combination used to compute SRT and LRT. For each subject, the mean SRT and LRT obtained from his/her 5 images was considered (Fig. 2). Differences between healthy and pathological subjects were evaluated by means of t-test for unpaired data. For both SRT and LRT, the obtained p-values (Table 1) revealed a significant statistical difference (< 0.05) between healthy and pathological subjects, in accordance with previous findings [5, 6].

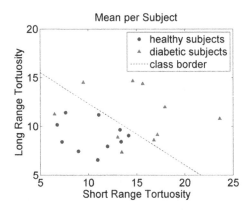

Fig. 2. Short Range Tortuosity (horizontal axis) and Long Range Tortuosity (vertical axis) obtained by the mean of the 5 images acquired from each healthy (blue dot) and diabetic (red triangle) subject. The dashed line represents the class border obtained by a Linear Classifier. (Color figure online)

A Linear Discriminant Analysis (LDA) was performed to evaluate the ability of each tortuosity index and of their linear combination to differentiate between healthy and diabetic subjects. The threshold that minimizes the number of classification errors is separately identified for SRT, LRT, and their linear combination. The accuracy obtained by SRT or LRT alone is 80% and 70%, respectively, whilst their linear combination provided an accuracy of 85% (Table 1).

Table 1. Statistical Analysis (t-test) and Linear Discriminant Analysis (LDA) conducted to evaluate the ability of Short Range Tortuosity (SRT), Long Range Tortuosity (LRT) and their linear combination (SRT & LRT) to differentiate between healthy and diabetic subjects.

	t-test p-value	LDA accuracy	LDA sensitivity	LDA specificity
SRT	0.014	80%	70%	90%
LRT	0.040	70%	90%	50%
SRT & LRT	0.007	85%	70%	100%

5 Discussion and Conclusions

Over the years, several approaches to quantify corneal nerve tortuosity have been proposed. However, most of them focused on quantifying a single, specific geometrical property. In order to improve the agreement between proposed measurements and graders' perception, two distinct forms of corneal nerve tortuosity have been identified, describing either short-range or long-range directional changes.

In this study, we proposed a mathematical description of these clinical perception of tortuosity. We recognized the multifaceted nature of tortuosity by using a combination of different geometrical measurements. We carefully designed each step of the computation, from the smoothing of automatic nerve tracing to the aggregation techniques, and tested for multiple alternatives. The proposed completely automated method provides tortuosity indexes that highly correlate with the clinical perception of experts, given by the ground truth orderings, for both SRT and LRT.

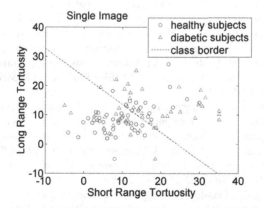

Fig. 3. Short Range Tortuosity (horizontal axis) and Long Range Tortuosity (vertical axis) obtained by each image acquired from healthy (blue dot) and diabetic (red triangle) subjects. The dashed line represents the class border obtained by a Linear Classifier. (Color figure online)

We also investigated if one or both forms of tortuosity exhibit differences between healthy and diabetic individuals with neuropathy. For each subject, the mean SRT and LRT values obtained by 5 images were considered. We showed that each index of tortuosity differentiates the two groups of subjects, but that the best accuracy is achieved by considering both indexes, SRT and LRT.

We also performed the computation of SRT and LRT in each single image (results shown in Fig. 3). This revealed a poor ability to differentiate between healthy and pathologic subjects (accuracy of 63%). This is probably due to the large variability of SRT and LRT in the different regions of the cornea and underlines the importance of standardizing the acquisition protocol, which should acquire images from a specific location of the cornea.

An exhaustive evaluation on images from a much larger number of subjects is currently in progress, as well as an investigation about the changes in one or the other index of nerve tortuosity exhibited by pathologies other than diabetes.

References

1. Krachmer, J.H., Mannis, M.J., Holland, E.J.: Cornea: Fundamentals, Diagnosis and Management, vol. 1. Elsevier Mosby, Philadelphia (2005)
2. Marfurt, C.F., Cox, J., Deek, S., Dvorscak, L.: Anatomy of the human corneal innervation. Exp. Eye Res. **90**(4), 478–492 (2010)
3. del Castillo, J.M.B., Wasfy, M.A., Fernandez, C., Garcia-Sanchez, J.: An in vivo confocal masked study on corneal epithelium and subbasal nerves in patients with dry eye. Invest. Ophthalmol. Vis. Sci. **45**(9), 3030–3035 (2004)
4. Parissi, M., Randjelovic, S., Poletti, E., et al.: Corneal nerve regeneration after collagen cross-linking treatment of keratoconus: A 5-year longitudinal study. JAMA Ophthalmol. **134**(1), 70–78 (2016)
5. De Cillà, S., Ranno, S., Carini, E., et al.: Corneal subbasal nerves changes in patients with diabetic retinopathy: an in vivo confocal study. Invest. Ophthalmol. Vis. Sci. **50**(11), 5155–5158 (2009)
6. Kallinikos, P., Berhanu, M., O'Donnell, C., et al.: Corneal nerve tortuosity in diabetic patients with neuropathy. Invest. Ophthalmol. Vis. Sci. **45**(2), 418–422 (2004)
7. Lagali, N., Poletti, E., Patel, D.V., et al.: Focused tortuosity definitions based on expert clinical assessment of corneal subbasal nerves. Invest. Ophthalmol. Vis. Sci. **56**(9), 5102–5109 (2015)
8. Guimarães, P., Wigdahl, J., Ruggeri, A.: Automatic estimation of corneal nerves focused tortuosities. In: Conference Proceedings of the IEEE Engineering in Medicine and Biology Society, pp. 1332–1335 (2016)
9. Guimarães, P., Wigdahl, J., Ruggeri, A.: A fast and efficient technique for the automatic tracing of corneal nerves in confocal microscopy. Transl. Vis. Sci. Technol. **5**(5), 7 (2016)
10. Smedby, O., Högman, N., Nilsson, S., et al.: Two-dimensional tortuosity of the superficial femoral artery in early atherosclerosis. J. Vasc. Res. **30**(4), 181–191 (1993)
11. Hart, W.E., Goldbaum, M., Cote, B., et al.: Measurement and classification of retinal vascular tortuosity. Int. J. Med. Inform. **53**(2), 39–252 (1999)
12. Scarpa, F., Zheng, X., Ohashi, Y., Ruggeri, A.: Automatic evaluation of corneal nerve tortuosity in images from in vivo confocal microscopy. Invest. Ophthalmol. Vis. Sci. **52**(9), 6404–6408 (2011)

A Comparative Study Towards the Establishment of an Automatic Retinal Vessel Width Measurement Technique

Fan Huang[1(✉)], Behdad Dashtbozorg[1], Alexander Ka Shing Yeung[2],
Jiong Zhang[1], Tos T.J.M. Berendschot[2], and Bart M. ter Haar Romeny[1,3]

[1] Department of Biomedical Engineering, Eindhoven University of Technology,
Eindhoven, The Netherlands
{F.Huang,B.DashtBozorg,J.Zhang1,B.M.TerHaarRomeny}@tue.nl
[2] University Eye Clinic Maastricht, Maastricht, The Netherlands
[3] Department of Biomedical and Information Engineering, Northeastern University,
Shenyang, China

Abstract. In this paper, we propose an automatic technique for the assessment of retinal vessel caliber in fundus images using a fully automatic technique exploiting a multi-scale active contour technique. The proposed method is compared with the well-known semi-automated IVAN software and the Vampire width annotation tool. Experimental results show that our approach is able to provide fast and fully automatic caliber measurements with similar caliber measurement and comparable system error as the IVAN software. It will benefit the analysis of quantitative retinal vessel caliber measurements in large-scale screening programs.

Keywords: Vessel width · Arteriolar-to-venular ratio · Fundus images · Active contour · Diabetes

1 Introduction

Many clinical studies have shown that the changes in retinal vessel caliber are associated with the progress of a variety of systemic diseases. In diabetic retinopathy (DR), the narrowing on arterioles and the widening on venules are observed, which result in a lower arteriolar-to-venular diameter ratio (AVR) [8,11]. Moreover, a decrease in generalized arteriolar diameter is associated with a higher risk of developing hypertension [7], and an increase on venular diameter is associated with renal failure, systemic inflammation and stroke [11].

Most works on assessing the change of vascular caliber on fundus images still rely on a semi-automatic tool: Eye-van (IVAN), which was developed at the University of Wisconsin, USA [3,4,10]. However, it takes approximate 7–10 min to obtain the precise width measurement of vessels, which includes the time of automatic vessel detection and classification, manual cropping, adding vessel segments and correcting their labels. Using IVAN in large-scale screening programs

© Springer International Publishing AG 2017
M.J. Cardoso et al. (Eds.): FIFI/OMIA 2017, LNCS 10554, pp. 227–234, 2017.
DOI: 10.1007/978-3-319-67561-9_26

is therefore too much time consuming, exhausting and prone to human error. Developing a fully automatic system for large-scale vessel caliber assessment is still an open challenge.

In this paper, we propose an automatic and precise quantitative width measurement for retinal blood vessels. We validate the technique by comparing the results with the IVAN software and the Vampire width annotation tool, where the former one is semi-automatic measurement and the latter is a manual measurement.

2   Methodology

The proposed method for automatic vessel caliber measurement uses the centerline of a segmented blood vessel for initializing a deformable enclosed contour. Then the contour is evolved iteratively and fitted to the boundaries of the vessel. Finally, the vessel caliber is measured by computing the distance from one detected vessel edge to the other one. The stages are summarized in Fig. 1.

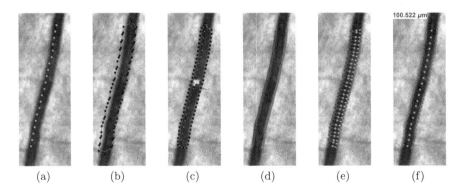

    (a)   (b)   (c)   (d)   (e)   (f)

Fig. 1. The stages of the proposed automatic width measurement technique: (a) centerline detection; (b) contour initialization; (c) active contour segmentation; (d) obtaining the left and right edges; (e) Euclidean distance calculation and (f) vessel caliber estimation.

(a) Vessel centerline extraction. The proposed method is initialized by automatically extracting the vascular tree. We used the vessel segmentation technique proposed in [12], which employs a set of multi-scale Gaussian derivative filters rotated to different directions in so-called 'orientation-scores'. This method provides an enhanced vessel map, which is then converted to a binary vascular map using a proper threshold value. The vessel segmentation is skeletonized by an iterative thinning algorithm to obtain the centerline of the vasculature. Junction points like vessel branchings and crossings are removed, resulting in a map of individual separated vessel segments.

(b) Artery/vein classification. The separated vessel segments are automatically classified into arteries and veins by a supervised classifier. In the training phase, a logistic regression classifier is trained by a dataset of 60 images, which are acquired by the same Canon camera. For each vessel centerline pixel, we extract in total 455 features including: the local intensity of RGB and HSB color channels; the mean, standard deviation, median, minimum and maximum of the intensities inside small, medium and large circular regions; the intensity values along each vessel centerline; and the intensity inside each vessel segment. After that, a genetic-search based feature selection approach is used to select a subset of features giving the highest classification accuracy. Finally, the classifier is trained with the selected features of the training data and used for the classification of arteries and veins in this study.

(c) Vessel caliber measurement. In this step, the geodesic active contour model proposed in [1] for solving a global optimization problem is exploited to locate the left and right edges for each vessel segment. First of all, an enclosed and deformable contour $\mathbf{x}(t) = (x(t), y(t))(t \in (0,1))$ is initialized using the extracted centerline pixels. Afterwards, the surface is iteratively deformed to minimize the energy function:

$$E(\mathbf{x}) = \int_0^1 E_{int}(\mathbf{x}(t)) + E_{ext}(\mathbf{x}(t)) + E_{con}(\mathbf{x}(t))dt \qquad (1)$$

where E_{int} (internal energy) is resulted by the force of the interaction between adjacent control points, which preserves the smoothness of the surface. While E_{ext} (external energy) is resulted by the image gradient which pulls the contour toward vessel boundary, and E_{con} (constraint energy) is resulted by a constraint for the external force. Therefore, at each iteration, the control points follow the contour evolution equation:

$$\frac{\partial \mathbf{x}(t))}{\partial t} = \alpha g(I)(c + \kappa)\overrightarrow{n} + \beta(\triangledown g(I) \cdot \overrightarrow{n})\overrightarrow{n} + \gamma \triangledown \mathbf{x}(t) \cdot \triangledown g(I), \qquad (2)$$

$$g(I) = \frac{1}{1 + \triangledown I^2}, \qquad (3)$$

where $I(x,y)$ is the image and $\triangledown I$ is the first-order Gaussian derivative of I, κ and $\overrightarrow{n}$ are the Euclidean curvature and the unit normal vector of $\mathbf{x}(t)$. $g(I)$ is the speed function given $\triangledown I$ and c, α, β and γ are weighting parameters. Contour evolution is terminated when a stop criterion (e.g. after a certain number of iterations) is satisfied, resulting in a smooth vessel edges detection.

Vessel caliber is then estimated using the evolved contour. The contour is split into left and right edges by removing the control points at the two ends of the vessel segments. For each control point on one side of the vessel, a corresponding nearest point is found on a B-spline interpolated curve of two nearest points on the other side. The Euclidean distance between each two points is computed and converted to micrometer μm using the pixel size of each image. We estimate the pixel size by taking the ratio between the general optic disc diameter (1800 μm) and the diameter in pixels measured by the method described in [2]. In order to prevent outliers, the measured distances with extreme values are eliminated and the vessel width is calculated as the average of the remained measurements.

(d) CRAE, CRVE and AVR measurement. The results are used for estimating the central retinal arterial equivalent (CRAE) and the central retinal venous equivalent (CRVE) (see Fig. 2). Firstly, the optic disc center and diameter are obtained using the super-elliptical convergence filters proposed in [2]. Then, the vessels within the standard area of 0.5 to 1.0 disc diameter around the disc center are selected and the width values are fed to the Knudtson's revised formulas [6]. Finally, the AVR value is defined as the ratio between the CRAE and CRVE.

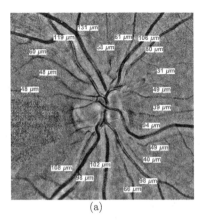 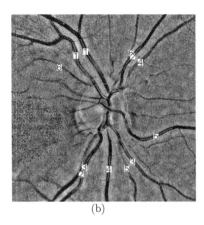

(a)   (b)

Fig. 2. The vessels within the standard region are selected for calculating the CRAE and CRVE values: (a) the widths of selected vessel are measured by the proposed method; (b) The six largest arteries and veins are then selected for the calculation of CRAE, CRVE and AVR values.

3   Experimental Result

3.1   Study Population

The study includes a group of 15 healthy volunteers (7 men and 8 women) with age between 20 and 60 years. For each subject, 5 optic-disc centered images were repeatedly acquired on the right eyes using a Canon Cr-1 Mark II fundus camera, with image resolution of 3627×2178 pixels. The images are used for the quantitative cross-sectional comparative study between the three caliber assessment methods.

3.2   Vessel Width Measurement Tools

IVAN Tool developed by the University of Wisconsin, USA, is a program for assessing the blood vessels caliber on fundus images (see Fig. 3(a)). First of all, it automatically locates the center of the optic disc and determines a standard area of 0.5 to 1.0 disc diameter around it. The vessels within the region-of-interest (ROI) are detected and their calibers are measured as the average distance between the vessel left and right edges. In addition, the detected vessels are classified as artery and vein for the measurement of CRAE and CRVE. After the automatic processing, a manual correction is performed by the user. It includes adjusting the position of the optic disc center, adding the miss-detected vessels, correcting the vessel labels and eliminating the wrongly detected vessel edges. When the manual correction is done, the tool computes the values of CRAE, CRVE and AVR using the Paired, the Parr-Hubbard [5], and the Knudtson's revised formulas [6].

Vampire Tool [9] developed by the University of Dundee, Scotland, is used for the manual measurement of vessel width (see Fig. 3(b)). The instructions of the program require clicking the vessels around the optic disc region to measure and determine their vessel type simultaneously. Then for each vessel, the left and right edges need to be clicked and the Euclidean distance between them is considered as the width of the vessel. Finally, the values of the CRAE, CRVE and AVR are computed using the Knudtson's revised formulas [6].

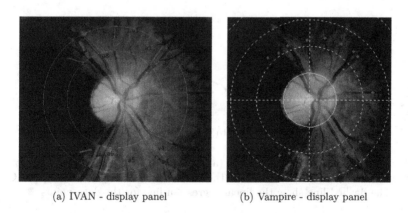

(a) IVAN - display panel   (b) Vampire - display panel

Fig. 3. The user interfaces for the IVAN and the Vampire tools. (a) The IVAN software measures vessel calibers by automatic processing and manual modification. (b) The Vampire annotation tool is used for measuring vessel calibers manually.

3.3   Results

The system error indicates the robustness of a tool on measuring biomarkers for the same vasculature acquired in multiple acquisitions. In this study, it is calculated by taking the average of the relative errors (mean/standard deviation)

Table 1. The relative error of the CRAE, CRVE and AVR values obtained by the proposed method, IVAN and Vampire tools.

Software	Relative error			
	CRAE	CRVE	AVR	Average
Our method	2.84%	2.40%	3.20%	2.81%
IVAN	2.32%	1.91%	2.65%	2.29%
Vampire	4.09%	3.63%	5.73%	4.48%

among 5 acquisitions on 15 subjects. The results are shown in Table 1. Comparing the error of three tools, as expected the Vampire annotation tool produces the largest variation among the three tools, which is two times larger than the other two tools. The calibers obtained by manual vessel annotation are clearly prone to human error.

We examined the correlation of the measurements obtained by our proposed method and the IVAN tool. Figure 4 shows the scatter plots for the CRAE, CRVE and AVR respectively by the two tools. pcc represents the Pearson's correlation coefficient and p is the corresponding p-value. Considering the confidence interval 95% ($p = 0.05$), the results of CRAE, CRVE and AVR obtained by two tools are significantly correlated. It implies that the proposed automatic tool produces similar caliber values compared to IVAN.

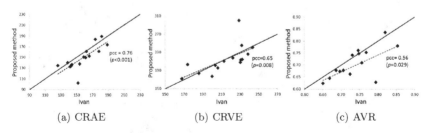

(a) CRAE   (b) CRVE   (c) AVR

Fig. 4. Scatter plots for comparing the (a) CRAE, (b) CRVE and (c) AVR obtained by our method and the IVAN tool on the retinal images acquired using the Canon camera. The dashed line show the linear regression line for the data points.

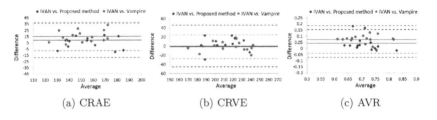

(a) CRAE   (b) CRVE   (c) AVR

Fig. 5. The Bland-Altman plots for comparing the (a) CRAE, (b) CRVE and (c) AVR values obtained by our method and the Vampire tool with the IVAN.

The Bland Altman plots in Fig. 5 compare the proposed method and the Vampire annotation tool using the IVAN software as the reference. The CRAE values measured by our method have better agreement with the values obtained from the IVAN, where it has a lower bias than the Vampire. In the case of measuring CRVE, the performance of both tools is similar, with almost zero bias, though the error of the Vampire is lower than our method. For measuring AVR, which is an important clinical relevant biomarker in large-scale setting, our fully automatic method produces much accurate results than the human annotation tool, with lower bias and variation.

The assessment of vascular caliber using the proposed method takes around 8 min on one image from the described dataset. In detail, the vessel segmentation, artery/vein classification and vessel caliber measurement steps respectively take 2, 4 and 2 min on a single core CPU. Since the full processing is automatic, the calculation time reduced to less than 1 min per image when we process the images in a parallel setting with a 12 cores 2.30 GHz CPU and 128 GB of RAM.

4   Conclusion

In conclusion, we propose an automatic technique for the vessel caliber measurement on retinal photographs, which will be used in a large-scale retinal screening program. We validate this method on a dataset consisting of images acquired on 15 healthy subjects, each of which receives 5 repeated acquisitions. In addition, we compare our tool with the semi-automatic tool - IVAN and the manual vessel annotation tool - Vampire. The result shows the superiority of the proposed automatic vessel caliber measurement. Additionally, IVAN requires time-consuming human attention to modify the automatic generated result, which prohibits analyzing great amounts of data. The proposed method is able to provide automatic caliber measurements with a comparable system error and similar CRAE, CRVE measurements to IVAN. It will enable fully quantitative retinal vessel caliber analysis in large-scale screening programs.

Acknowledgments. The work is part of the Hé Programme of Innovation Cooperation, which is financed by the Netherlands Organization for Scientific Research (NWO), dossier No. 629.001.003.

References

1. Caselles, V., Kimmel, R., Sapiro, G.: Geodesic active contours. Int. J. Comput. Vision **22**(1), 61–79 (1997)
2. Dashtbozorg, B., Zhang, J., Huang, F., ter Haar Romeny, B.M.: Automatic optic disc and fovea detection in retinal images using super-elliptical convergence index filters. In: Campilho, A., Karray, F. (eds.) ICIAR 2016. LNCS, vol. 9730, pp. 697–706. Springer, Cham (2016). doi:10.1007/978-3-319-41501-7_78
3. Drobnjak, D., Munch, I.C., Glümer, C., Faerch, K., Kessel, L., Larsen, M., Veiby, N.C.: Retinal vessel diameters and their relationship with cardiovascular risk and all-cause mortality in the inter99 eye study: a 15-year follow-up. J. Ophthalmol. **2016**, 1–8 (2016)

4. Frydkjaer-Olsen, U., Soegaard Hansen, R., Simó, R., Cunha-Vaz, J., Peto, T., Grauslund, J., et al.: Correlation between retinal vessel calibre and neurodegeneration in patients with type 2 diabetes mellitus in the european consortium for the early treatment of diabetic retinopathy (eurocondor). Ophthalmic Res. **56**(1), 10–16 (2016)
5. Hubbard, L.D., Brothers, R.J., King, W.N., Clegg, L.X., Klein, R., Cooper, L.S., Sharrett, A.R., Davis, M.D., Cai, J., Atherosclerosis Risk in Communities Study Group, et al.: Methods for evaluation of retinal microvascular abnormalities associated with hypertension/sclerosis in the atherosclerosis risk in communities study. Ophthalmology **106**(12), 2269–2280 (1999)
6. Knudtson, M.D., Lee, K.E., Hubbard, L.D., Wong, T.Y., Klein, R., Klein, B.E.: Revised formulas for summarizing retinal vessel diameters. Curr. Eye Res. **27**(3), 143–149 (2003)
7. Neubauer, A.S., Luedtke, M., Haritoglou, C., Priglinger, S., Kampik, A.: Retinal vessel analysis reproducibility in assessing cardiovascular disease. Optom. Vis. Sci. **85**(4), E247–E254 (2008)
8. Nguyen, T.T., Wong, T.Y.: Retinal vascular changes and diabetic retinopathy. Curr. Diab.Rep. **9**(4), 277–283 (2009)
9. Perez-Rovira, A., MacGillivray, T., Trucco, E., Chin, K., Zutis, K., Lupascu, C., Tegolo, D., Giachetti, A., Wilson, P., Doney, A., et al.: Vampire: vessel assessment and measurement platform for images of the retina. In: 2011 Annual International Conference of the IEEE Engineering in Medicine and Biology Society, EMBC, pp. 3391–3394. IEEE (2011)
10. Shin, Y.U., Lee, S.E., Cho, H., Kang, M.H., Seong, M.: Analysis of peripapillary retinal vessel diameter in unilateral normal-tension glaucoma. J. Ophthalmol. **2017**, 1–7 (2017)
11. Sun, C., Wang, J.J., Mackey, D.A., Wong, T.Y.: Retinal vascular caliber: systemic, environmental, and genetic associations. Surv. Ophthalmol. **54**(1), 74–95 (2009)
12. Zhang, J., Bekkers, E., Abbasi, S., Dashtbozorg, B., ter Haar Romeny, B.M.: Robust and fast vessel segmentation via Gaussian derivatives in orientation scores. In: Murino, V., Puppo, E. (eds.) ICIAP 2015. LNCS, vol. 9279, pp. 537–547. Springer, Cham (2015). doi:10.1007/978-3-319-23231-7_48

Automatic Detection of Folds and Wrinkles Due to Swelling of the Optic Disc

Jason Agne[1]($\boxtimes$), Jui-Kai Wang[1], Randy H. Kardon[2,3],
and Mona K. Garvin[1,2]($\boxtimes$)

[1] Department of Electrical and Computer Engineering,
The University of Iowa, Iowa City, IA, USA
{jason-agne,mona-garvin}@uiowa.edu
[2] Iowa City VA Health Care System, Iowa City, IA, USA
[3] Department of Ophthalmology and Visual Sciences,
The University of Iowa, Iowa City, IA, USA

Abstract. We propose a method for detecting mechanically induced wrinkles that present themselves around the optic disc as a result of swelling. Folds and wrinkles have recently been found to be useful features for diagnosing optic disc swelling and for differentiating papilledema (optic nerve swelling due to raised intracranial pressure) from pseudopapilledema. A total of 22 patients were diagnosed with varying degrees and causes of optic disc swelling, with 3D spectral domain optical coherence tomography (SD-OCT) images obtained. The images were used to create fold-enhanced 2D images. Features were extracted pertaining to the orientation, Gabor responses, Fourier responses, and coherence to train a pixel-level classifier to distinguish between folds, vessels, image artifacts, and background. An area under the curve of 0.804 was achieved for the classification.

1 Introduction

The optic disc is the region of the back of the eye which gathers and funnels information from the optical receptors of the eye into the optic nerve via the retinal ganglion cell axons, and ultimately to the brain. While its healthy function is critical for the sake of vision, due to its direct connection to the brain, there are abnormalities which can result in signs visible at the optic disc. In this paper, we are specifically concerned with swelling of the optic disc (Fig. 1). A swollen optic disc can be indicative of a number of problems, such as ischemic optic neuropathy [1], optic neuritis, and papilledema [2]. The retinal area around the optic disc can respond to the biomechanical physical stress of a swelling and result in wrinkles (or folds) of the tissue around the optic disc [3].

Additionally, there is a benign condition, known as pseudopapilledema, that causes the optic disc to appear swollen. Little is known about the cause of pseudopapilledema, apart from that it is congenital and often correlates to the presence of calcified deposits in the optic nerve head known as drusen. However, it is postulated that, since pseudopapilledema is a congenital condition, there is

© Springer International Publishing AG 2017
M.J. Cardoso et al. (Eds.): FIFI/OMIA 2017, LNCS 10554, pp. 235–242, 2017.
DOI: 10.1007/978-3-319-67561-9_27

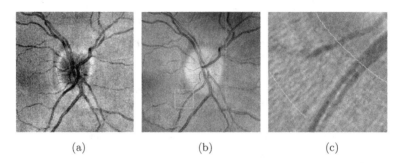

(a)   (b)   (c)

Fig. 1. The SD-OCT is a 3D greyscale image, and it is common to take an average of values in the posterior/anterior direction (known as an *en face* image). Shown here is the *en face* image (a) of a swollen disc and the corresponding 2D fundus image cropped to show the optic disc (b). Folds are barely visible but are indicated with a green box, which is also shown magnified (c), with lines drawn parallel to the folds. (Color figure online)

no stress from the apparent swelling on the tissue around the optic disc to cause retinal folds. As such, we expect that a definitive way of determining if something is a true case of optic disc swelling is if there are folds present — although the absence of folds does not rule out true optic disc swelling. Additionally, it is likely that different causes of optic disc swelling cause different types of folds. However, because folds have only been investigated relatively recently, there are not yet any automated approaches to detecting or quantifying them. We propose an algorithm to isolate and detect folds in the region around the optic disc, using spectral domain optical coherence tomography (SD-OCT) *en face* images.

2   Methods

There were two main components to this work, which were image generation (Sect. 2.1) and feature extraction (Sect. 2.2). We use an *en face* rendering (ILM in Fig. 2) of only the top surface and an *en face* image of the RPE complex for fold, vessel, and artifact classification. The feature extraction includes Gabor filter responses, coherence, orientation, and Fourier results, with straightforward variants of these features also being used (Sect. 2.2).

2.1   Image Generation

The layers in the SD-OCT images of the optic disc were first segmented [4] using a graph-based method developed for optic disc swelling (Fig. 2). The layer segmentation algorithm has a smoothing feature that can complicate its direct use to visualize folds, as the smoothed surface cuts through the local average of minor fluctuations along the ILM (Fig. 3). As such, we generate a fold-enhanced 2D image by taking the average pixel value within 7 pixels of the ILM (a total span of about 29.3 microns). The result is a 2D image in which folds appear to be thin, tube-like structures. One obstacle is that there are other thin, tube-like

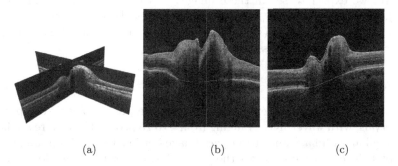

(a)   (b)   (c)

Fig. 2. A 3D rendering of the SD-OCT image (a), depicting a captured optic disc image, along with two slices (b/c) from our dataset. The green line indicates the ILM and the red line indicates the bottom of the RPE complex. (Color figure online)

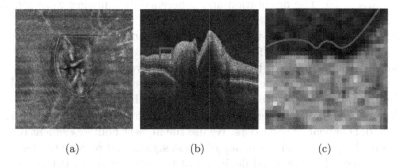

(a)   (b)   (c)

Fig. 3. The (ILM) fold-enhanced *en face* image (a) with cross section shown (b) to highlight a visible wrinkle. Red area is magnified (c) to show it more closely. An outline of the surface is suspended over the surface to accentuate the folds. (Color figure online)

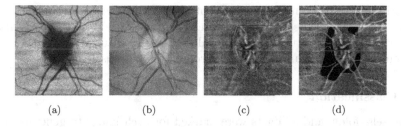

(a)   (b)   (c)   (d)

Fig. 4. Vessel image, which is the *en face* image of the RPE complex (a), along with the cropped fundus image (b) to underscore the likeness. The fold-enhanced 2D image from the 3D SD-OCT (c) along with a version (d) with marked folds (red), vessels (blue), and artifacts (green). (Color figure online)

structures we expect to see in these images — the blood vessels and artifacts (Fig. 4). In order to robustly account for blood vessels, we also generate an *en face* image of the RPE layer (where vessels are most pronounced). Features from both images are used for classification.

2.2 Feature Extraction

The full feature list can be seen in Table 1. Gabor responses [5] were computed at 15° intervals, with wavelengths ranging from 4 to 25 pixels. These were applied to the fold-enhanced image and the *en face* image of the RPE, each upsampled by a factor of 4 since we do not expect the physical wavelength of the folds to always be a whole integer value. In physical space, this means the Gabor wavelengths ranged between 30 and 187.5 microns. The maximum Gabor response across all wavelengths and orientation angles, M_G, for each pixel location in the fold-enhanced image was extracted and summed to the maximum Gabor response from the inverse of the fold-enhanced image, M_G'. In this paper, we define the sum of $M_G + M_G' = I_G$. The orientation and coherence [6,7] images were computed for I_G, M_G, and M_G' (Fig. 5).

A line of 29 sample points was extracted from each pixel location in I_G spanning 435 microns (roughly half-pixel intervals), perpendicular to the orientation. In regions with folds present, this sample would have a sinusoidal element to it. We quantify this by taking the Fourier transform of each sample, and the derivative of each sample (to remove linear components). Disregarding the 0th Fourier coefficient, the highest Fourier response should correspond to the frequency of the sinusoidal element, if one exists. We use the highest Fourier element to create the magnitude, phase, and frequency of a test signal, and remove the test signal from the sample. The standard deviation of the leftover signal is then taken as a feature to determine how dominant the sinusoidal element was. Additionally, the Fourier magnitudes were used as features, directly.

As the artifacts we are looking to detect tend to occur across the image, rather than in isolated areas, we use the horizontal average of the vertical derivative as a feature. This means all locations along a horizontal slice have the same feature value, in a given image. Additionally, as the artifacts often appear to be the result of a horizontal shift when the image is captured, the displaced location of the minimum average vertical derivative when each horizontal slice is shifted across its full range was used as a feature. Finally, local, 5 × 5 contrast measures, such as local maximum, local minimum, and the difference, were also used as features.

2.3 Classification

The vessels, folds, and artifacts were marked for each image to generate truths (Fig. 4). These were classified using a common feature set, but were trained as separate classifiers. The features were extracted from the fold-enhanced and RPE complex images, and trained in three leave-one-patient out random forest regression analyses with 10,000 trees, each 10 decisions deep, with a true set to 1 and a false set to 0. Once trained, the entire feature set from the left-out image

Table 1. Complete list of features used for classification.

Feature count	Description
1	RPE complex image
2	Radial distance from center
3–24	Coherence of Gabor responses to upsampled fold-enhanced images (each pixel-wavelength used as a separate feature)
25	Coherence of average Gabor response across all wavelengths
26	Gaussian filter applied to 25
27–48	Coherence of Gabor responses to upsampled inverse of fold-enhanced image
49	Coherence of average Gabor response to inverse fold-enhanced image
50	Gaussian filter applied to 49
51	Local maximum in 7×7 window of fold-enhanced image
52	Local minimum in 7×7 window of fold-enhanced image
53	Range in a 7×7 window (i.e. features $52 - 51$)
54	Normalized version of feature 53 (i.e. $(52 - 51)/(52 + 51)$)
55	M_G
56	M'_G
57–78	Gabor responses of RPE complex image
79–100	Gabor responses of inverse of RPE complex image
101	Average of 57–78
102	Average of 79–100
103	Orientation of I_G (sum of average Gabor responses)
104	Coherence of I_G
105	Standard deviation of cross section after top frequency removed
106	Standard deviation of derivative of cross section after top frequency removed
107–120	Sorted magnitude of Fourier response of cross section
121–133	Sorted magnitude of Fourier response of derivative of cross section
134	Maximum Fourier response of cross section
135	Difference between max and second rank Fourier responses of cross section
136	Difference between max and third rank Fourier responses of cross section
137–139	Features 134–136 repeated for derivative of cross section
140	Vertical displacement measure of fold-enhanced image
141	Local max of 140
142	Vertical displacement measure of RPE complex image
143	Local max of 142
144	Vertical derivative of fold-enhanced image
145	Vertical derivative of RPE complex image
146	Product of features 144 and 145
147	Locally normalized I_G
148	Coherence of thresholded and skeletonized I_G
149	11×11 median filter applied to I_G

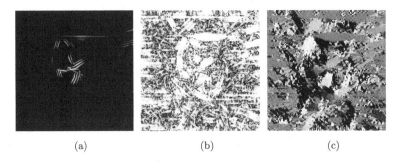

(a)	(b)	(c)

Fig. 5. (a) I_G (max Gabor response), along with the coherence (b) and orientation (c). The orientation ranges from $-90°$ to $90°$ with respect to the horizontal.

was tested for each of the three classifiers, resulting in a pixel-level probability map. The results from the vessel and artifact classifications are used to mask (omit) positive results from the fold classification, while the vessel and artifact truths were used to mask the fold truth.

3   Experimental Methods

A total of 22 images were obtained with varying causes of optic disc swelling. From these, the *en face* images of 200×200 pixels, spanning 6×6mm, were made and marked for classification. The classifier was trained on 100 samples taken from each feature set of the 22 patients (minus 1 left-out patient) at random, to

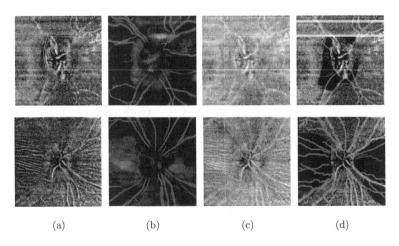

(a)	(b)	(c)	(d)

Fig. 6. Example of fold-enhanced images (a) and classification results (b), alongside an overlay (c) and the ground truth (d). Note that the heavier green areas correspond to artifact location, blue corresponds to vessels, and brighter red areas correspond to the location of folds. (Color figure online)

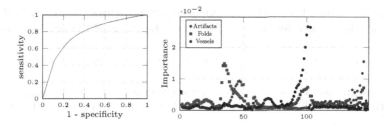

Fig. 7. Resulting ROC curve of the classification. Area under the curve is 0.804. Additionally a plot of average importance for each feature, for each classifier. For example, the highest point is at feature 100, with a value of 0.0296. This corresponds to the longest wavelength Gabor response to the RPE complex image, which one would expect to be significant for the detection of vessels.

include an equal mix of each possible classification (folds, vessels, artifacts, and background) available for each image. A set of fold probability maps (Fig. 6) were produced for each combination of vessel and artifact thresholds. The ROC curves associated with each set of fold probability maps were compiled to generate the overall ROC curve (Fig. 7).

4   Results

We achieved an AUC of 0.804. The right-most plot in Fig. 7 also shows the average importance for each feature, listed in order of Table 1. The average processing time for feature extraction was 9 min and 17 s per image, using unoptimized Matlab. For regression training, the average time was 2 min and 21 s.

5   Discussion and Conclusion

The automatic detection of folds in the ILM is instrumental for determining if an optic disc is truly swollen or only appears to be. Moreover, extracting attributes of detected folds is expected to be useful for determining the cause of the swelling. Some of the most important features for the detection of folds includes the coherence of the Gabor responses to the inverse of the fold-enhanced image. This is due to the fact that in the inverse image, vessels are dark instead of bright, thus diminishing the effects of the Gabor response and reducing false positives. Additionally, the Gabor responses to the inverse of the RPE complex image were of high importance, which is sensible as we expect a high-coherence location in the fold-enhanced image and a low-coherence location in the RPE complex image to be the most basic indication of a fold on the ILM. Other attributes of the folds (orientation, spatial wavelength, size) are expected to be meaningful to the classification of the cause of the optic disc swelling that resulted in folds, and such attributes are among the features. As such, should a correlation between fold attributes and edema type be clinically quantified, our algorithm should be useful for extracting the features to classify folds, and then using those same features to determine the cause of the swelling, directly. Future work may include inpainting vessels, instead of masking them, as folds can theoretically overlap vessels without existing elsewhere to be detected.

Acknowledgments. This study was supported, in part, by the National Institutes of Health R01 EY023279 and the Department of Veterans Affairs Merit Award I01 RX001786.

References

1. Hayreh, S.S.: Ischemic optic neuropathy. Int. Ophthalmol. **1**(1), 9–18 (1978)
2. Hayreh, S.S.: Optic disc edema in raised intracranial pressure, V. Pathogenesis. Arch. Ophthalmol. **97**(9), 1553–1565 (1977)
3. Sibony, P.A., Kupersmith, M.J., Feldon, S.E., Wang, J.K., Garvin, M., The OCT Substudy Group for the NORDIC IIHTT: Retinal and choroidal folds in papilledema. Invest. Ophthalmol. Vis. Sci. **56**, 5670–5680 (2015)
4. Wang, J.K., Kardon, R.H., Kupersmith, M.J., Garvin, M.K.: Automated quantification of volumetric optic disc swelling in papilledema using spectral-domain optical coherence tomography. Invest. Ophthalmol. Vis. Sci. **53**(7), 4069–4075 (2012)
5. Batool, N., Chellappa, R.: Fast detection of facial wrinkles based on Gabor features using image morphology and geometric constraints. Pattern Recogn. **48**(3), 642–658 (2015)
6. Püspöki, Z., Storath, M., Sage, D., Unser, M.: Transforms and operators for directional bioimage analysis: a survey. In: De Vos, W.H., Munck, S., Timmermans, J.-P. (eds.) Focus on Bio-Image Informatics. AAECB, vol. 219, pp. 69–93. Springer, Cham (2016). doi:10.1007/978-3-319-28549-8_3
7. Rezakhaniha, R., Agianniotis, A., Schrauwen, J., Griffa, A., Sage, D., Bouten, C., van de Vosse, F., Unser, M., Stergiopulos, N.: Experimental investigation of collagen waviness and orientation in the arterial adventitia using confocal laser scanning microscopy. Biomech. Model. Mechanobiol. **11**(3–4), 461–473 (2012)

Representation Learning for Retinal Vasculature Embeddings

Luca Giancardo[1,2(✉)], Kirk Roberts[1], and Zhongming Zhao[1,2]

[1] School of Biomedical Informatics, University of Texas Health Science Center
at Houston (UTHealth), Houston, USA
luca.giancardo@uth.tmc.edu
[2] Center for Precision Health, UTHealth, Houston, USA

Abstract. The retinal vasculature imaged with fundus photography has
the potential of encoding precious information for image-based retinal
biomarkers, however, progress in their development is slow due to the
need of defining vasculature morphology variables *a priori* and developing algorithms specific to these variables. In this paper, we introduce a
novel approach to learn a general descriptor (or embedding) that cap-
tures the vasculature morphology in a numerically compact vector with
minimal feature engineering. The vasculature embedding is computed by
leveraging the internal representation of a new encoder-enhanced fully
convolutional neural network, trained end-to-end with the raw pixels and
manually segmented vessels. This approach effectively transfers the vasculature patterns learned by the network into a general purpose vasculature embedding vector. Using Messidor and Messidor-2, two publicly
available datasets, we test the vasculature embeddings on two tasks:
(1) an image retrieval task, which retrieved similar images according to
their vasculature; (2) a diabetic retinopathy classification task, where we
show how the vasculature embeddings improve the classification of an
algorithm based on microaneurysms detection by 0.04 AUC on average.

1 Introduction

The retina is an important direct or indirect indicator of some of the most
common diseases in the industrialized world, such as cardiovascular conditions,
diabetes complications and neurodegeneration [1]. Fundus imaging is an inexpensive and non-invasive optical imaging technique to monitor retinas in the
general population, thus allowing for screening medical risk factors, tracking
progression or diagnosis. Multiple research groups have focused on the development of automatic or semi-automatic tools to estimate candidate image based
biomarkers based on the vasculature morphology such as: vessel width, vessel
tortuosity, artery to vein ratio or even fractal analysis [2–5]. While effective,
all of these methods require different algorithmic pipelines and data representations for each of vasculature variables. Inspired by transfer learning [6] and recent
advances in convolutional networks for segmentation [7,8], we introduce a new
approach to learn a general purpose vasculature descriptor or "embedding" from

© Springer International Publishing AG 2017
M.J. Cardoso et al. (Eds.): FIFI/OMIA 2017, LNCS 10554, pp. 243–250, 2017.
DOI: 10.1007/978-3-319-67561-9_28

the image data itself with minimal feature engineering. Such descriptor has the potential of significantly reducing the time required for algorithm development (by avoiding manual feature engineering) and allowing the creation of candidate vasculature based biomarkers without a priori information.

Figure 1 diagrammatically illustrates how our method learns a compact vasculature representation by leveraging a new encoder-enhanced fully convolutional neural network. We test the vasculature embeddings on an image retrieval task and on a diabetic retinopathy classification task.

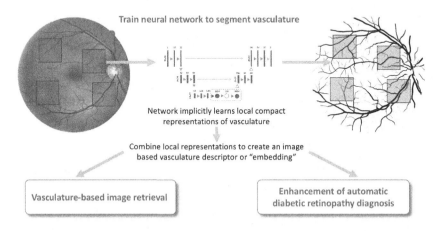

Fig. 1. Diagram of the analysis presented in this manuscript. We train an encoder-enhanced fully convolutional neural network to segment the retinal vasculature and at the same time to implicitly learn a compact representation of such vasculature. This representation is then used for two experiments, firstly for image retrieval, then to evaluate if the vasculature information can benefit diabetic retinopathy diagnosis algorithms.

2   Methods

Preprocessing. The image undergoes minimal preprocessing. First, the image is converted to a single channel and rescaled to 584 pixels of height (maintaining the aspect ratio), then its luminosity and contrast are adjusted by subtracting the global mean and diving by the standard deviation. Finally, the image contrast is enhanced by contrast limited adaptive histogram equalization [9]. The image is then divided into overlapping patches that are subsequently used as input for the neural network.

Neural Network. Fully convolutional networks such as U-Net are recent neural network-based techniques able to be trained on inputs of arbitrary size and produce correspondingly-sized output with efficient inference and learning [10,11]. As shown in Fig. 2, our network works on local image patches of 48×48 pixels and it consists of the typical U-shaped contracting and expanding of fully convolutional network approaches with the addition of encoding layers (see dashed lines). While not strictly necessary, we decided to work with local image patches for computational reasons (i.e. keeping a small parameter space and manageable training time). The contracting path consists in repeated 3×3 convolutions, followed by rectifier linear units and max pooling operations with a stride of 2 for downsampling, which reduce the spatial resolution and increase the number of filters. The expanding path works in a similar fashion but with upsampling operations and 3×3 "up-convolutions", which decrease the number of filters and increase image resolution until reaching the final layer. This last layer is mapped to a tensor with two channels in its third dimension. These channels represent the likelihood of each pixel of being a vessel or background and use a softmax activation.

In our network, we relax the fully convolutional network approach and add three fully connected non-convolutional layers on the saddle point of the network, where the imaging scale is lowest and the number of filters is highest. These fully connected layers continue the U-shaped paradigm but act as an implicit encoder to compress the relevant information flowing through the convolutional filters. While similar to autoencoders, the encoding layers differ because they do not try to reconstruct their own input. We train the network end-to-end using stochastic gradient descent (SGD) using a 0.1 learning rate, dropout regularization with 0.2 ratio after each of the convolutional layers and cross entropy as loss function.

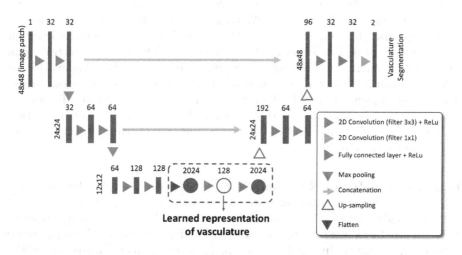

Fig. 2. Neural network architecture. The dashed box represent the encoding layers allowing the creation of the vasculature embedding and are the main changes over a typical U-Net architecture [10]. Each blue box represents a 3D dimensional tensor. The tensors dimensions are shown on the left and on the top of the box, displaying the first two dimensions (i.e. image x-y) and last dimension (number of filters) respectively. Each round box represent a vector with a number showing its size. The arrows represent different operations. (Color figure online)

The cross entropy loss function is computed uniquely between the target vessel segmentation and final layer. The result is then back-propagated using SGD to all layers, including the in the encoding layers.

Once trained, the network receives an image patch as input and it outputs a vessel segmentation map at the end layer. Importantly, we also generate a vector $\mathbf{a} \in \mathbb{R}^{128}$ by retrieving the activation of 128 neurons in the lowest layer of the encoder (shown as empty circle in Fig. 2). In order to generate an image wide vessel embedding $\mathbf{e} \in \mathbb{R}^{256}$ we combine the n image patches as follow:

$$\mathbf{A} = [a_{p=1}, a_{p=2} \cdots a_{p=n}], \qquad \mathbf{e} = \begin{bmatrix} f_{\mathrm{med}}(\mathbf{A}_1) \\ f_{\mathrm{iqr}}(\mathbf{A}_1) \\ \vdots \\ f_{\mathrm{med}}(\mathbf{A}_n) \\ f_{\mathrm{iqr}}(\mathbf{A}_n) \end{bmatrix}$$

where a_p is the vector containing the encoder activations for image patch p, f_{iqr} is the function to compute the interquantile range and f_{med} is the function to compute the median.

3   Experiments and Results

We trained our network on the DRIVE datasets [12] using a randomly sampled set of 190,000 patches extracted from the 20 images (in the training set), leaving out 10% patches as validation set. We trained with mini batches of 320 patches for 150 epochs. The final network weights are retrieved from the training epoch that provided the best accuracy on the validation set. The network was trained in less than 24 h and it was able to generate a full vasculature embedding in 3.16 s on a Nvidia Titan X GPU without any code optimization. The code for our experiments was implemented in Python using Keras (https://keras.io), Tensorflow (https://www.tensorflow.org) and scikit-learn (http://scikit-learn.org) libraries. Part of the implementation is based on the retina-unet GitHub project (https://github.com/orobix/retina-unet).

Experiment 1: Image Retrieval. Here, we used the Messidor dataset which contains 1,200 fundus images annotated with a diabetic retinopathy diagnosis and risk for macular edema [13]. This dataset was not used for any training purposes. We compute the 4 closest samples for all 1,200 candidates using Euclidean distance between the vectors $\mathbf{e}$. In Fig. 3, we show on the left the "query" image and on the right the 4 closest samples. In order to avoid any selection bias, we show the first 5 groups of images sorted according to ascending "in-group distance". This distance is computed as $|\mathbf{e_0} - \mathbf{e_1}| + |\mathbf{e_0} - \mathbf{e_2}| + \cdots + |\mathbf{e_0} - \mathbf{e_4}|$ where $\mathbf{e_0}$ is the query vector and $\mathbf{e_i}$s are the i-closest vectors. We observed that the vessel embedding appeared to be insensitive to the retina orientation and that each row has approximately similar vessel morphology especially of the main vasculature arches. Unexpectedly, we found some duplicated images in the dataset (see Fig. 3, first two columns in

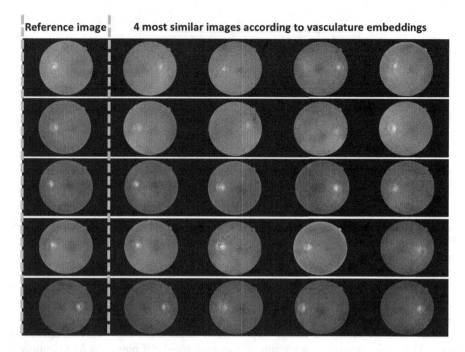

Fig. 3. Example of the images retrieval task according to the similarity to the query image (left column). The similarity is computed using the euclidean distance between vasculature embeddings vectors. Best viewed electronically.

row 3, 4 and 5). To our knowledge, it has never been reported before. This further builds our confidence in the potential of our approach.

In order to further investigate the performance of the vasculature embeddings for image retrieval, we evaluated the ability of matching left to right retinas with a realistic public dataset, Messidor-2. This dataset contains 874 retinal examinations of both eyes (for a total of 1748 images) [13] which were not used for any training purposes. For each subject, we used his/her right retina as reference image and computed the euclidean distance to all 874 left retinas in the vasculature embedding vector space. Figure 4 shows the ratio of correct matches as a function of the number closest neighbors taken into account. The vasculature embedding allow for identifying the correct image pairs significantly better than chance. Other works on vasculature biomarkers showed a significant group level correlation between left and right eye [1], however, the vasculature morphology can vary significantly at subject level and perfect matching is not to be expected, as indicated by our results.

Experiment 2: Diabetic Retinopathy Classification. Obvious changes in retinal vasculature are typically visible at late stage of diabetic retinopathy, when neovascularization occurs. Still, it is plausible for different vasculature

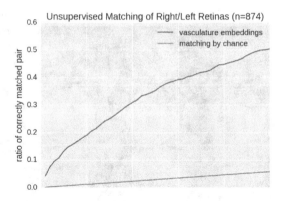

Fig. 4. Unsupervised matching of right/left retinas based on the vasculature embeddings on the Messidor-2 dataset. The vasculature embeddings allow for identifying the correct image pairs significantly better than chance.

Table 1. Diabetic retinopathy classification performance on the Messidor dataset with different feature vectors. All results expressed as areas under the receiving operating curve (AUC). No hyperparameter tuning was performed. Of note, the AUC improves when the vasculature embedding are included in the feature vector, regardless of the severity of the disease. ***p<0.001, **p<0.01, *p<0.5 for a two-sided Mann-Whitney U test to reject the null hypothesis that the healthy and DR samples come from the same distribution.

Healthy vs. Diabetic retinopathy (DR) (n=1,200)			
	Vasculature embed.	*Microaneurysm feat.*	*Combination*
Logistic Regr. (L1 reg.)	0.680***	0.842***	0.863***
Logistic Regr. (L2 reg.)	0.683***	0.845***	0.863***
Linear SVM	0.678***	0.803***	**0.865*****
Healthy vs. High DR (n=801)			
	Vasculature embed.	*Microaneurysm feat.*	*Combination*
Logistic Regr. (L1 reg.)	0.806***	0.947***	0.962***
Logistic Regr. (L2 reg.)	0.819***	0.947***	**0.965*****
Linear SVM	0.808***	0.951***	0.964***
Healthy vs. Mild DR (n=700)			
	Vasculature embed.	*Microaneurysm feat.*	*Combination*
Logistic Regr. (L1 reg.)	0.558*	0.666***	0.685***
Logistic Regr. (L2 reg.)	0.566*	0.667***	**0.692*****
Linear SVM	0.533	0.504	0.679***

morphologies to be correlated with earlier stage of diabetic retinopathy as they are associated with myocardial infarction [1].

In this experiment, we evaluated whether the vasculature embeddings can be used to classify diabetic retinopathy (DR) and if they are able to enhance the DR classification performance of an algorithms trained to identify microaneurysms [14], which are the pathological hallmarks used by ophthalmologists to diagnose DR from its early stage.

For each image in the Messidor dataset, we computed three features vectors: the standalone vasculature embedding $\mathbf{e}$, the microaneurym-based feature vector $\mathbf{m}$ and a combination of the two $\mathbf{c} = \begin{bmatrix} \mathbf{e} \\ \mathbf{m} \end{bmatrix}$. The microaneurym-based feature vector $m \in \mathbb{R}^3$ represents the microaneurysms probability histogram computed with a radon based operator trained on a separate dataset [14]. In these experiments, we are not much interested in the absolute classification performance, rather we focus on the relative performance change using the different feature vectors. Therefore, we used a set of common linear machine learning classifiers without any hyper-parameter tuning (the default hyper-parameters provided by the scikit-learn 0.18.1 library were used). The tests were performed with a 50-fold cross-validation on the Messidor dataset.

Table 1 shows the diabetic retinopathy classification performance with the various combination of classifiers and feature vectors. The most relevant result to highlight is that the vasculature embeddings consistently improved the classification performance regardless of the severity of the disease. The average improvement across classifiers is 0.04 AUC points.

4   Conclusions

We have introduced a new approach to learn vasculature embeddings from vessel segmentation data without the need of defining vasculature morphology variables a priori. The vasculature embeddings have been tested on two separate tasks, image retrieval and diabetic retinopathy classification enhancement. In the former task, we retrieved similar images according to their vasculature, in the latter task we showed how the vasculature embeddings improve the classification of an algorithm based on microaneurysms detection by 0.04 AUC on average. The results obtained are encouraging but further work is needed to test repeatability and validity as candidate image based biomarker as well as direct comparison with alternative methods to characterize vasculature. The methodology developed is not inherently specific to retina images, we will explore other imaging modalities in future work.

Acknowledgement. This work has been supported by the Center for Precision Health and School of Biomedical Informatics at University of Texas Health Science Center at Houston. We would like to thank Daniele Cortinovis for the initial implementation of U-Net on https://github.com/orobix/retina-unet. The Messidor and Messidor-2 datasets are kindly provided by the LaTIM laboratory (see http://latim.univ-brest.fr/) and the Messidor program partners (see http://messidor.crihan.fr/)".

References

1. MacGillivray, T.J., Cameron, J.R., Zhang, Q., El-Medany, A., Mulholland, C., Sheng, Z., Dhillon, B., Doubal, F.N., Foster, P.J., Trucco, E., Sudlow, C.: Suitability of UK biobank retinal images for automatic analysis of morphometric properties of the vasculature. PLoS ONE **10**(5), 1–10 (2015)
2. Trucco, E., Giachetti, A., Ballerini, L., Relan, D., Cavinato, A., MacGillivray, T.: Morphometric measurements of the retinal vasculature in fundus images with vampire. In: Biomedical Image Understanding: Methods and Applications, pp. 91–111 (2015)
3. Fiorin, D., Ruggeri, A.: Computerized analysis of narrow-field ROP images for the assessment of vessel caliber and tortuosity. In: Proceedings of EMBS, pp. 2622–2625 (2011)
4. Xu, X., Niemeijer, M., Song, Q., Sonka, M., Garvin, M.K., Reinhardt, J.M., Abramoff, M.D.: Vessel boundary delineation on fundus images using graph-based approach. IEEE Trans. Med. Imaging **30**(6), 1184–1191 (2011)
5. Azemin, M.Z.C., Kumar, D.K., Wong, T.Y., Kawasaki, R., Mitchell, P., Wang, J.J.: Robust methodology for fractal analysis of the retinal vasculature. IEEE Trans. Med. Imaging **30**(2), 243–250 (2011)
6. Bengio, Y., Courville, A., Vincent, P.: Representation learning a review and new perspectives. IEEE Trans. Pattern Anal. Mach. Intell. **35**(8), 1798–828 (2013)
7. Fu, H., Xu, Y., Lin, S., Kee Wong, D.W., Liu, J.: DeepVessel: Retinal vessel segmentation via deep learning and conditional random field. In: Ourselin, S., Joskowicz, L., Sabuncu, M.R., Unal, G., Wells, W. (eds.) MICCAI 2016. LNCS, vol. 9901, pp. 132–139. Springer, Cham (2016). doi:10.1007/978-3-319-46723-8_16
8. Maninis, K.-K., Pont-Tuset, J., Arbeláez, P., Van Gool, L.: Deep retinal image understanding. In: Ourselin, S., Joskowicz, L., Sabuncu, M.R., Unal, G., Wells, W. (eds.) MICCAI 2016. LNCS, vol. 9901, pp. 140–148. Springer, Cham (2016). doi:10.1007/978-3-319-46723-8_17
9. Pizer, S.M., Amburn, E.P., Austin, J.D., Cromartie, R., Geselowitz, A., Greer, T., Ter Haar Romeny, B., Zimmerman, J.B., Zuiderveld, K.: Adaptive histogram equalization and its variations. Comput. Vis. Graph. Image Process. **39**(3), 355–368 (1987)
10. Ronneberger, O., Fischer, P., Brox, T.: U-Net: Convolutional networks for biomedical image segmentation. In: Navab, N., Hornegger, J., Wells, W.M., Frangi, A.F. (eds.) MICCAI 2015. LNCS, vol. 9351, pp. 234–241. Springer, Cham (2015). doi:10.1007/978-3-319-24574-4_28
11. Long, J., Shelhamer, E., Darrell, T.: Fully convolutional networks for semantic segmentation. In: Proceedings of CVPR, pp. 3431–3440 (2015)
12. Staal, J., Abramoff, M.D., Niemeijer, M., Viergever, M.A., van Ginneken, B.: Ridge-based vessel segmentation in color images of the retina. IEEE Trans. Med. Imaging **23**(4), 501–509 (2004)
13. Decencière, E., Zhang, X., Cazuguel, G., Laÿ, B., Cochener, B., Trone, C., Gain, P., Ordóñez-Varela, J.R., Massin, P., Erginay, A., Charton, B., Klein, J.C.: Feedback on a publicly distributed image database: The Messidor database. Image Anal. Stereology **33**(3), 231–234 (2014)
14. Giancardo, L., Meriaudeau, F., Karnowski, T.P., Tobin, K.W., Chaum, E.: Validation of microaneurysm-based diabetic retinopathy screening across retina fundus datasets. In: Proceedings of CBMS, pp. 125–130 (2013)

Author Index

Printed in the United States
By Bookmasters

Printed in the United States
By Bookmasters